Phlebotomy Essentials

Phlebotomy Essentials

RUTH E. McCALL, MT(ASCP), CLS (NCA)

Director of Phlebotomy Program
Instructor, MLT Program
Albuquerque Technical-Vocational Institute
Albuquerque, New Mexico

CATHEE M. TANKERSLEY, MT(ASCP), CLS (NCA)

Director of Phlebotomy, EKG, and EEG Programs
Phoenix College
Phoenix, Arizona

J. B. Lippincott Company   *Philadelphia*

Sponsoring Editor: Andrew Allen
Coordinating Editorial Assistant: Miriam Benert
Project Editor: Amy P. Jirsa
Indexer: Vicki Boyle
Design Coordinator: Kathy Kelley-Luedtke
Interior Designer: Arlene Putterman
Cover Designer: Ilene Griff
Production Manager: Helen Ewan
Production Coordinator: Nannette Winski
Compositor: G&S Typesetters, Inc.
Printer/Binder: R.R. Donnelley and Sons Company
Cover Printer: New England Book Components, Inc.
Color Insert Printer: Princeton Polychrome Press

Library of Congress Cataloging-in-Publication Data
McCall, Ruth E.
    Phlebotomy essentials / Ruth E. McCall and
  Cathee M. Tankersley.
       p.   cm.
    Includes bibliographical references and index.
    ISBN 0-397-54929-6
    1. Phlebotomy.   I. Tankersley, Cathee M.
    II. Title.
    [DNLM: 1. Bloodletting.   WB 381 M478p]
RB45.15.M33 1993
616.07′561—dc20
DNLM/DLC
for Library of Congress   92-48817
                                                CIP

6   5   4

Any procedure or practice described in this book
should be applied by the health-care practitioner
under appropriate supervision in accordance with
professional standards of care used with regard to
the unique circumstances that apply in each practice
situation. Care has been taken to confirm the
accuracy of information presented and to describe
generally accepted practices. However, the authors,
editors, and publisher cannot accept any
responsibility for errors or omissions or for any
consequences from application of the information in
this book and make no warranty express or implied,
with respect to the contents of the book.

Every effort has been made to ensure drug selections
and dosages are in accordance with current
recommendations and practice. Because of ongoing
research, changes in government regulations and the
constant flow of information on drug therapy,
reactions and interactions, the reader is cautioned to
check the package insert for each drug for
indications, dosages, warnings and precautions,
particularly if the drug is new or infrequently used.

Selected figures (illustrations) in this text were
reproduced with permission from the following J. B.
Lippincott sources: Craven RF, Hirnle CJ:
Fundamentals of Nursing: Human Health & Function,
1992; Jones SA, Weigel A, White RD, McSwain NE,
Breiter M: *Advanced Emergency Care for Paramedic
Practice,* 1992; Memmler RL, Cohen BJ, Wood DL:
The Human Body in Health and Disease, 7th edition,
1992; Metheny NM: *Fluid and Electrolyte Balance:
Nursing Considerations,* 2nd edition, 1992; Rosdahl C:
Textbook of Basic Nursing, 5th edition, 1991; Timby
BK, Lewis LW: *Fundamental Skills and Concepts in
Patient Care,* 5th edition, 1992.

---

*To my parents Charles and Marie Ruppert, my husband John,
and my sons Chris and Scott for their encouragement,
patience, and support of this effort.*

Ruth E. McCall

*To my loving family, Tank, Todd, and Jaime, and two special moms,
Mary and Lucille, for their understanding and support.*

Cathee M. Tankersley

Preface

Phlebotomy Essentials was designed to provide accurate, up-to-date, practical information and instruction in phlebotomy procedures and techniques, as well as a comprehensive background in the theory and principles behind them. Outstanding features include a list of key terms and objectives at the beginning of each chapter plus study questions and suggested laboratory activities at the end of each chapter. The early chapters offer a brief history of how the practice of phlebotomy has evolved to the present day along with an introduction to the health care profession, orienting the phlebotomist to the American health care system. Medical terminology and an overview of anatomy and physiology—with special emphasis on the circulatory system—are included to enhance understanding and provide a foundation of related information on which phlebotomy skills can be built. Chapters containing information on basic computer terminology and laboratory information systems, quality assurance, and total quality management acquaint the student with emerging laboratory practice. This book is intended to be an instructional text in phlebotomy basics for those students with no prior experience in the subject, as well as a reference for technique for practicing phlebotomists who wish to update their skills or pass a national certification exam. It was written with input from both employers in the health care community concerning expected duties and performance of phlebotomy personnel, and phlebotomy educators throughout the United States concerning necessary content. All procedures were written to conform to standards developed by the National Committee for Clinical Laboratory Standards (NCCLS), when applicable, and to meet standards for phlebotomy training developed by the National Accrediting Agency for Clinical Laboratory Sciences (NAACLS). The authors wish to express their gratitude to the reviewers: Barbara J. Cohen, BA, MS; Beverly M. Kovanda, PhD, MT(ASCP) MS; Janice LaReau, MS, MT(ASCP) SH; Mary Ellen O'Rorke, MEd, MT(ASCP); Glen Parnell, MT(ASCP), CLS(NCA); and Susan Szucs, BS, MBA, RN; the photographers: Christopher McCall and Lou Hodges; New Mexico Oncology Hematology Consultants, for their fax machine; and to all others who assisted and supported this effort.

Ruth E. McCall, MT(ASCP)
Cathee M. Tankersley, MT(ASCP)

Contents

**List of Color Plates
Following page**   *84*

Color Plate 1   Heart and great vessels
Color Plate 2   Common color coded evacuated tube stoppers
*Color Plate 3   Blood vessels constitute the closed system for the flow
                  of blood*

Phlebotomy: Past and Present

1

OBJECTIVES

On successful completion of this chapter, the reader should be able to:

1 Describe the evolution of phlebotomy to present day.
2 List the duties of a phlebotomist.
3 Describe traits that form the professional image.
4 Contrast certification, licensure, and accreditation.
5 Identify national organizations that support phlebotomy as a profession.
6 List the important points in the Patient's Bill of Rights.
7 Define tort, negligence, and malpractice; compare criminal and civil law.
8 Describe how to avoid litigation as a phlebotomist.

KEY TERMS

accreditation
approval
ASCP
ASMT
ASPT
assault
battery
breach of confidentiality
certification
civil law
continuing education units (CEUs)
essentials
informed consent
licensure
malpractice
NAACLS
NCA
NCCLS
negligence
Patient's Bill of Rights
phlebotomy
professionalism
reciprocity
risk management
tort

McCall: PHLEBOTOMY ESSENTIALS. © 1993
J. B. Lippincott Company.

AN HISTORICAL PERSPECTIVE ON PHLEBOTOMY

Since very early times, man has been fascinated by blood and has believed in some connection between the blood racing through his veins and his well-being. From this belief, certain medical principles and procedures dealing with blood evolved, some surviving to the present day. An early medical theory developed by Hippocrates (460–377 B.C.) stated that disease was the result of excess substances, such as blood, phlegm, black bile, and yellow bile, within the body. It was thought that removal of the excess would restore balance. The process of removal or extraction became the treatment and could either be done by expelling disease materials through the use of drugs or by direct removal during surgery. One important surgical technique was phlebotomy—the process of bloodletting. Bloodletting involved cutting into a vein with a sharp instrument and releasing blood in an effort to rid the body of evil spirits, to cleanse the body of impurities, or, as in Hippocrates' time, to bring the body into proper balance. Literal translation of the word **phlebotomy** comes from the Greek words *phlebos*, meaning vein and *tome*, meaning incision.

Some authorities believe phlebotomy dates back to the last period of the Stone Age when crude tools were used to puncture vessels to allow excess blood to drain out of the body. Bloodletting in Egypt around 1400 B.C. is evidenced by a painting in a tomb showing the application of a leech to a patient. In 13th century Europe, it was often the barber who practiced surgery and, consequently, bloodletting. Public bathhouses often had this barber–surgeon bleed patrons for preventive purposes at the same time they received their shave and haircut. The once familiar barber pole evolved from this period as it symbolized the staff grasped by the patron during the procedure. The often blood-stained staff was wrapped with white bandages after use, thus giving it the characteristic red-and-white-striped appearance.

During the 17th and 18th centuries, phlebotomy was considered a major therapeutic (treatment) process. Anyone willing to claim medical training could perform phlebotomy. The lancet, a tool used for cutting the vein, was promoted, but antisepsis was unknown as lancets were passed from patient to patient without cleansing. The usual amount of blood withdrawn was approximately 10 ml but excessive phlebotomy was common. In fact, it was thought to have contributed to George Washington's death in 1799, when he was diagnosed with a throat infection and the physician removed 9 pints of blood in 24 hours.

During this same period, phlebotomy was accomplished by three procedures: cupping, venesection, and leeches. Cupping involved the application of a special suction apparatus to the skin to draw blood to the surface. This process was called *dry cupping* when performed prior to cutting the skin, and *wet cupping* if performed after cutting the skin. Venesection involved slicing a vein in the forearm and collecting the specimen in what was called a "bleeding bowl" (Fig. 1-1). The use of leeches involved making a small cut in the skin to entice the leech to bite. Once the leech was engorged with blood, it was removed by dusting it with ashes or ground salt.

Two bloodletting instruments were developed during this period: the schnapper and the scarificator (Fig. 1-2). The crudely designed schnapper, a spring-activated lancet, was an ancestor of similar devices used in laboratories today. The scarificator had several crescent-shaped, spring-loaded blades concealed within a boxlike case which,

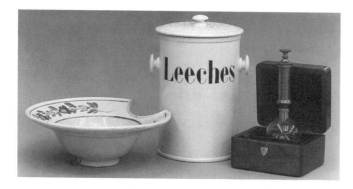

Figure 1–1 Early phlebotomy equipment (left to right): bleeding bowl, leech jar, and 19th century cupping glass and evacuating pump. (Courtesy Robert Kravetz, MD, FACP, FACG, Phoenix, AZ.)

when activated, instantaneously created a series of parallel cuts. Like the spring lancet, the scarificator has its modern-day counterpart in the devices used for bleeding time tests.

Historically, therapeutic phlebotomy was defended well into the 1920s. During that time, studies suggested that the immune system functioned more efficiently and red blood cells carried oxygen better after small amounts of blood were removed. In spite of such studies, bloodletting for therapeutic purposes eventually declined. Meanwhile, the practice of phlebotomy to obtain blood specimens for diagnostic purposes, which establish the cause and nature of illness, began to gain favor.

PHLEBOTOMY TODAY

The practice of phlebotomy continues to this day; however, principles and methods have improved dramatically. Today, the main purpose of phlebotomy is to obtain blood for diagnostic testing. Phlebotomy procedures also are used to remove blood for transfusion purposes. Phlebotomy for therapeutic purposes is still practiced for special cases, such as in patients with polycythemia, a disease involving overproduction of

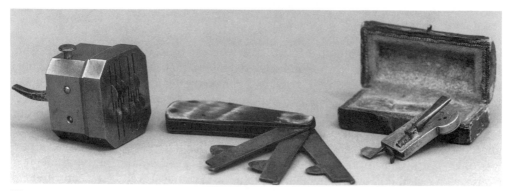

Figure 1–2 Octagonal multiple scarificator, set of fleams (lancets), and schnapper with leather-covered wooden case. (Courtesy Robert Kravetz, MD, FACP, FACG, Phoenix, AZ.)

red blood cells. The use of leeches has reemerged with a new purpose: that of reducing hemostatic swelling during microsurgery procedures.

Phlebotomy today is accomplished by one of two procedures: 1) venipuncture, which involves collecting blood by penetrating a vein with a needle and syringe or other collection apparatus; and 2) skin puncture, which involves collecting blood after puncturing the skin with a lancet or similar skin puncture device.

THE ROLE OF THE PHLEBOTOMIST

Today, phlebotomy is one of the fastest-growing health care occupations. The term *phlebotomist* is applied to a person who has been trained to perform phlebotomy procedures. The primary responsibility of a phlebotomist is to collect blood for laboratory analysis, which is necessary for the diagnosis and care of a patient. Manual skills required are those necessary to obtain blood specimens by venipuncture and skin puncture techniques. Mental skills required are the ability to organize efficiently, perform under pressure, and follow written standardized procedures. Thorough knowledge of laboratory test requirements and departmental policies is also necessary.

The Duties of a Phlebotomist

1. Collect routine capillary and venous specimens for testing as required.
2. Prepare specimens for transport to ensure stability of sample.
3. Transport specimens to the laboratory.
4. Comply with new or revised procedures instituted in the procedure manual.
5. Promote good public relations with patients and hospital personnel.
6. Assist in collecting and documenting monthly workload and recording data.
7. Maintain safe working conditions.
8. Perform laboratory computer operations.
9. Participate in continuing education programs.

Phlebotomy is considered a profession with a standardized educational curriculum or "body of knowledge" and accepted routes for national certification that have led to increased recognition for phlebotomists.

Professionalism

Phlebotomists, as all other health care workers, must practice professionalism. **Professionalism** is defined as the conduct and qualities that characterize a professional person. The overall impression conveyed by a person creates an image. The professional image is the way in which an occupation or a member of that occupation is perceived. This image is formed by two levels of traits. One level concerns the superficial aspects, for example, the way people dress or their manner of speaking. In fact, general appearance and grooming reflect directly on whether the phlebotomist is perceived as a professional. The proper attire for the phlebotomist is defined by institution guidelines. Conservative clothing, proper personal hygiene, and physical well-being contribute to a professional appearance.

The other level of traits that forms a professional image comes from public recognition of the education level the individual has achieved and the assumption that there is regulation of the profession. It is through national accrediting and certifying agencies that professions ensure adherence to the standards expected of them. Because there are different philosophies concerning standards for phlebotomy curriculum and certification, a number of agencies have evolved offering the phlebotomist options for professional recognition.

CERTIFICATION

Today, health care facilities are finding it advantageous to require national certification of their phlebotomists to satisfy changing requirements by state and federal agencies. **Certification** is a process which indicates the completion of defined academic and training requirements and the attainment of a satisfactory score on a national examination. This is verified by the awarding of a title signified by initials, which a phlebotomist is allowed to display after his or her name. The purpose of certification is to protect the public through control of personnel working at a specified level of responsibility. Agencies that certify phlebotomists and the title each awards include the following:

- *American Society of Clinical Pathologists (**ASCP**):* Phlebotomy Technician, PBT(ASCP)
- *American Society for Phlebotomy Technology (**ASPT**):* Certified Phlebotomy Technician, CPT(ASPT)
- *National Certification Agency for Medical Laboratory Personnel (**NCA**):* Clinical Laboratory Phlebotomist, CLPlb (NCA)
- *National Phlebotomy Association (**NPA**):* Certified Phlebotomy Technician, CPT(NPA)

LICENSURE

Licensure is defined as a process similar to certification but at the state or local level. A license to practice a specific trade is granted through examination to a person who can meet the requirements for education and experience in that field. For example, barbers, beauticians, and nurses are licensed by the state in which they practice. Licensure **reciprocity**, which is the recognition by one state of the license or certificate granted by another state, may be granted to a professional who moves from one state to another.

PROGRAM ACCREDITATION/APPROVAL

Accreditation and **approval** of health care training programs provides an individual with an indication of the quality of the program or institution. The accreditation process involves external peer review of the educational program, including an on-site survey to determine if the program meets certain established qualifications or educational standards referred to as "**Essentials**." Most medical technology, medical laboratory technician, and histology programs seek accreditation. For phlebotomy programs, approval, rather than accreditation, is offered. The approval process is similar to accreditation; however, programs must meet educational—"Standards" and "Competencies,"—rather than Essentials, and an on-site survey is not required. Examples of approval agencies for phlebotomy programs include the following:

- *The American Society of Phlebotomy Technicians (ASPT)*
- *The National Accrediting Agency for Clinical Laboratory Sciences (NAACLS)*
- *The National Phlebotomy Association (NPA)*

CONTINUING EDUCATION

To remain current in the increasingly complex field of laboratory medicine, it is important for a phlebotomist to participate in workshops and seminars to continually upgrade skills and knowledge. Some certification agencies require proof of such "**continuing education**" to renew certification. Employers may offer in-service education or funds to attend off-site programs. National organizations that offer the phlebotomist continuing education units (CEUs) are the following:

- *The American Society of Clinical Pathologists (ASCP)*
- *The American Society for Medical Technology (ASMT)*
- *The American Society of Phlebotomy Technicians (ASPT)*
- *The National Phlebotomy Association (NPA)*

NATIONAL STANDARDS

A national, nonprofit organization formed by representatives from the profession, industry, and government called the **National Committee for Clinical Laboratory Standards (NCCLS)** develops guidelines and sets standards for all areas of the laboratory. Phlebotomy program approval as well as certification examination questions are based on these important national standards.

Another agency that affects the standards of phlebotomy is the College of American Pathologists (CAP). This national organization is an outgrowth of the American Society for Clinical Pathologists (ASCP). The membership in this specialty organization is made up of board-certified pathologists only and offers, among other services, a continuous form of laboratory inspection by pathologists. The CAP Inspection and Accreditation Program does not compete with the Joint Commission on Accreditation of Health Care Organizations (JCAHO) accreditation for health care facilities, because it was designed for pathology services only. A CAP-certified laboratory also meets Medicare/Medicaid standards because JCAHO grants reciprocity to CAP in the area of laboratory inspection.

Public Relations

As a member of the clinical laboratory team, the phlebotomist plays an important role in public relations for the laboratory. Positive public relations involves promoting good will and a harmonious relationship with staff, visitors, and especially patients. The phlebotomist is often the only real contact the patient has with the laboratory. A confident phlebotomist with a professional manner and a neat appearance helps to put the patient at ease and helps establish a positive relationship. In many cases, the patient equates this encounter with the caliber of care they receive while in the hospital.

DIPLOMACY AND ETHICAL BEHAVIOR

A phlebotomist should demonstrate diplomacy and ethical behavior at all times. Diplomacy means the phlebotomist uses effective communication skills and tact while dealing with the patient, even in stressful situations. Ethical behavior entails conforming to a standard of right and wrong conduct to avoid harming the patient in any way. Based on a system of principles called **ethics**, the professional can identify conduct that is morally desirable. A **code of ethics**, while not enforceable by law, leads to uniformity and defined expectation by the members of that profession.

Ethical decisions made every day in health care facilities inevitably focus on the most complex application of modern medicine. Such decisions touch on a variety of management and patient concerns, including patient confidentiality, informed consent, treatment of the terminally ill, care for the poor, and allocation of funds for special procedures. As in the Hippocratic Oath, the primary objective in any health care professional's code of ethics must always be the patient's welfare. *Primum non nocere*, or "first, do no harm."

PATIENT RIGHTS

The phlebotomist, as any other member of the health care team, must recognize the rights or privileges a patient has while in a hospital or other health care facility. These rights have been clearly defined in a document originally published in 1975 by the American Hospital Association called **A Patient's Bill of Rights**. This document, while not legally binding, is an accepted statement of principles that guides health care workers in their dealings with patients. It states that all health care professionals, including phlebotomists, have a primary responsibility for quality patient care, while at the same time maintaining the patient's personal rights and dignity. Two rights especially pertinent to the phlebotomist are the right of the patient to refuse to have blood drawn and the right to have results of lab work remain confidential. (See the complete *Patient's Bill of Rights* in Box 1-1.)

Legal Considerations

Due to consumer awareness, lawsuits have increased in all areas of society, but this is especially true in the health care industry where the physicians and providers were once considered above reproach. As phlebotomists go about their daily activities, there are many practices that, if performed without reasonable care and skill, could result in a lawsuit. It has been proven in past lawsuits that phlebotomists can and will be held legally accountable for their actions.

For example, misidentification of patient samples that ultimately result in a patient's death or prolonged recovery time have led to filing of civil action suits against phlebotomists and their employers. Strict adherence to accepted procedures and accurate and legible medical records, including documentation at the time of incidents, are the best defenses against lawsuits. Documentation in the form of "incident or occurrence reports" plays an important part in identifying trends that are putting employees or patients at risk. A new area called "risk management" has evolved out of these concerns.

RISK MANAGEMENT

Risk is defined as "the chance of loss or injury." Because there are risks inherent in the health care profession, it is important for phlebotomists to know about these risks and know how to minimize them. Careful planning, in the form of objectives, will reduce hazards and benefit the employee as well as the patient. Steps in risk management involve: *identification* of the risk; *treatment* of the risk using policies and procedures al-

(text continues on page 10)

BOX 1–1. A PATIENT'S BILL OF RIGHTS

Introduction

The American Hospital Association presents *A Patient's Bill of Rights* with the expectation that observance of these rights will contribute to more effective patient care and greater satisfaction for the patient, his physician, and the hospital organization. Further, the Association presents these rights in the expectation that they will be supported by the hospital on behalf of its patients, as an integral part of the healing process. It is recognized that a personal relationship between the physician and the patient is essential for the provision of proper medical care. The traditional physician–patient relationship takes on a new dimension when care is rendered within an organizational structure. Legal precedent has established that the institution itself also has a responsibility to the patient. It is in recognition of these factors that these rights are affirmed.

Bill of Rights

1. The patient has the right to considerate and respectful care.
2. The patient has the right to obtain from his physician complete current information concerning his diagnosis, treatment, and prognosis in terms the patient can be reasonably expected to understand. When it is not medically advisable to give such information to the patient, the information should be made available to an appropriate person in his behalf. He has the right to know, by name, the physician responsible for coordinating his care.
3. The patient has the right to receive from his physician information necessary to give informed consent prior to the start of any procedure and/or treatment. Except in emergencies, such information for informed consent should include but not necessarily be limited to the specific procedure and/or treatment, the medically significant risks involved, and the probable duration of incapacitation. Where medically significant alternatives for care or treatment exist, or when the patient requests information concerning medical alternatives, the patient has the right to such information. The patient also has the right to know the name of the person responsible for the procedures and/or treatment.
4. The patient has the right to refuse treatment to the extent permitted by law and to be informed of the medical consequences of his action.
5. The patient has the right to every consideration of his privacy concerning his own medical care program. Case discussion, consultation, examination, and treatment are confidential and should be conducted discreetly. Those not directly involved in his care must have the permission of the patient to be present.
6. The patient has the right to expect that all communications and records pertaining to his care should be treated as confidential.

BOX 1–1 *Continued*

7. The patient has the right to expect that, within its capacity, a hospital must make reasonable response to the request of a patient for services. The hospital must provide evaluation, service and/or referral as indicated by the urgency of the case. When medically permissible, a patient may be transferred to another facility only after he has received complete information and explanation concerning the needs for and alternatives to such a transfer. The institution to which the patient is to be transferred must first have accepted the patient for transfer.
8. The patient has the right to obtain information as to any relationship of his hospital to other health care and educational institutions insofar as his care is concerned. The patient has the right to obtain information as to the existence of any professional relationships among individuals, by name, who are treating him.
9. The patient has the right to be advised if the hospital proposes to engage in or perform human experimentation affecting his care or treatment. The patient has the right to refuse to participate in such research projects.
10. The patient has the right to expect reasonable continuity of care. He has the right to know, in advance, what appointment times and physicians are available and where. The patient has the right to expect that the hospital will provide a mechanism whereby he is informed by his physician or a delegate of the physician of the patient's continuing health care requirements following discharge.
11. The patient has the right to examine and receive an explanation of his bill, regardless of source of payment.
12. The patient has the right to know what hospital rules and regulations apply to his conduct as a patient.

Conclusion

No catalog of rights can guarantee for the patient the kind of treatment he has a right to expect. A hospital has many functions to perform, including the prevention and treatment of disease, the education of both health professionals and patients, and the conduct of clinical research. All these activities must be conducted with an overriding concern for the patient, and, above all, the recognition of his dignity as a human being. Success in achieving this recognition assures success in the defense of the rights of the patient.

Reaffirmed by the Institutional Practices Committee in 1990. *A Patient's Bill of Rights* was first adopted by the American Hospital Association in 1973. ©1990 by the American Hospital Association. Used with permission.

ready in place; *education* for employees and patients; and *evaluation* of what should be done in the future. Continuing education and communication are necessary to manage risk and keep employees informed of changes made to improve safety.

CRIMINAL VERSUS CIVIL LAW

In the United States, the legal system encompasses two areas of law: criminal and civil. **Criminal law** is concerned with acts committed in violation of laws established by state governmental agencies such as the legislature. A person convicted of a criminal offense can be imprisoned, fined, or both. **Civil law** is concerned with actions between two private parties and is based on **tort**, a legal term referring to any wrongful act resulting in injury or damage willfully committed by a private party against another party. A claim of malpractice is a tort action, which may result in monetary awards for damages.

MALPRACTICE

A patient is legally entitled to compensation for injuries caused by improper or careless actions by a health care provider. **Malpractice** is a claim of improper treatment or negligence brought against a professional person by means of a civil lawsuit. To support a claim of malpractice, it must be proven that there was negligence on the part of the health care provider. **Negligence** is defined as the failure to exercise a reasonable amount of care in a situation that causes harm to someone or something. It can involve doing something carelessly or failing to do something that should have been done. There are various levels of negligence including slight (not much), ordinary (failing to act as a reasonable, careful person), or gross (reckless and willfull).

For negligence to be claimed there must be:

1. a legal *duty* or obligation owed by one person to another.
2. a breaking or *breach of duty*.
3. harm done as a direct result of the action.

INFORMED CONSENT

Informed consent means that the a patient must be given adequate information as to the method, risks, and consequences concerning a procedure before consenting to it. An individual has a constitutional right to refuse medical treatment. A phlebotomist who attempts a procedure without the patient's consent is violating this right and can be charged with **assault and battery**. Assault is defined as the threat to touch a person. Actually touching a person without their consent is called battery. It is, therefore, mandatory for the health care provider to obtain the patient's permission or consent before initiating any medical procedure.

CONFIDENTIALITY

The role of confidentiality is seen by many as the ethical cornerstone of professional behavior in the health care field. It serves to protect both the patient and the practitioner. As a professional, the phlebotomist should recognize that all patient information is absolutely private or confidential. **Confidentiality** or maintaining privacy of information, whether patient or employee, must always be maintained, especially when dealing with sensitive areas such as drug screens, sexually transmitted diseases, or celebrity patients. Patient information, such as a patient's test results, treatment, or condition are not to be discussed with a coworker on an elevator, in the lunchroom, or anywhere where the information might be overheard by friends or family of the patient. In addition, patient information should not be released to unauthorized persons. Any questions relating to patient information, such as from a reporter in the case of a celebrity, should be referred to the proper person in administration. Unauthorized release of information concerning a patient can lead to a claim of **breach of confidentiality** or **invasion of privacy**.

Study & Review Questions

1. Early equipment used for bloodletting includes all of the following EXCEPT the:
   a. hemostat
   b. lancet
   c. schnapper
   d. scarificator

2. A factor which contributes to the phlebotomist's professional image is:
   a. personal hygiene
   b. national certification
   c. a pleasant smile and a positive attitude
   d. all of the above

3. After successful completion of the National Certification Agency phlebotomy examination, the initials for the title granted are:
   a. CLPlb
   b. CLT
   c. CPT
   d. PBT

4. The principles of right and wrong conduct as they apply to professional problems are called:
   a. certification
   b. ethics
   c. esteem
   d. tort

5. Necessary elements of risk management are all of the following EXCEPT:
   a. education
   b. evaluation
   c. identification
   d. obligation

6. Which of the following is NOT a phlebotomist's duty?
   a. collect routine capillary specimens
   b. promote good public relations with patients
   c. obtain blood pressures and temperatures of patients
   d. perform laboratory computer operations

7. Which of the following is a patient right?
   a. to watch your test being performed in the laboratory
   b. to read other patients' medical charts
   c. to refuse treatment
   d. to be disruptive to other patients

8. Informed consent means a:
   a. phlebotomist tells the patient what is ordered and the implications of the test results
   b. patient agrees to a procedure after being told of the consequences associated with it
   c. patient has the right to look at all his or her medical records
   d. nurse has the right to perform a procedure on a patient even if the patient refuses

Suggested Lab Activities

1. Write an article on phlebotomy history from a library resource.

2. Spend a day in a health care setting where phlebotomy is performed.

3. Review case studies involving patients' rights and discuss them in class.

BIBLIOGRAPHY AND SUGGESTED READINGS

Chamberlain RT: "Professional Negligence and the Clinical Laboratory," *Journal of Medical Tech-nology*, May/June 1987.
Haller J: "The Glass Leech: Wet and Dry Cupping Practices in the Nineteenth Century," *New York Journal of Medicine*, February 15, 1973.
Murdock S, Murdock J: "From Leeches to Luers: The History of Phlebotomy," *Journal of Medical Technology*, September/October 1987.
Oran D: *Dictionary of Law*. Los Angeles: West Publishing Co., 1991.
Stanfield PS: *Introduction to the Health Professions*. Boston: Jones and Bartlett Publishers, 1990.
Wilbur, KC: *Antique Medical Instruments*. West Chester, PA: Schiffer Publishing Ltd., 1987.

The Health Care Setting

2

OBJECTIVES

On successful completion of this chapter, the reader should be able to:

1 List types of health care facilities.
2 Compare third party payer types of coverage and methods of payment.
3 Explain prospective payment system (PPS) and diagnostic-related groups (DRGs).
4 Describe hospital organization and identify the health care providers in hospitals.
5 List clinical analysis areas of the laboratory and types of laboratory procedures performed in the different areas.
6 Describe the different levels of personnel found in the clinical laboratory.

KEY TERMS

accepting assignment
CLIA '88
cost shifting
diagnostic-related groups
entitlements
health maintenance
　organizations
inpatient care
Medicaid
Medicare
outpatient/ambulatory
　care
preferred provider
　organizations
prospective payment
　system
third party payer

McCall: PHLEBOTOMY ESSENTIALS. © 1993
J. B. Lippincott Company.

STUDENTS in health care, as well as professionals, must be familiar with the organization of health care in the United States. Health providers, such as phlebotomists, benefit from this knowledge by recognizing different types of health care facilities, understanding how health care is financed, and recognizing the changing roles of personnel.

TYPES OF HEALTH CARE FACILITIES

The recent expansion of the health care system and increased specialization has led to many types of health care facilities. The two main types are inpatient and outpatient (or ambulatory). Inpatient facilities are places where patients stay overnight. Outpatient facilities are places where patients receive treatment or care and go home the same day. Some health care facilities provide both inpatient and outpatient care.

Institutions that provide inpatient services include nursing homes, extended care facilities, rehabilitation centers, and hospitals. Facilities offering outpatient care include doctor and dentist offices, clinics, day-surgery and health centers, and hospitals.

Inpatient care is care that is performed in a hospital setting. Hospitals can be classified in one of three ways: based on length-of-stay, predominant type of service offered, or according to ownership. Box 2-1 shows some categories of ownership and types of hospitals that fall under this classification.

Outpatient or **ambulatory care** is the primary source of health care services for most people. Outpatient service is defined as the care provided outside of inpatient institutions or "care for the walking patient." As noted previously, there is a wide range of outpatient care service provided through many settings and providers, each with its own advantages and limitations. Most of the outpatient care that people receive is provided in office-based practices.

Box 2–1. CLASSIFICATION OF INPATIENT FACILITIES

Government, federal	**Government, nonfederal**
Air Force	state
Army	county
Navy	city
Public Health Indian Service	
Veterans Administration	
Nongovernment, not-for-profit	**Investor-owned, for-profit**
church-operated	individual
community	partnership
	corporation

FINANCING HEALTH CARE

Health care is expensive and the cost continues to escalate. The consumer must make choices based on financial as well as medical need, and can no longer afford to be passive in the process. The health care professional, such as the phlebotomist, in addition to being a consumer, is also an employee of an institution that relies on third party payers (health insurers) for a large portion of its income. Consequently, a health professional needs to understand the financing of health care.

Third Party Payers

Insurance is a way of pooling or distributing the risk (probability) of incurring a financial loss due to health problems and is made available through a third party payer. A third party payer can be an insurance company or government program that pays for health care services on behalf of a patient.

TYPES OF COVERAGE

Basic health insurance provides limited coverage for the most expensive services, primarily inpatient hospital and physician services. **Major medical insurance** extends coverage to include doctor visits, outpatient mental health care, medication, equipment used, ambulances, and more. **Comprehensive insurance** covers both basic and major medical plans.

METHODS OF PAYMENT

Third party payers have greatly influenced the direction of medical care. In the past decade, there have been major changes in health care payments and third party reimbursements.

PPS and DRGs. Due to the rapid rise in health care costs, the government put into place the **prospective payment system (PPS)**. The PPS, begun in 1983, attempted to standardize the Medicare/Medicaid payments made to hospitals. This plan, originally designed by the American Hospital Association, reimburses hospitals a set amount for each patient procedure using established disease categories called **diagnostic-related groups (DRGs)**. This means that the third party payer, Medicare, rather than paying on the basis of services actually used by the patient, reviews the patient's diagnosis and gives the provider a predetermined amount based on that diagnosis. Additional costs must be covered by the patient or supplemental insurance or they must be absorbed by the health care facility.

Accepting assignment. Many private insurers have followed this example and also have fixed amounts they are willing to reimburse for given services. A provider who is willing to take the amount offered as payment in full is said to "**accept assignment**." Providers who will not accept assignment reserve the right to bill the patient for the difference between what the provider's fee is and what the insurer pays.

Cost shifting. Additional methods of covering costs have been termed "**cost shifting**." This term is used to describe how providers attempt to make up for reduced reimbursements from government-paid programs by charging more to other payers.

Types of Insurance Based on Employment Status

Health insurance can be divided into three categories related to employment status: voluntary enrollment, social entitlement, and public welfare.

VOLUNTARY HEALTH INSURANCE

Voluntary health insurance was first available in 1929. Today two-thirds of those insured in the United States rely on voluntary, private insurance, which is most often linked to employment. Major categories of voluntary insurance are Blue Cross/Blue Shield; private or commercial insurance companies, such as Hartford Life and Aetna; and alternative delivery systems, such as **health maintenance organizations (HMOs) and preferred provider organizations (PPOs)**.

HMOs. Group practices that are reimbursed on a prepaid, rather than a fee-for-service basis are an increasingly popular alternative design in health care plans and are called HMOs. Members usually pay a flat fee for all defined services. Basic elements of HMOs include a legal responsibility for financing and arranging to deliver a complete package of health care services to members. HMOs compete for members, and therefore they have incentives to provide efficient, economical services. If expenditures exceed revenues, the HMO may incur a loss, which is often shared with its participating doctors and hospitals. HMOs have been on the health care scene for some time, recently moving to center stage. Large numbers of employees and their dependents are drawn to HMO company benefit options with no deductibles. HMOs are capable of commanding sizable discounts on hospital beds and service. Besides their emphasis on preventative care, HMOs control member hospital usage by encouraging outpatient surgery for certain procedures, screening proposed hospital admission, closely monitoring length of stay, and providing alternative care at home or in skilled nursing facilities (nursing homes). Some very large HMOs, such as Kaiser-Permanente, even run their own hospitals.

PPOs. Another form of alternative delivery system, a PPO is an independent group of doctors and hospitals that offer its services to employers at discounted rates in exchange for a steady supply of patients. PPOs are a blend of standard health insurance and HMOs. They encourage but do not require members to use specified providers who have agreed to offer service, usually at a set fee. The member is frequently offered a financial incentive for using a preferred provider, that is, his or her out-of-pocket expense will be greater if he or she chooses a provider who is not participating in the PPO.

SOCIAL INSURANCE PROGRAMS/ENTITLEMENTS

Two major programs fall under the category of social insurance programs: Worker's Compensation and Medicare. These programs are called **entitlements** because they are a right earned by individuals through employment. This means the employee or employer has consistently contributed a portion of earnings to a government fund to take care of future unforeseen costs.

Workers Compensation.   Workers Compensation is designed to compensate for costs, as well as pain and suffering due to work-related accidents. Benefits are paid for wages lost or medical care necessary.

Medicare.   **Medicare**, first enacted in 1965, is a federally funded program that provides health care to people over the age of 65 and the disabled, regardless of financial status. Medicare is financed through Social Security payroll deductions. Benefits provided through Medicare are divided into two categories: part A, called hospital services, and part B, called supplementary medical insurance (SMI). Virtually all of the aged population in the United States is included in Part A. Part A benefits are geared to hospital stays or "benefit periods." Benefit periods begin when the Medicare recipient is admitted to a hospital or skilled nursing facility and ends 60 days after discharge. Benefits include 90 days of inpatient care per year, and 100 days of posthospitalization skilled nursing care per year. Part B, which requires a monthly participant payment, not only complements the program, but is becoming increasingly necessary. Benefits from SMI provide payments for physician services, diagnostic tests, medical therapy, rural clinic services, home health care, and other expenses not covered by Part A.

PUBLIC WELFARE
Medicaid is a state and federal program that provides medical assistance for the indigent. It has no entitlement features. Consequently, recipients must prove their eligibility. The funds used for reimbursement purposes come from federal grants and are administered by the state. Medicaid payments are closely tied to the economic status of the beneficiary. Benefits cover inpatient care, outpatient and diagnostic services, skilled nursing facilities, and home health and physician services. Medicare and Medicaid provide more than half the funding for health care for the older population in the United States. Because these programs are administered by individual states, they vary from one state to another. Arizona is the only state that does not have Medicaid. It has a program called Arizona Health Care Cost Containment Systems (AHCCCS) which works with previously established health plans to provide medical services to those that qualify.

The Changing Health Care System
Health care systems are undergoing major revisions. The driving force behind these changes is the government's move from retrospective payments (payments made to the health provider after care is completed) to a PPS and the use of DRGs. With the implementation of the PPS, the length of patient stay has decreased and fewer admissions have been noted.

Health care facilities are struggling to survive. Additional sources of income must be found to head off an apparent disaster in health care financing. The cutbacks in reimbursement payments made by the federal government to hospitals are made to encourage the development of alternatives to inpatient care. To create additional income, hospitals are now providing a more comprehensive range of services. Some of these include:

- *Outpatient surgery services:* provides an efficient way of performing limited surgical procedures without incurring other hospital costs.
- *Long-term care and skilled nursing facilities:* used as extensions of the hospital, as medium-care facilities for short stays, or until the patient is ready to go home.
- *Home care services:* provided by hospitals for patients who require care after discharge from the hospital, decreasing the possibility of readmission to the hospital.
- *Wellness clinics:* provided by hospitals, these facilities are often located in community centers and churches. They offer health screening and monitoring, education programs, and a referral mechanism to hospital services. These services lead to reduced costs for health care.
- *Mobile vans:* equipped with the latest technology, mobile van services allow even the smallest health care facility to offer the latest technology, such as ultrasonic lithotripsy (the use of ultrasound waves to break up kidney stones), and magnetic resonance imaging, at reasonable prices.

Noting the need for change in today's health care climate, the hospital is drastically modifying services to cut costs while still meeting community needs. These changes must be successful to ensure hospital survival. Other suggested changes involve establishing "clinical-treatment protocols" whereby administration and clinicians would work together on health care management to make certain the care provided is appropriate. Cost-containment also involves tackling the issue of physician preferences for certain medical supplies and pharmaceuticals (*ie,* controlling costs means selecting the right drug for the patient, not just the most current drug on the market).

MEDICAL SPECIALTIES

The scope of the physician's profession has expanded dramatically in the last few decades due to advancements in technology. New technologies are creating entirely new areas of medical practice. Some of the health care specialties by which a doctor of medicine (MD) or doctor of osteopathy (DO) can be classified are listed below.

- *Dermatology:* treats diseases and injuries of the skin and, more recently, skin cancer.
- *Endocrinology:* diagnoses and treats disorders of the endocrine glands, such as sterility, diabetes, and thyroid problems.
- *Family Practice:* similar to general practice but now qualifies as a specialty.
- *Gastroenterology:* a subspecialty of internal medicine; treats digestive tract diseases.
- *Geriatrics:* treats disorders of old age.
- *Gerontology:* treats disorders of the aging physiologically, as well as psychologically and pathologically.
- *Hematology:* treats disorders of the blood and blood-forming organs.
- *Internal Medicine:* a general practitioner (with the exception of surgery and obstetrics) for adults.
- *Neurology:* treats disorders of the brain, spinal cord, and nerves.
- *Obstetrics/Gynecology:* deals with the female reproductive tract including prenatal

care, labor and delivery, gynecologic surgery, and menstrual and menopausal disorders.

- *Oncology:* treats patients with tumors.
- *Ophthalmology:* treats eye diseases and performs eye examinations and surgery.
- *Orthopedics:* deals with disorders of the musculoskeletal system.
- *Pediatrics:* diagnoses and treats diseases of children from birth to adolescence, does wellness checks, and gives vaccinations.
- *Urology:* treats urinary tract diseases and disorders of the male reproductive organs.

DEPARTMENTS WITHIN THE HOSPITAL

Hospitals are often large organizations whose internal structure is complex. Figure 2-1 shows one example of a hospital organization chart. The following is a description of some of the major departments in a hospital and their services.

Patient Care Services

- *Nursing:* one of the major services in the hospital involves direct patient care. This includes careful observation to assess patient condition and administration of medications and treatments as prescribed by the physician. Types of nurses found in a hospital setting include nursing assistant (NA); licensed practical nurse (LPN); registered nurse (RN), which can be either an associated degree nurse (ADN) or bachelor's degree nurse (BSN); and nurse specialists, such as nurse practitioner, nurse clinician, or nurse anesthetist. A newly emerging category of personnel in the nursing service area is the patient care technician (PCT), usually an NA who has been trained to do phlebotomy and electrocardiograms (ECGs).
- *Emergency Room (ER)/ Emergency Department (ED):* the department designed to handle medical emergencies that call for immediate assessment and management of injured or acutely ill patients, staffed by specialists such as emergency medical technicians (EMTs) and MDs who specialize in emergency medicine.
- *Intensive Care Unit:* an area of the hospital designed for increased bedside care due to the fragile condition of the patient. Intensive care units (ICUs) are found in many areas of the hospital and are named for the patient care they provide (*ie,* trauma ICU, pediatric ICU, medical ICU).

Support Services

- *Central Supply:* this unit prepares and dispenses all the necessary supplies required for patient care including surgical packs for the operating room, intravenous pumps, bandages, syringes, and other inventory controlled by computer for close accounting.
- *Dietary:* selects foods and supervises food services to coordinate diet with medical treatment.
- *Environmental Services:* includes housekeeping and grounds keepers whose services maintain a clean and attractive facility.
- *Medical Records:* maintains accurate and orderly records for inpatient medical history, test results and reports, treatment plans and notes from doctors and nurses to be used for insurance claims, legal actions, and utilization reviews.

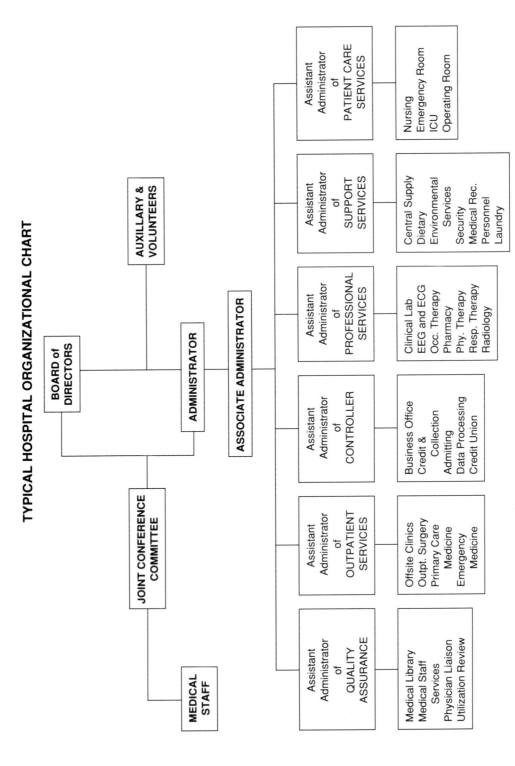

TYPICAL HOSPITAL ORGANIZATIONAL CHART

Figure 2–1 Typical hospital organization flow chart.

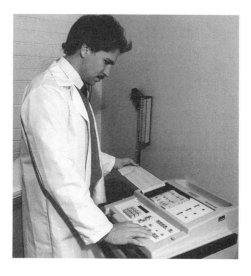

Figure 2–2   ECG technician reviews a patient tracing.

Professional Services

- *Cardiodiagnostics/Electrocardiography (ECG or EKG):* performs ECGs, Holter monitoring and stress testing for diagnosis and monitoring therapy in cardiovascular patients (Fig. 2-2).
- *Clinical Laboratory:* performs laboratory testing on blood and other body fluids to detect and diagnose disease, monitor treatments and, more recently, assess health. Highly automated, the laboratory performs complicated testing in several specialized areas of the laboratory called departments (see the following section "Departments in the Clinical Laboratory").
- *Electroneurodiagnostics/Electroencephalography (EEG):* uses techniques such as ambulatory EEG monitoring, evoked potential, polysomography (sleep studies), and brain wave mapping to diagnose and monitor neurophysiological disorders (Fig. 2-3).

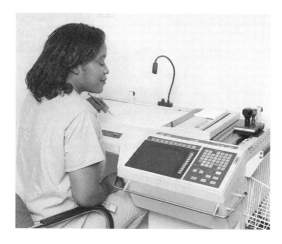

Figure 2–3   Technologist monitors an EEG.

- *Occupational Therapy (OT):* uses techniques designed to develop and/or assist patients who are mentally, physically, or emotionally disabled to maintain daily living skills.
- *Pharmacy:* prepares and dispenses drugs ordered by physicians, advises the medical staff on selection and harmful side effects of drugs, therapeutic drug monitoring, and drug use evaluation.
- *Physical Therapy (PT):* diagnoses impairment to determine the extent of the disability, and provides therapy to restore mobility through individually designed treatment plans.
- *Respiratory Therapy (RT):* diagnoses, treats, and manages patients' lung deficiencies; *ie,* analyzes arterial blood gases (ABGs), tests capacity of the lungs, and administers oxygen therapy.
- *Radiology:* diagnoses medical conditions by taking x-ray films of all parts of the body; latest procedures involve powerful forms of imaging that do not involve radiation hazards, such as ultrasound machines, magnetic resonance scanner, and positron emission scanners.

Departments in the Clinical Laboratory

There are two major divisions in the clinical laboratory: clinical analysis, and anatomic and surgical pathology. The clinical analysis area is divided into subunits including specimen processing, hematology, chemistry, microbiology, blood bank or immunohematology, immunology/serology, and education. In the larger facilities, specimens of blood and other body fluids are analyzed using automation and advanced technology. Anatomic and surgical pathology procedures include performance of autopsies, tissue analysis, cytologic examination, surgical biopsy, and frozen sections.

CLINICAL ANALYSIS AREA

Hematology. The hematology department performs laboratory analysis to identify diseases associated with blood and blood-forming tissues. Hematology tests aid the physician in diagnosing infections, leukemia, polycythemia, anemia, and other blood dyscrasias (abnormalities). The most commonly ordered hematology test is the complete blood count (CBC), which is routinely performed on automated instruments, such as the Coulter counter, that electronically count the cells and calculate results (Fig. 2-4). A complete blood count is actually a multipart assay that usually includes:

1. hematocrit (Hct)
2. hemoglobin (Hgb)
3. red blood cell (RBC) count
4. white blood cell (WBC) count
5. platelet count
6. differential white count (Diff)

Other tests performed in the hematology department include: platelet and reticulocyte counts, erythrocyte sedimentation rate (ESR), sickle cell testing, and red cell indices, which include mean corpuscular hemoglobin (MCH), mean corpuscular volume (MCV), and mean corpuscular hemoglobin concentration (MCHC).

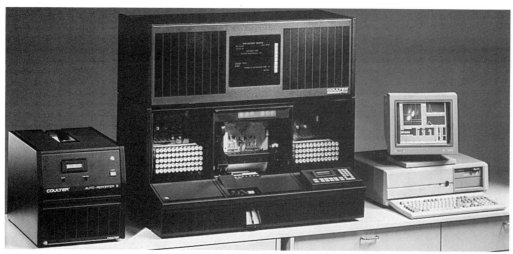

Figure 2–4   Coulter STKS System, introduced in 1989, is a fully automated, high-volume hematology analyzer. (Courtesy Coulter Electronics, Inc., Hialeah, FL.)

Coagulation.   This department is often housed in the hematology area. Coagulation deals with the study of defects in the blood clotting mechanism and the monitoring of medication given to patients as "blood thinners" or anticoagulant therapy. (An anticoagulant is a chemical that prevents the blood from clotting.) The two most common coagulation tests are the prothrombin time (PT) and the activated partial thromboplastin time (APTT or PTT). The type of specimen required is whole blood with the anticoagulant sodium citrate added. Special tests for clotting factors and platelets are also performed in this area. Disease conditions, such as hemophilia and disseminated intravascular coagulation are commonly diagnosed in this department.

Urinalysis (UA).   This department may be housed in the hematology or chemistry area. Urinalysis is a routine test performed on urine that involves chemical tests to screen for substances such as sugar and protein, and a microscopic examination to identify the presence or absence of blood cells, bacteria, crystals, and other substances. Urine culture, a very common test, is often delivered to the urinalysis area but must be taken to the microbiology department first for culture and then returned to the urinalysis section for further testing.

Microbiology.   The microbiology department analyzes body fluids and tissues for the presence of microorganisms primarily by means of culture and sensitivity (C&S) testing (Fig. 2-5). Results of a C&S tell the physician the type of organisms present, as well as the particular antibiotic that would be most effective for treatment. Collecting and transporting microbiology specimens is very important in the identification of microorganisms. Subsections of microbiology are bacteriology (study of bacteria), parasitology (study of parasites), mycology (study of fungi), and virology (study of viruses). These subsections are growing rapidly in the number of tests performed due to the in-

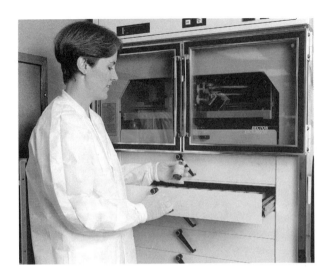

Figure 2–5 Microbiologist reviews blood cultures processed by the BACTEC NR-860.

creased numbers of contagious diseases (such as acquired immunodeficiency syndrome [AIDS] and herpes) and the increase in international travel, which exposes people to a wider range of microorganisms.

Chemistry. The chemistry department performs the majority of laboratory tests. Automated chemistry, a subsection of this department, performs most of the chemistry panels or profiles done in the laboratory. Large computerized instruments are capable of performing multiple tests from one sample. These analyzers can be programmed to do discrete (individualized) tests ordered by the physician, making this a much more efficient and cost-effective method than running all tests on all samples. Examples of tests normally performed in the automated clinical laboratory section include: glucose, triglycerides, cholesterol, electrolytes (sodium, potassium, chloride, CO_2), uric acid, creatinine, blood urea nitrogen, bilirubin, serum proteins, iron, and liver and cardiac enzymes. Subsections of clinical chemistry are **special chemistry** where tests such as lipoprotein and hemoglobin electrophoresis are performed, and a section called **immunoassay** which includes the techniques of radioimmunoassay (RIA) and enzyme immunoassay (EIA). Radioimmunoassay uses radioactively labeled antibodies and antigens while enzyme immunoassay uses enzymes in color reactions to test for hormones, hepatitis, and drugs. Chemistry tests impact other areas of laboratory analysis and are commonly involved in confirming diagnoses, as well as assessing health.

Serology or immunology. Serology literally means the study of serum. These tests deal with the body's response to the presence of bacterial, viral, fungal, or parasitic diseases, which stimulate antigen–antibody reactions and can easily be demonstrated in the laboratory. Testing is done by means of EIA, agglutination, complement fixation, or precipitation to determine the antibody or antigen present and to assess the concentration or titer. Common testing includes: rapid plasma reagin (RPR) for syphilis, cold agglutinins for atypical pneumonia, "spot tests" for mononucleosis and rheumatoid arthritis, and Antistreptolysin O (ASO) titer to demonstrate infection from *Streptococcus* bacteria.

Blood bank or immunohematology.   Routine antibody–antigen testing on red cells is performed in this department. This includes blood typing, crossmatching/compatibility testing, and antibody screening. Blood samples from all donors and the recipient's blood must be carefully tested before a transfusion can be administered so that incompatibility and transfusion reactions can be avoided. Correct patient identification and proper specimen labeling is the keystone of this department. The blood bank technologist relies on the phlebotomist to perform identification without error.

ANATOMIC AND SURGICAL PATHOLOGY
Histology.   This department is literally defined as the study of the microscopic structure of cells and tissues. Before the pathologist studies samples of tissue from autopsy or surgery, they must be processed and stained. This is the role of the histologist. Tissues can be evaluated as normal or pathologic (diseased).

Cytology.   Cytology and histology are often confused. In cytology, histologists process and prepare body fluids and tissues for a pathologist or cytologist to examine carefully for signs of disease, such as cancer. The Pap smear, a test for early detection of cancer cells, primarily of the cervix and vagina, is one of the most common examinations performed by this department.

Cytogenetics.   An area found in larger labs is cytogenetics. In this section, samples are examined for chromosomal deficiencies that relate to genetic disease. Each day, new discoveries are being made in genetic research and the study of hereditary variations. Consequently, it is predicted that this area of the laboratory will be very important in the future. Specimens used for chromosomal studies include tissue, blood, bone marrow, and amniotic fluid.

SUPPORT SERVICES
Education.   Large laboratories may have their own training programs or may serve as clinical sites for college and university programs in clinical laboratory science areas, such as medical laboratory technician, medical technologist, histologist, cytologist, phlebotomist, or pathologist. Coordination of these programs and continuing education offerings for the staff is the responsibility of this department.

Outreach programs.   This newly emerging area has become more predominant in many laboratories recently. Due to the changes in health care financing described earlier in this chapter, hospitals are being encouraged to offer laboratory services to ambulatory care facilities. The purpose of this department is to market and maintain accounts for doctors' offices and smaller labs that need diagnostic testing. This patient-oriented service uses technical people in the laboratory to offer quality lab testing to produce revenue and assist physicians in maintaining consistent patterns in patient lab results.

CLINICAL LABORATORY PERSONNEL

Laboratory Director/Pathologist

The pathologist is a physician who is a specialist in diagnosing disease from lab findings. It is his or her duty to direct lab services so they benefit both the physician and patient. This includes establishing policies and protocols; providing consultation services to medical staff; teaching in educational programs; interpreting lab results; evaluating tissues from surgery and autopsies; and performing cytology evaluations and bone marrow examinations.

Laboratory Administrator/Laboratory Manager

The lab administrator is usually a technologist with an advanced degree and several years of experience. Duties of the administrator include overseeing all operations involving physician and patient services; establishing policies and procedures; hiring new personnel; developing and maintaining operational and capital budgets; ensuring that all standards are maintained; directing all inspection processes; providing continuing education for the clinical and supervisory staff; and setting goals and objectives for the lab.

Technical Supervisors

For each laboratory section or subsection, there may be a technical supervisor who is responsible for the administration of the area and who reports to the laboratory administrator. The following responsibilities fall under this job description: ensuring adequate coverage and the best use of personnel; evaluating technical procedures and specimen requirements; ensuring that procedures are followed by all section personnel; providing continuing education, instruction, and training for the section staff; maintaining and revising procedural manuals; and contributing to preparation of the budget.

Medical Technologist/Clinical Laboratory Scientist

The medical technologist (MT) or clinical laboratory scientist (CLS) usually has a bachelor's degree in a chemical/biological science with study in an MT program for 1 year or more. Some states require licensing for MTs but will often give reciprocity to those MTs who are nationally certified. The responsibilities of the MT include performing all levels of testing, including chemical, hematologic, microbiological, and immunologic procedures pertaining to patient diagnosis; reporting results; performing quality control; conducting preventative maintenance; and troubleshooting equipment.

Medical Laboratory Technicians/Clinical Laboratory Technicians

The medical laboratory technician (MLT) or clinical laboratory technician (CLT) is an individual with an associate degree from a 2-year college or certification from a military or proprietary (private) school. As with MTs, states requiring licensing for medical/clinical laboratory technician level personnel may offer reciprocity to nationally certified technicians. The technician is responsible for performing routine testing; operating all equipment; performing basic instrument maintenance; recognizing instrument problems; and assisting in problem-solving.

Phlebotomist

The phlebotomist is trained to collect blood specimens for lab analysis necessary for the diagnosis and care of the patient. A number of facilities use phlebotomists as clerical assistants or specimen processors (see page 4 for duties).

CLINICAL LABORATORY PERSONNEL AS PROPOSED BY CLIA '88

The Clinical Laboratory Improvement Amendments of 1988 **(CLIA '88)** were signed into law on October 31, 1988, and mandated that all laboratories must be regulated using the same standards regardless of their location, type, or size. Laboratories which fall under the new regulations include more than 200,000 sites with 130,000 physician office laboratories (POL) now being included. The regulations put into force by this law deal with, among other things, laboratory standards. The standards are designed for two types of laboratory facilities. The lab type is determined by the complexity of testing done at that facility, *ie*, moderately complex or highly complex. Personnel qualifications for each of the types are stated in the regulations.

Moderately complex laboratories must have employees who can serve as director, technical consultant, clinical consultant, testing personnel, and general supervisor.

Director

The director must oversee the complete functioning of the laboratory and must periodically evaluate the competencies of the technical personnel. The director must be one of the following:

- MD, DO, pathologist
- MD or DO with 1 year of training or experience
- A person with a PhD
- A person with an MS degree with 2 years of experience or training
- A person with a BS degree with 4 years of training or experience

Technical Consultant

The technical consultant is responsible for overseeing the technical aspects of the laboratory. The technical consultant must be one of the following:

- MD, DO, pathologist
- MD or DO with 1 year of training or experience
- A person with a PhD or MS, 1 year of training or experience
- A person with a BS degree with 2 years of training or experience

Clinical Consultant

The clinical consultant serves as a liaison between the lab and its clients when reporting and interpreting results. The clinical consultant must be one of the following:

- MD, DO, pathologist
- MD or DO with 1 year of training or experience

- A person with a PhD, board certified
- MD, DO, state licensed

Testing Personnel

Testing personnel are the people who are qualified to perform the procedures at that specified laboratory level. Testing personnel in a moderately complex lab must have any one of the following credentials:

- MD, DO
- PhD, MS, bachelor's degree in an appropriate science
- Associate degree in a science
- High school diploma and appropriate training specified in the regulations

The highly complex laboratory is staffed by the same four types of personnel but the training and experience requirements are more specialized, depending on the types of testing performed. An additional category for highly complex laboratory is general supervisor.

General Supervisor

The general supervisor must be accessible to testing personnel at all times and must provide direct supervision to personnel with only high school diplomas. The general supervisor must have one of the following credentials:

- Lab director or technical supervisor
- MD or DO
- PhD, MS, bachelor's degree, and 1 year of training or experience
- Associate degree, 2 years of experience

Because of the varied job categories now in effect with CLIA '88, phlebotomists should obtain a detailed job description on employment, which could serve as legal documentation of their job responsibilities. Care should be taken to ensure that phlebotomists do not perform tasks out of their realm of responsibility because legal consequences may result.

Study & Review Questions

1. An institution that provides inpatient services is a:
   - a. clinic
   - b. doctor's office
   - ✓c. hospital
   - d. day-surgery

2. An example of a third party payer is:
   - ✓a. Medicare
   - b. DRGs
   - c. OSHA
   - d. none of the above

3. When a provider does not bill the patient for costs exceeding those covered by insurance, it is called:
   - ✓a. accepting assignment
   - b. ambulatory care
   - c. cost shifting
   - d. prospective payment system

4. State and federally funded insurance is called:
   a. OSHA
   b. PPO
   c. ASCP
   d. Medicaid

5. The specialty that treats disorders of old age is called:
   a. cardiology
   b. gerontology
   c. pathology
   d. psychiatry

6. The department in the hospital that records brain waves for diagnosis is:
   a. electroneurodiagnostics
   b. occupational therapy
   c. physical therapy
   d. radiology

7. The microbiology department in the laboratory performs:
   a. typing and crossmatching
   b. enzyme-linked immunoassay
   c. electrolyte monitoring
   d. blood culture testing

8. The abbreviation for the routine hematology test that includes hemoglobin, hematocrit, red blood count, and white blood count determinations is called:
   a. CDC
   b. CRP
   c. CBC
   d. CPK

Suggested Laboratory Activities

1. Tour a major hospital or other health care facility.

2. Summarize a news article concerning health issues.

3. Spend a day with a health care worker in a field other than phlebotomy.

4. Form class debate teams and discuss current hot topics in health care.

5. Tour a laboratory with a check-off list of terms related to departments and tests.

BIBLIOGRAPHY AND SUGGESTED READINGS

Stanfield PS: *Introduction to the Health Professions.* Boston: Jones and Bartlett Publishers, 1990.

Williams S, Torrens P: *Introduction to Health Services,* (3rd ed.). New York: Delmar Publishers, Inc., 1988.

"CLIA '88: Final Standard is Published," *Clinical Chemistry News,* March 1992.

Medical Terminology

3

OBJECTIVES

On successful completion of this chapter, the reader should be able to:

1 Describe how the meaning of a medical term is determined.
2 Define the terms word root, prefix, suffix, combining vowel, and combining form.
3 State the meanings of common word roots, prefixes, and suffixes.
4 List common medical abbreviations and give their meanings.

McCall: PHLEBOTOMY ESSENTIALS. © 1993
J. B. Lippincott Company.

INTRODUCTION

All professions have a special vocabulary of scientific or technical terms necessary to speak or write effectively and exactly. Medical terminology is the special language of the health care professions. Medical terminology is based on an understanding of a few basic elements derived from Greek and Latin words that form the foundation of nearly all medical terms. These elements are: **word roots**, **prefixes**, **suffixes**, **combining vowels**, and **combining forms**.

WORD ROOTS

The foundation of all medical terms is a **word root**. A word root usually signifies the tissue, organ, or body system involved, such as *nephr*, meaning kidney. Some medical terms have more than one word root. An example is cardiopulmonary, which is made up of two word roots: *cardio*, meaning heart and *pulmonary*, meaning lung. See Table 3-1 for a list of common medical word roots.

Table 3–1.
Common Word Roots

Root	Meaning	Example
angi	vessel	angiogram
arteri	artery	arteriosclerosis
arthr	joint	arthritis
broncho	bronchus	bronchitis
cardi	heart	electrocardiogram
cephal	head	cephalic
cyst	bladder	cystitis
cyt	cell	cytology
derm	skin	dermabrasion
encephal	brain	encephalitis
esophag	esophagus	esophagitis
gastr	stomach	gastrectomy
glyc	sugar	glycolysis
hem	blood	hematology
hepat	liver	hepatitis
lip	fat	liposuction
onco	tumor	oncologist
oste	bone	osteochondritis
phleb	vein	phlebotomy
pulmon	lung	pulmonary
scler	hard	sclerotic
thromb	clot	thrombosis
thorac	chest	thoracic
vas	vessel	vasectomy
ven	vein	venipuncture

homeostasis – balance

Table 3–2.
Common Prefixes

Prefix	Meaning	Example
a-, an-, ar-	without	afebrile
aero-	air	aerobic
aniso-	unequal	anisocytosis
anti-	against	antiseptic
cyto-	cell	cytometer
cysto-	bladder	cystocele
hemo-	blood	hemostasis
hemi-	half	hemiplegia
hetero-	different	heterosexual
homo-	same	homogeneous
hyper-	too much, high	hypertension
hypo-	low, under	hypoactive
intra-	within	intramuscular
inter-	between	intercellular
iso-	equal, same	isothermal
macro-	large, long	macrocyte
micro-	small	microcyte
poly-	many, much	polyuria

stop bleeding

PREFIXES

A **prefix** precedes a word root and modifies its meaning. A term is never made up of a prefix alone.

Example: A   / NUCLEAR
            prefix   root
        (without)   (nucleus)

The prefix "a" means "without"; the word root "nuclear" means "nucleus." The word anuclear means "without a nucleus." Table 3-2 lists common prefixes.

SUFFIXES

A **suffix**, often referred to as a "word ending," follows a word root and either changes the meaning of the word root or adds to it. A word meaning is best determined by starting with the suffix. As with a prefix, a suffix never stands alone.

Example: GASTR /   IC
            root   suffix
        (stomach)   (pertaining to)

The word root "gastr" means stomach. The suffix "ic" means "pertaining to." Thus the word gastric means "pertaining to the stomach." Table 3-3 lists common suffixes.

Table 3-3.
Common Suffixes

Suffix	Meaning	Example
-algia	pain	neuralgia
-centesis	surgical puncture to remove a fluid	thoracentesis
-coccus	berry-shaped bacteria	*Streptococcus*
-cyte	cell	erythrocyte
-emia	blood condition	anemia
-gram	recording, writing	electrocardiogram
-itis	inflammation	tonsillitis
-logist	specialist in the study of	cardiologist
-lysis	breakdown, separation	hemolysis
-megaly	enlargement	acromegaly
-oma	tumor	hepatoma
-ometer	instrument that measures or counts	thermometer
-osis	condition	necrosis
-pathy	disease	cardiomyopathy
-penia	deficiency	leukopenia
-stasis	stopping, controlling	hemostasis
-tomy	cutting, incision	phlebotomy

COMBINING VOWELS

A **combining vowel** (usually an "o") joins the word root to a suffix or another word root. A combining vowel eases pronunciation.

Example: HEMAT /   O   / LOGY
          root   combining vowel   suffix
          (blood)   (study of)

The word root "hemat" meaning "blood" is joined by the combining vowel "o" to "logy" meaning "the study of." Hematology thus means "the study of blood."

The combining vowel is usually dropped when the suffix begins with a vowel.

Example: PHLEB /   ITIS
          root   suffix
          (vein)   (inflammation)

Because the suffix "itis" begins with a vowel, a combining vowel is not used after the word root "phleb." Phlebitis means "inflammation of a vein."

The combining vowel is kept between word roots even if the second root begins with a vowel.

Example: GASTR / O / ENTER / O / LOGY
          root   root   suffix
          (stomach)   (intestines) (study of)

The combining vowel after "gastr" remains even though the second root "enter" begins with a vowel. Gastroenterology means "study of the stomach and intestines."

COMBINING FORMS

A word root along with a combining vowel is called a **combining form**. A combining form can be attached to a suffix or another word root.

Example: LEUK /   O   / CYTE
                    combining form
         root + combining vowel
         (white)   (cell)

The word "leuk," meaning "white" combined with the word "cyte," meaning "cell" combines to form leukocyte, meaning "white blood cell."

MEDICAL TERMINOLOGY REMINDERS

1. When defining a medical term, begin at the suffix and read back through the word to the beginning.
2. When a suffix starts with a vowel, drop the combining vowel before the suffix.
3. A combining vowel remains between word roots, even when the root begins with a vowel.

ABBREVIATIONS AND SYMBOLS

Some of the most common medical abbreviations and symbols are listed in Table 3-4.

Table 3–4.
Common Medical Abbreviations and Symbols

ABO	blood group system
a.c.	before meals
ACTH	adrenocorticotropic hormone
ADH	antidiuretic hormone
ad lib	as desired
AIDS	acquired immunodeficiency syndrome
ALL	acute lymphocytic leukemia
alk phos	alkaline phosphatase
ALT	alanine transaminase (see SGPT)
AML	acute myelocytic leukemia
aq	water (*aqua*)
AST	aspartate aminotransferase (see SGOT)
b.i.d.	twice a day (*bis in die*)
BP	blood pressure
BUN	blood urea nitrogen
Bx	biopsy

(continued)

Table 3–4.
Common Medical Abbreviations and Symbols (*Continued*)

c̄	with (*cum*)
Ca	calcium, cancer
CAD	coronary artery disease
CBC	complete blood count
cc	cubic centimeter
CCU	coronary care unit
Chemo	chemotherapy
CK	creatine kinase
cm	centimeter
CML	chronic myelogenous leukemia
CNS	central nervous system
CO_2	carbon dioxide
COPD	chronic obstructive pulmonary disease
CPR	cardiopulmonary resuscitation
crit	hematocrit (see Hct)
C-section	cesarean section
CSF	cerebrospinal fluid
CT scan	computed tomography scan
CVA	cerebrovascular accident (stroke)
CXR	chest x-ray
DIC	disseminated intravascular coagulation
diff	differential count of white blood cells
dil	dilute
DNA	deoxyribonucleic acid
DOB	date of birth
Dx	diagnosis
EBV	Epstein-Barr virus
ECG	electrocardiogram (see EKG)
EEG	electroencephalogram
EKG	electrocardiogram (see ECG)
ENT	ear, nose, and throat
Eos	eosinophils
ER	emergency room
ESR	erythrocyte sedimentation rate (see Sed rate)
exc	excision
FBS	fasting blood sugar
Fe	iron
FSH	follicle stimulating hormone
FUO	fever of unknown origin
GI	gastrointestinal
Gm, gm	gram
GTT	glucose tolerance test
GYN	gynecology
h	hour
Hb, Hgb	hemoglobin
HCG	human chorionic gonadotropin

(continued)

Table 3–4.
Common Medical Abbreviations and Symbols (*Continued*)

HCL	hydrochloric acid
Hct	hematocrit (see crit)
HDL	high-density liproprotein
Hg	mercury
HIV	human immunodeficiency virus
h/o	history of
H_2O	water
h.s.	at bedtime (*hora somni*)
hx	history
ICU	intensive care unit
IM	intramuscular
IV	intravenous
IVP	intravenous pyelogram
K^+	potassium
Kg	kilogram
L	liter; left
Lat	lateral
LD, LDH	lactic dehydrogenase
LDL	low-density lipoprotein
LE	lupus erythematosus (lupus)
lymphs	lymphocytes
lytes	electrolytes
m	meter
MCH	mean corpuscular hemoglobin
MCHC	mean corpuscular hemoglobin concentration
MCV	mean corpuscular volume
mets	metastases
mg	milligram
Mg^{++}	magnesium
MI	myocardial infarction
ml	milliliter
mm	millimeter
mono	monocyte
MRI	magnetic resonance imaging
MS	multiple sclerosis
Na^+	sodium
neg	negative
NG	nasogastric
NPO	nothing by mouth (*nulla per os*)
O_2	oxygen
OB	obstetrics
OR	operating room
P	pulse; phosphorus
Path	pathology
p.c.	after meals
PCO_2	pressure of carbon dioxide in the blood

(continued)

Table 3–4.
Common Medical Abbreviations and Symbols (*Continued*)

Peds	pediatrics
pH	hydrogen ion concentration (measure of acidity or alkalinity)
PKU	phenylketonuria *FOR infants.*
PMNs	polymorphonuclear leukocytes
PO_2	pressure of oxygen in the blood
p/o	postoperative
p.o.	orally (*per os*)
polys	polymorphonuclear leukocytes
pos	positive
post-op	after operation
PP	after meals (postprandial)
pre-op	before operation
prep	prepare for
PRN (p.r.n.)	as necessary (*pro re nata*)
PT	prothrombin time/protime
PTT	partial thromboplastin time
pt	patient
PVC	premature ventricular contraction
q.n.s.	quantity not sufficient
R	right
RA	rheumatoid arthritis
RBC (rbc)	red blood cell
req	requisition
RIA	radioimmunoassay
R/O	rule out
RT	respiratory therapy
RR	recovery room
Rx	treatment
s̄	without
Sed rate	erythrocyte sedimentation rate (ESR)
segs	segmented white blood cells
SGOT (AST)	serum glutamic-oxaloacetic transminase
SGPT (ALT)	serum glutamic-pyruvic transaminase
SLE	systemic lupus erythematosus
sol	solution
Staph	*Staphylococcus*
stat (STAT)	immediately
Strep	*Streptococcus*
Sx	symptoms
T	temperature
T_3	triiodothyronine (a thyroid hormone)
T_4	thyroxine (a thyroid hormone)
TB	tuberculosis
T-cells	lymphocytes from the thymus
T & C	type and cross-match (type & x)
TIBC	total iron binding capacity

(*continued*)

Table 3–4.
Common Medical Abbreviations and Symbols (*Continued*)

TPN	total parenteral nutrition (intravenous feeding)
TPR	temperature, pulse, and respiration
Trig	triglycerides
TSH	thyroid-stimulating hormone
Tx	treatment
U	unit
UA, ua	urinalysis
URI	upper respiratory infection
UTI	urinary tract infection
UV	ultraviolet
VCU	voiding cystourethrogram
VD	venereal disease
VDRL	venereal disease research laboratory
W	water reactive
WBC, wbc	white blood cell
wd	wound
WT, wt	weight
y/o	years old

Study & Review Questions

1. What is the meaning of the term "dermatosis"?
   - a. abnormal condition of the skin
   - b. examination of the skin
   - c. inflammation of the skin
   - d. study of the skin

2. Which of the following terms means "inflammation of a vein"?
   - a. phlebitis
   - b. phlebology
   - c. phlebotomize
   - d. phlebotomy

3. To what part of the body does the word root "hepat" refer?
   - a. head
   - b. heart
   - c. liver
   - d. lung

4. A hematologist specializes in the study of:
   - a. blood
   - b. heart
   - c. liver
   - d. stomach

5. Which part of gastr/o/enter/o/logy is the suffix?
   - a. gastr
   - b. enter
   - c. o
   - d. logy

6. Of the following word parts, which is a prefix?
   - a. arthro
   - b. hyper
   - c. oste
   - d. emia

7. What does the suffix "-algia" mean?
   - a. between
   - b. condition
   - c. disease
   - d. pain

8. Which of the following is the medical term for a red blood cell?
   a. erythrocyte
   b. hepatocyte
   c. leukocyte
   d. thrombocyte

Suggested Laboratory Activities

1. Make flash cards with word parts and meanings.

2. Have a spelling or "meaning of the term" bee.

3. Do matching exercises with medical terminology lists supplied by the instructor.

4. Write a fictional case study using a list of assigned terms.

BIBLIOGRAPHY AND SUGGESTED READINGS

Cohen BJ: *Medical Terminology: An Illustrated Guide*. Philadelphia: JB Lippincott Company, 1989.
Thomas C: *Taber's Cyclopedic Medical Dictionary*, 16th ed. Philadelphia: F.A. Davis Company, 1989.

An Overview of the Anatomy and Physiology of the Human Body

4

OBJECTIVES

On successful completion of this chapter, the reader should be able to:

1 List and define body planes and cavities.
2 Identify parts of the body based on their relationship to one of the body planes.
3 Define homeostasis and the primary processes of metabolism.
4 Name all body systems and identify the following: (a) components or major structures; (b) basic function of the system; (c) disorders related to the system; and (d) diagnostic tests associated with each system.
5 Define basic terminology associated with anatomy and physiology of the body.
6 Describe body system disorders and list diagnostic tests associated with those disorders.

KEY TERMS
anabolism
anatomic position
anterior
body cavities
body plane
catabolism
distal
dorsal cavities
frontal plane
homeostasis
inferior
metabolism
proximal
sagittal plane
superior
transverse plane
ventral cavities

McCall: PHLEBOTOMY ESSENTIALS. © 1993
J. B. Lippincott Company.

INTRODUCTION

Anatomy is the branch of science that deals with the structure of living things. **Physiology** is the branch of science that deals with the functions of living things. A basic understanding of the structure and functions of the human body is helpful to the phlebotomist.

ANATOMIC POSITION

Anatomic position is a way of referring to the body regardless of actual body position. Although a patient is usually in a **supine** (lying on the back) position when examined, medically speaking, parts of the body are referred to as if the patient is standing erect, arms at the side with palms facing forward. This is called the **anatomic position**.

BODY PLANES

A **body plane** (Fig. 4-1) is a flat surface resulting from a real or imaginary cut through a body in the anatomic position. Areas of the body are often referred to according to their location with respect to one of the following body planes: frontal, sagittal, or transverse.

The **frontal** (or **coronal**) **plane** divides the body vertically into front and back portions. The **sagittal plane** divides the body vertically into right and left portions. A vertical division resulting in equal right and left portions is called a **midsagittal** (or **medial**) **plane**. The **transverse plane** divides the body horizontally into upper and lower portions.

A procedure called **computerized axial tomography (CT** or **CAT scan)** produces an x-ray of the body in a transverse plane of the body. **Magnetic resonance imaging (MRI)** can produce images of the body in all three planes using magnetic waves instead of x-rays.

BODY DIRECTIONAL TERMS

Areas of the body are also identified using **directional terms**. Directional terms describe the relationship of an area or part of the body with respect to the rest of the body or body part. Directional terms are often paired with a term that means the opposite. The following are some of the more common paired directional terms:

Anterior (ventral) refers to the front. **Posterior (dorsal)** refers to the back.
Medial means toward the midline or middle. **Lateral** means toward the side.
Proximal means nearest to the center of the body, origin, or point of attachment. **Distal** means farthest from the center of the body, origin, or point of attachment.
Superior (cranial) means higher, above, or toward the head. **Inferior (caudal)** means beneath, lower, or away from the head.

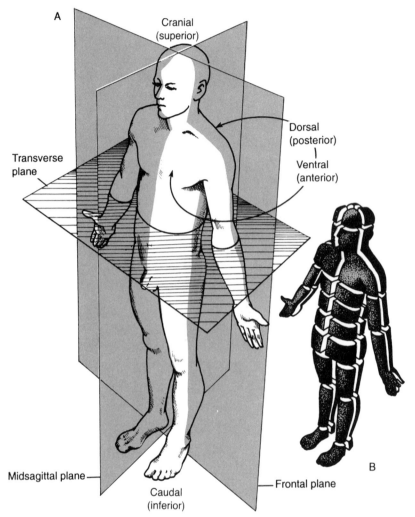

Figure 4–1   Body planes and directions (Rosdahl C).

BODY CAVITIES

Various organs of the body are housed in large hollow spaces called **body cavi-ties** (Fig. 4-2). These body cavities are divided into the following two groups, according to their location within the body.

Dorsal cavities are located in the back of the body and include:

1. the **cranial cavity**, which houses the brain
2. the **spinal cavity**, which encases the spinal cord.

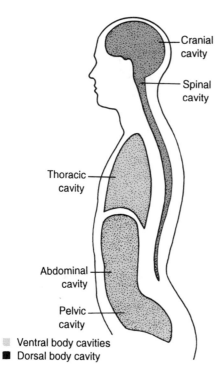

Cranial cavity

Spinal cavity

Thoracic cavity

Abdominal cavity

Pelvic cavity

▨ Ventral body cavities
■ Dorsal body cavity

Figure 4–2   Side view of body cavities (Rosdahl C).

Ventral cavities are located in the front of the body and include:

1. the **thoracic cavity**, which houses primarily the heart and lungs
2. the **abdominal cavity**, which houses numerous organs including the stomach, liver, pancreas, gallbladder, spleen, and kidneys (it is separated from the thoracic cavity by a muscle called the **diaphragm**)
3. the **pelvic cavity**, which houses primarily the urinary bladder and reproductive organs.

BODY FUNCTIONS

Homeostasis

The human body constantly strives to maintain its internal environment in a state of equilibrium or balance. This balanced or "steady state" condition is called **homeostasis** (ho'me-o-sta'sis), which literally translated means "staying the same." Homeostasis enables all the cells of the body to obtain the nutrients and oxygen necessary to maintain life.

Metabolism

Metabolism (me-tab'o-lizm) is the sum of all the chemical reactions necessary to sustain life. There are two primary processes of metabolism: catabolism and anabolism.

Catabolism/Anabolism

Catabolism (kah-tab'o-lizm) is the process by which complex substances in food are broken down into simple substances. **Anabolism** (ah-nab'o-lizm) is the process by which the body converts simple compounds into complex substances needed to carry out the cellular activities of the body.

BODY SYSTEMS

Body structures and organs which are related to one another and function together are called **body systems**. The following are 10 commonly recognized body systems.

Skeletal System

The **skeletal system** (Fig. 4-3) is comprised of all the bones (206) and joints of the body. It is the framework which gives the body shape and support, protects internal organs, and, along with the muscular system, provides movement and leverage. In addition, the skeletal system is responsible for calcium storage and **hemopoiesis** (he'mo-poy-e'sis), also called **hematopoiesis** (hem'a-to-poy-e'-sis), the production of blood cells.

TYPES OF BONES

The bones of the skeletal system are categorized by shape into four groups.

1. **Flat bones**, such as rib and most skull (cranial) bones.
2. **Irregular bones**, such as back bones (vertebrae) and some facial bones.
3. **Long bones**, such as leg (femur, tibia, fibula), arm (humerus, radius, ulna), and finger and toe bones (phalanges).
4. **Short bones**, such as wrist (carpals) and ankle (tarsals) bones.

SKELETAL SYSTEM DISORDERS

- *Arthritis* (ar-thri'tis): a common joint disorder characterized by inflammation, usually accompanied by pain and swelling.
- *Bursitis* (bur-si'tis): inflammation of the fluid-filled sac (bursa) between muscle attachments and bone.
- *Gout* (gowt): a disorder of the joints (most commonly those of the feet), caused by faulty uric acid metabolism. It is a form of arthritis.
- *Osteomyelitis* (os'te-o-mi'el-i'tis): inflammation of the bone, especially the bone marrow, caused by bacterial infection.
- *Osteochondritis* (os'te-o-kon-dri'tis): inflammation of the bone and cartilage.
- *Osteoporosis* (os'te-o-por-o'sis): disorder involving loss of bone density.
- *Rickets* (rik'ets): abnormal bone formation indirectly resulting from lack of vitamin D, which is necessary for calcium absorption.
- *Tumors:* abnormal bone growths.

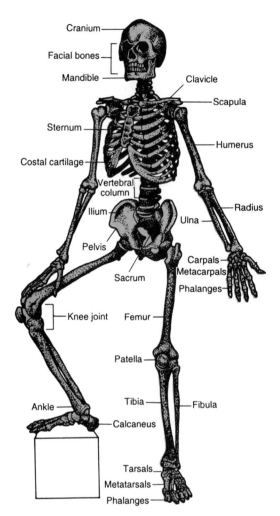

Figure 4-3   The human skeleton
(Rosdahl C).

DIAGNOSTIC TESTS

- Alkaline phosphatase
- Calcium
- Complete blood count
- Erythrocyte sedimentation rate
- Phosphorus
- Synovial fluid analysis
- Uric acid
- Vitamin D

Muscular System

The muscular system is comprised of all the muscles of the body. It includes not only those attached to the skeletal system but also those that form the walls of the heart and those that line the walls of blood vessels and the digestive tract. Muscles give the body the ability to move, maintain posture, and produce heat.

TYPES OF MUSCLES

Muscles are classified according to their location, histologic (microscopic) structure, and how they are controlled (Fig. 4-4).

Skeletal muscle is attached to bone, has **striated** (stri'a-ted) or banded muscle fibers, and is under **voluntary** (conscious) control. **Visceral** (vis'er-al) **muscle** lines the walls of blood vessels and most internal organs, is **nonstriated**, and is under **involuntary** or unconscious control. Visceral muscle is often called **smooth** muscle.

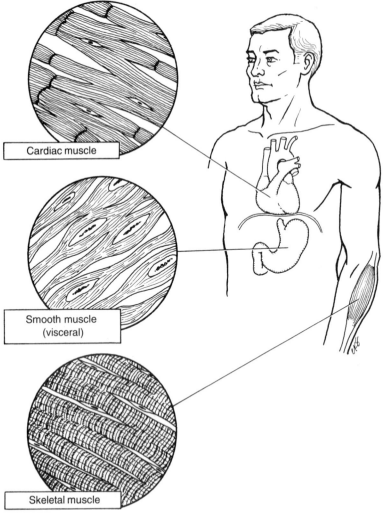

Cardiac muscle

Smooth muscle
(visceral)

Skeletal muscle

Figure 4–4 Types of muscle tissue.

Cardiac muscle forms the wall of the heart, is a special kind of **striated** muscle, and is under **involuntary** control.

MUSCULAR SYSTEM DISORDERS

- *Atrophy* (at'ro-fe): wasting (a decrease in size) of a muscle usually caused by inactivity.
- *Muscular dystrophy* (dis'tro-fe): a genetic disease in which the muscles waste away or atrophy.
- *Myalgia* (mi-al'je-ah): painful muscle.
- *Tendinitis* (ten'di-ni'tis): inflammation of muscle tendons usually due to overexertion.

DIAGNOSTIC TESTS

- Autoimmune antibodies
- Creatine phosphokinase (CPK/CK)
- CPK/CK isoenzymes
- Lactic acid
- Lactic dehydrogenase (LDH/LD)
- Myoglobin
- Electromyography

Reproductive System

The reproductive system (Fig. 4-5) produces the **gametes** (gam'eets), or **sex cells**, that are needed to form a new human being. In males, the gametes are called **spermatozoa** (sper'mat-o-zo'a) or sperm. In females, the gametes are called **ova** (o'va) or eggs. The reproductive system consists of glands called **gonads** (go'nads) and their associated structures and ducts. The gonads manufacture and store the gametes and produce the hormones (see "Endocrine System" section) that regulate the reproductive process. The male gonads are the **testes**. The female gonads are the **ovaries**. Reproduction occurs when an **ovum** (singular of ova) is fertilized by a sperm.

Structures of the female reproductive system include the ovaries, **fallopian** (fa-lo'pe-an) **tubes, uterus, cervix, vagina,** and **vulva.** Structures of the male reproductive system include the **testes, seminal vesicles, prostate, epididymis** (ep'i-did'i-mis), **vas deferens** (vas def'er-enz), **seminal ducts, urethra, penis, spermatic cords,** and **scrotum.**

REPRODUCTIVE SYSTEM DISORDERS

- *Cervical cancer:* cancer of the cervix.
- *Infertility:* a lower-than-normal ability to reproduce.
- *Ovarian cancer:* cancer of the ovaries.
- *Ovarian cyst:* a usually nonmalignant growth in an ovary.
- *Prostate cancer:* cancer of the prostate gland.
- *Sexually transmitted diseases:* diseases such as syphilis, gonorrhea, and genital herpes, which are usually transmitted by sexual contact.
- *Uterine cancer:* cancer of the uterus.

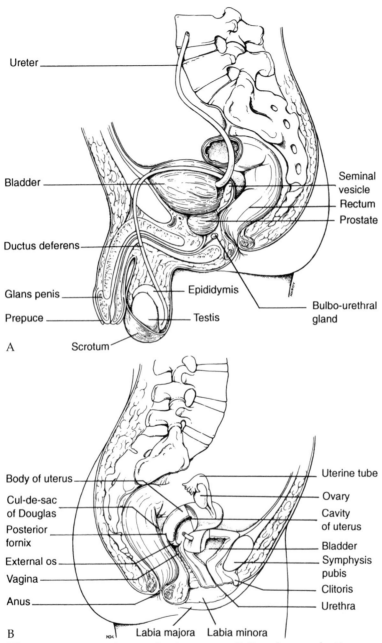

Ureter

Bladder

Ductus deferens

Glans penis

Prepuce

Epididymis

Testis

Scrotum

A

Seminal vesicle

Rectum

Prostate

Bulbo-urethral gland

Body of uterus

Cul-de-sac of Douglas

Posterior fornix

External os

Vagina

Anus

Uterine tube

Ovary

Cavity of uterus

Bladder

Symphysis pubis

Clitoris

Urethra

B   Labia majora Labia minora

Figure 4–5   *A*. Male reproductive system; *B*. Female reproductive system (Rosdahl C).

- Acid phosphatase
- Estrogen
- Follicle-stimulating hormone (FSH)
- Human chorionic gonadotropin (HCG)
- Luteinizing hormone (LH)
- Microbiologic cultures
- Pap smear
- Rapid plasmin reagin
- Testosterone
- Viral tissue studies

Digestive System

The **digestive system** (Fig. 4-6) provides the means by which the body takes in food, breaks it down into usable components for absorption, and eliminates waste products from this process.

The digestive system components form a continuous passageway called the **digestive tract**, which extends from the mouth to the anus. The digestive tract is often called the **gastrointestinal (GI) tract**. The GI tract components include the **mouth, pharynx, throat, esophagus, stomach**, and **small** and **large intestines**.

The digestive system also includes and is assisted by a number of accessory organs and structures: **lips, teeth, tongue, salivary glands, liver, pancreas**, and **gallbladder**.

DIGESTIVE SYSTEM DISORDERS

- *Appendicitis* (a-pen'di-si'tis): inflammation of the appendix.
- *Cholecystitis* (ko'le-sis-ti'tis): inflammation of the gallbladder.
- *Colitis* (ko-li'tis): inflammation of the colon.
- *Diverticulosis* (di'ver-tik'u-lo-sis): pouches in the walls of the colon.
- *Gastritis* (gas-tri'tis): inflammation of the stomach lining.
- *Gastroenteritis* (gas'tro-en-ter-i'tis): inflammation of the stomach and intestinal tract.
- *Hepatitis* (hep'a-ti'tis): inflammation of the liver.
- *Pancreatitis* (pan'kre-a-ti'tis): inflammation of the pancreas.
- *Peritonitis* (per'i-to-ni'tis): inflammation of the abdominal cavity lining.
- *Ulcer:* open sore or lesion.

DIAGNOSTIC TESTS

- Amylase
- Bilirubin
- Carcinoembryonic antigen
- Carotene
- Cholesterol
- Complete blood count
- Glucose
- Lipase

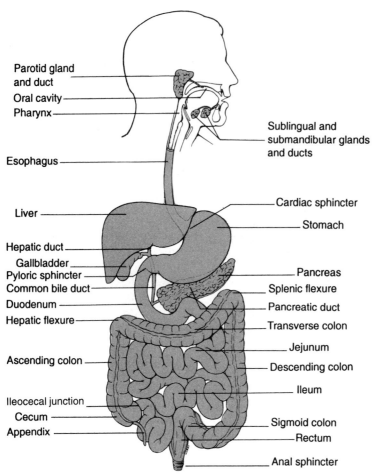

Figure 4–6 The digestive system (Rosdahl C).

- Occult blood
- Ova and parasite
- Triglycerides

Endocrine System

The word **endocrine** comes from the Greek words *endon,* meaning "within" and *krinein,* meaning "to secrete," and is used to describe a type of gland that secretes substances called hormones directly into the bloodstream. Glands of this type, also known as ductless glands, comprise the **endocrine system** (Fig. 4-7). The hormones secreted by these glands are powerful chemical substances that have a profound effect on metabolism, growth and development, reproduction, personality, and the ability of the body to react to stress and resist disease.

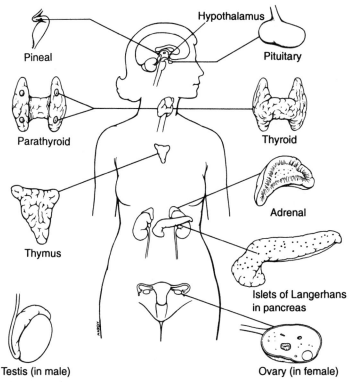

Figure 4–7   Glands of the endocrine system (Rosdahl C).

GLANDS OF THE ENDOCRINE SYSTEM

The **pituitary** (pi-tu'i-tar-ee) **gland**, located in the brain, is often called the master gland because it releases hormones that stimulate other glands. Examples of hormones released by the pituitary gland are **adrenocorticotropic** (ad-re'no-kor'ti-ko-trop'ik) **hormone (ACTH)**, which stimulates the **adrenal** (ad-re'nal) **glands; antidiuretic** (an'ti-di-u-ret'ik) **hormone (ADH)**, which decreases urine secretion; **follicle-stimulating hormone (FSH),** which affects the ovaries; **growth hormone (GH),** which is important in regulating growth; and **thyroid** (thi'royd)**-stimulating hormone (TSH),** which controls thyroid activity.

The **pineal** (pin'e-al) **gland** is located posterior to the pituitary. The endocrine function of the pineal gland is not yet fully understood. A number of hormones have been isolated from this gland, but only **melatonin** (mel'a-to'nin) is known to be a major secretory product. Release of melatonin is inhibited by light and enhanced by darkness, causing melatonin levels in the blood to follow a **diurnal** (daily) **rhythm** with levels lowest around noon and peaking at night.

The **thyroid gland** is located in the throat near the larynx. The thyroid produces **calcitonin** (kal'si-to'nin), which regulates the amount of calcium in the blood and **thy-**

roxine (thi-roks'in) or **T₄**, which increases the metabolic rate. Production of thyroid hormones requires the presence of iodine.

There are four **parathyroid** (par-a-thi'royd) **glands** located behind the thyroid gland, two on each side. The parathyroid glands produce **parathyroid hormone (PTH)**, which regulates calcium and phosphorous metabolism.

The **thymus** (thi'mus) is located in the chest behind the sternum (breastbone). The thymus produces the hormone **thymosin** (thi'mo-sin), which is necessary for the maturation of **T-lymphocytes** (specialized white blood cells) and the development of immunity. This gland is most active before birth and during childhood.

There are two **adrenal glands**, one located on top of each kidney. The inner portion of each adrenal gland produces the hormones **epinephrine** (ep-i-nef'rin) and **norepinephrine**, also called **adrenalin** (a-dren'a-lin), and **noradrenaline**. These hormones are known as the "fight-or-flight" hormones because of their effects when the body is under stress.

The outer portion of the adrenal glands produces numerous hormones. The major ones are **cortisol** (kor'ti-sol), which has the ability to suppress inflammation, and **aldosterone** (al-dos'ter-on), which is involved in regulating the amount of sodium and potassium in the bloodstream.

Special cells of the pancreas, known as **islets** (i'lets) **of Langerhans** (lahng'er-hanz), also perform endocrine activity. The islet cells secrete **insulin**, which is necessary for the normal movement of glucose from the blood into the cells, thus reducing the amount of glucose in the bloodstream. Islet cells also secrete **glucagon** (gloo'ka-gon), which stimulates the liver to release stored glucose into the bloodstream, counterbalancing the effect of insulin and increasing blood glucose levels.

The **testes** secrete the hormone **testosterone** (tes-tos'ter-on), which is responsible for the growth and functioning of the male reproductive system, as well as the development of male sexual characteristics.

The **ovaries** secrete the hormones **estrogen** (es'tro-jen) and **progesterone** (pro'jester-on), which are responsible for the growth and functioning of the female reproductive system, as well as the development of female sexual characteristics.

Other structures such as the **lining of the stomach**, the **placenta**, and the **kidneys** also have endocrine function. For example, the kidneys secrete **renin**, which increases blood pressure, and **erythropoietin** (e-rith'ro-poi'e-tin), which stimulates red blood cell formation.

ENDOCRINE SYSTEM DISORDERS

Endocrine disorders are most commonly caused by tumors, which can cause either **hypersecretion** (secreting too much) or **hyposecretion** (secreting too little) of the gland.

Pituitary disorders

- *Dwarfism:* the condition of being abnormally small, one cause of which is GH deficiency in infancy.
- *Acromegaly* (ak'ro-meg'a-le): the overgrowth of the bones in the hands, feet, and face caused by excessive GH in adulthood.
- *Gigantism:* excessive development of the body or of a body part due to excessive GH.

- *Diabetes insipidus* (di'a-be'tez in-sip'id-us): a condition characterized by increased thirst and increased urine production, caused by inadequate secretion of **ADH**, also called **vasopressin** (vas'o-pres'in).

Thyroid disorders

- *Congenital hypothyroidism:* insufficient thyroid activity in a newborn, either from a genetic deficiency or maternal factors such as lack of dietary iron during pregnancy.
- *Cretinism:* severe untreated congenital hypothyroidism in which the development of the child is impaired, resulting in a short disproportionate body, thick tongue and neck, and mental handicap.
- *Goiter* (goy'ter): an enlargement of the thyroid gland.
- *Hyperthyroidism (Graves' disease):* a condition characterized by weight loss, nervousness, and protruding eyeballs, due to an increased metabolic rate caused by excessive secretion of the thyroid gland.
- *Hypothryoidism:* a condition characterized by weight gain and lethargy, due to a decreased metabolic rate caused by decreased thyroid secretion.
- *Myxedema (hypothyroid syndrome):* a condition characterized by anemia, slow speech, mental apathy, drowsiness, and sensitivity to cold, resulting from decreased functioning of the thyroid gland.

Parathyroid disorders

Hypersecretion of the parathyroids can lead to kidney stones and bone destruction. Hyposecretion can cause muscle spasms and convulsions.

Adrenal disorders

- *Addison's disease:* a condition characterized by weight loss, dehydration, and hypotension (abnormally low blood pressure), caused by decreased glucose and sodium levels due to hyposecretion of the adrenal glands.
- *Aldosteronism:* a condition characterized by hypertension (high blood pressure) and edema caused by excessive sodium and water retention due to hypersecretion of aldosterone.
- *Cushing's syndrome:* a condition characterized by swollen "moon-shaped" face and redistribution of fat to the abdomen and back of the neck caused by an excess of cortisone.

Pancreatic disorders

- *Diabetes mellitus:* a condition in which there is impaired carbohydrate, fat, and protein metabolism due to a deficiency of insulin.
- *Diabetes mellitus type I* or *insulin-dependent diabetes mellitus (IDDM):* a type of diabetes mellitus in which the body is totally unable to produce insulin. This type is often called juvenile-onset diabetes because it usually appears before 25 years of age.
- *Diabetes mellitus type II* or *noninsulin-dependent diabetes mellitus (NIDDM):* a type of diabetes mellitus in which the body is able to produce insulin, however, either the amount produced is insufficient or there is impaired use of the insulin produced. This type of diabetes occurs predominantly in adults.

- *Hyperinsulinism:* a condition in which there is too much insulin in the blood due to excessive secretion of insulin or an overdose of insulin (insulin shock).
- *Hypoglycemia* (hi'po-gli-se'me-a): a condition in which the glucose (blood sugar) is abnormally low due to hyperinsulinism.

DIAGNOSTIC TESTS

- Adrenocorticotropic hormone (ACTH)
- Aldosterone
- Antidiuretic hormone (ADH)
- Cortisol
- Erythropoietin
- Glucagon
- Glucose tolerance test (GTT)
- Growth hormone (GH)
- Insulin level
- Renin
- Serotonin
- Thyroid function studies (*ie*, T_3, T_4, thyroid-stimulating hormone [TSH])

Nervous system

The **nervous system** (Fig. 4-8) controls and coordinates activities of the various body systems by means of electrical impulses and chemical substances sent to and received from all parts of the body. The fundamental unit of the nervous system is the **nerve cell** or **neuron**. Neurons are highly complex cells that are capable of conducting messages in the form of nerve impulses. There are two main structural divisions of the nervous system: the **central nervous system** and the **peripheral nervous system**.

The **central nervous system (CNS)** consists of the **brain** and **spinal cord**, both of which are completely enclosed and protected by three layers of connective tissue called the **meninges** (me-nin'jez). The brain and spinal cord are surrounded, cushioned, and separated from the meninges by a space filled with a clear, plasmalike fluid called **cerebrospinal** (ser'e-bro-spi'nal) **fluid (CSF)**.

The CNS functions as command center of the nervous system by interpreting information and dictating responses. Every part of the body is in direct communication with the CNS by means of its own set of nerves. All of these nerves come together in one large trunk which forms the spinal cord.

The **peripheral nervous system (PNS)** consists of all the nerves that connect the CNS to every part of the body. Two functional divisions of the peripheral nervous system are the **sensory** or **afferent** (a'fer-ent) **division** and the **motor** or **efferent** (ef'fer-ent) **division**. **Sensory nerves** carry impulses *to* the CNS from sensory receptors in various parts of the body. **Motor nerves** carry impulses *from* the CNS to organs, glands, and muscles.

The motor division can be further subdivided into the **somatic** (so-mat'ik) or **voluntary nervous system** and the **autonomic** (aw-to-nom'ik) or **involuntary nervous system (ANS)**. The somatic nervous system conducts impulses from the CNS that allow an individual to consciously control skeletal muscles. The ANS plays an important role in maintaining homeostasis by conducting impulses that affect involuntary activities of smooth muscle, cardiac muscle, and glands.

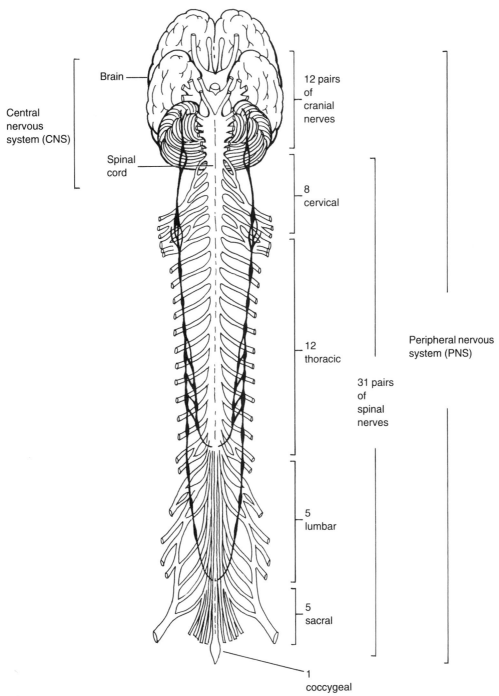

Brain

Central
nervous
system (CNS)

Spinal
cord

12 pairs
of
cranial
nerves

8
cervical

12
thoracic

5
lumbar

5
sacral

1
coccygeal

31 pairs
of
spinal
nerves

Peripheral nervous
system (PNS)

Figure 4–8   The nervous system.

- *Amyotrophic lateral sclerosis (ALS):* a disease involving muscle weakness and atrophy due to degeneration of portions of the brain and spinal cord.
- *Encephalitis:* inflammation of the brain.
- *Epilepsy:* recurrent pattern of seizures.
- *Hydrocephalus:* accumulation of CSF in the brain.
- *Meningitis:* inflammation of the membranes of the spinal cord or brain.
- *Multiple sclerosis:* disease causing destruction of the myelin sheath (fatlike covering) of the nerves of the brain.
- *Neuralgia* (nu-ral'je-a): severe pain along a nerve.
- *Parkinson's disease:* chronic nervous disease characterized by fine muscle tremors and muscle weakness.
- *Shingles:* acute eruption of herpes blisters along the course of a peripheral nerve.

DIAGNOSTIC TESTS

- Acetylcholine receptor antibody
- CSF analysis
    Cell count
    Glucose
    Protein
    Culture
- Cholinesterase
- Drug levels

Urinary system

The **urinary system** (Fig. 4-9) is responsible for filtering waste products of metabolism from the blood and eliminating them from the body. It also plays an important role in the regulation of body fluids. The urinary system is composed of two **kidneys**, two **ureters**, a **bladder**, and **urethra**.

The kidneys function to maintain water and electrolyte balance. **Electrolytes** are substances that conduct electricity when dissolved in water. Electrolytes include sodium, potassium, chloride, and bicarbonate. The kidneys also eliminate urea, a waste product of protein metabolism. In addition, the kidneys are responsible for the production of several hormones including erythropoietin.

Water and solutes filter out of the blood as it passes through the kidneys. Necessary water and substances are later reabsorbed into the bloodstream. What is left forms urine, which collects in the kidneys and travels through the ureters to the bladder. Urine is stored in the bladder and later excreted through the urethra, which leads to the exterior of the body.

URINARY SYSTEM DISORDERS

- *Renal failure:* a sudden and severe impairment of renal function.
- *Nephritis:* inflammation of the kidneys.

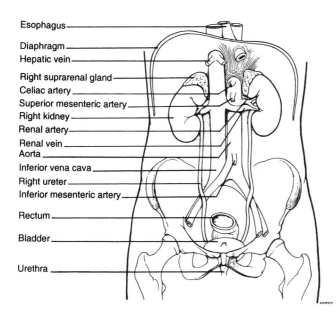

Esophagus
Diaphragm
Hepatic vein
Right suprarenal gland
Celiac artery
Superior mesenteric artery
Right kidney
Renal artery
Renal vein
Aorta
Inferior vena cava
Right ureter
Inferior mesenteric artery
Rectum
Bladder
Urethra

Figure 4–9 The urinary system (Rosdahl C).

- *Uremia:* impaired kidney function with a build-up of waste products in the blood.
- *Kidney stones:* uric acid, calcium phosphate, or oxalate stones in the kidneys, ureter, or bladder.
- *Cystitis:* bladder inflammation.
- *Urinary tract infection (UTI):* infection involving organs or ducts of the urinary system.

DIAGNOSTIC TESTS

- Albumin
- Ammonia
- Blood urea nitrogen (BUN)
- Creatinine clearance
- Electrolytes
- Osmolality
- Urinalysis
- Urine culture and sensitivity (C&S)

Integumentary System

Integument (in-teg'u-ment) means covering or skin. The **integumentary system** (Fig. 4-10) is made up of the **skin** and its appendages: the **hair** and **nails**. The skin is sometimes referred to as the largest organ of the body. It is the cover that protects the body from bacterial invasion, dehydration, and the harmful rays of the sun. The skin also functions in the regulation of body temperature, the elimination of small amounts of waste (through sweat), the reception of environmental stimuli (sensation of heat, cold, touch, and pain), and the manufacture of vitamin D from sunlight.

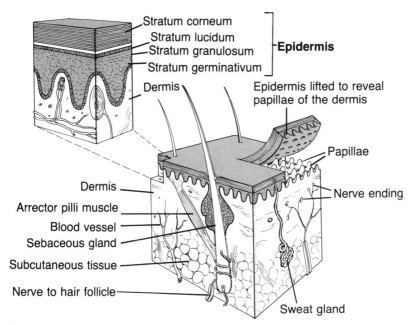

Stratum corneum
Stratum lucidum
Stratum granulosum
Stratum germinativum
Epidermis
Dermis
Epidermis lifted to reveal papillae of the dermis
Papillae
Nerve ending
Dermis
Arrector pilli muscle
Blood vessel
Sebaceous gland
Subcutaneous tissue
Nerve to hair follicle
Sweat gland

Figure 4–10   Cross-section of the skin (Rosdahl C).

LAYERS OF THE SKIN

There are two main layers of the skin: the **epidermis** (ep′i-der′mis) and the **dermis**. They are connected to a layer of **subcutaneous tissue**, which connects the skin to surface muscles and bone.

The epidermis is the outermost and thinnest layer of the skin. It is primarily made up of **stratified** (layered), **keratinized** (hardened) **epithelial** (ep′i-the′le-al) cells. The epidermis is avascular, meaning it contains no blood vessels. The only living cells of the epidermis are in its deepest layer, which is called the **stratum germinativum** (ger-mi-na-ti′vum). The stratum germinativum is the only layer of the skin where **mitosis** (cell division) occurs. It is also the layer where the skin pigment melanin is produced. The cells of the stratum germinativum are nourished by diffusion of nutrients from the dermis.

The **dermis**, also called **corium** or true skin, is the inner layer of the skin. It is much thicker than the epidermis and is composed of elastic and fibrous connective tissue. **Papillae** (pah-pil′e) or elevations and depressions in the dermis where it meets the epidermis give rise to the ridges and grooves that form fingerprints. The dermis contains blood and lymph vessels, nerves, **sebaceous** (se-ba′shus) glands and **sudoriferous** (su-dor-if′er-us) glands, and hair follicles. These structures can also extend into the subcutaneous layer.

The **subcutaneous** (under the skin) layer is composed of connective, as well as adipose (fat) tissue that connects the skin to the surface of muscles.

MAJOR STRUCTURES OF THE SKIN

Hair follicles are the sheaths from which hair develops. Hair is nonliving and is primarily composed of **keratin** (ker'a-tin), a tough protein substance.

Nails are also nonliving and made of keratin. Nails grow continuously as new cells form from the nail root located at the proximal end of the nail.

Sebaceous glands are connected to hair follicles. They are also referred to as oil glands because they secrete an oily substance called **sebum** (se'bum). Sebum helps lubricate the skin and hair and keeps it from drying out.

Sudoriferous glands, commonly called *sweat glands,* are coiled structures located in the dermis with ducts extending through the epidermis and ending in a pore on the surface of the skin. The sweat or perspiration produced by these glands is a mixture of water, salts, and waste.

Arrector pili are tiny smooth muscles attached to hair follicles. These muscles are responsible for the formation of "goose bumps" as they react to pull the hair up straight when a person is cold or frightened.

SKIN DISORDERS

- *Acne:* inflammatory disease of the sebaceous gland and hair follicles.
- *Cancer:* basal cell, squamous, melanoma.
- *Dermatitis:* skin inflammation.
- *Fungal infections:* tinea = ringworm.
- *Herpes:* cold sore = viral infection.
- *Impetigo: Staphylococcus* or *Streptococcus* infection.
- *Keloid:* fibrous tissue growth at scar area.
- *Pediculosis:* lice infestation.
- *Pruritus:* itching.
- *Psoriasis:* a chronic skin disease of unknown origin, characterized by clearly defined red patches of scaly skin.

DIAGNOSTIC TESTS

- Biopsy
- Skin scrapings for fungal culture
- Tissue cultures
- Microbiology cultures

Respiratory System

The respiratory system (Fig. 4-11) functions along with the circulatory system to deliver a constant supply of oxygen (O_2) to all the cells of the body and to remove carbon dioxide (CO_2), a waste product of cell metabolism.

These functions are accomplished through **respiration**. Respiration permits the exchange of O_2 and CO_2 between the blood and the air and involves two processes: **external respiration** and **internal respiration**. External respiration is the process by which O_2 from the air enters the bloodstream in the lungs, and CO_2 leaves the bloodstream and is breathed into the air from the lungs. Internal respiration involves the process by which

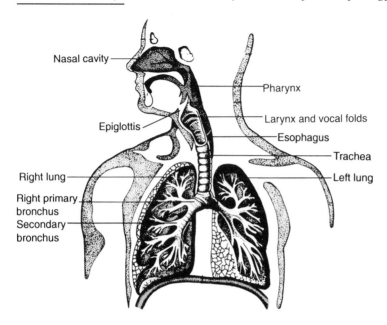

Nasal cavity

Pharynx

Larynx and vocal folds

Epiglottis

Esophagus

Trachea

Right lung

Left lung

Right primary bronchus

Secondary bronchus

Figure 4–11   The respiratory system (Rosdahl C).

O_2 leaves the bloodstream and enters the cells, and CO_2 from the cells enters the bloodstream.

The major structures of the respiratory system are the **nose, pharynx (throat), larynx (voice box), trachea (windpipe), bronchi,** and **lungs.**

The **nose** provides the main airway for respiration. (Some air enters and leaves through the mouth.) The nose also warms, moistens, and filters entering air. In addition, the nose provides a resonance chamber for the voice and contains receptors for the sense of smell.

From the nose, the air moves into the **pharynx,** a funnel-shaped passageway for both food and air. The pharynx connects with the **larynx** leading to the **lungs,** as well as to the esophagus, which leads to the stomach. The larynx acts as a switching mechanism, routing food and air into the proper pathway. The larynx also produces the sounds of the voice.

Air from the larynx then moves into the **trachea,** which branches into two main airways called **bronchi,** which lead into the lungs. Once the bronchi enter the lungs they divide into two branches, which, in turn, divide many more times into smaller and smaller branches until they reach the **terminal bronchioles.** The terminal bronchioles branch into **respiratory bronchioles,** which are attached to **alveolar** (al-ve-o-lar) **ducts.** The respiratory bronchioles, as well as the alveolar ducts have cup-shaped outpouchings called **alveoli** (al-ve'o-li). The alveoli at the ends of the alveolar ducts are clustered together into **alveolar sacs.** Gas exchange between the air and the blood occurs across the walls of the alveoli.

The walls of the alveoli are composed of a singular layer of epithelium surrounded by a thin membrane. The thinness of the walls would ordinarily leave them prone to collapse. However, a coating of fluid called **surfactant** lowers the surface tension (or pull) on the walls and helps to stabilize them. (A deficiency of surfactant in premature babies allows their alveoli to collapse and is often involved in a condition called **infant respiratory distress syndrome** or IRDS.)

Under normal conditions, oxygen and carbon dioxide are able to diffuse (go from an area of higher concentration to an area of lower concentration) through the walls of the alveoli and the tiny one-cell thick blood vessels (capillaries) of the lungs. Because the blood in lung capillaries is low in O_2 and high in CO_2, O_2 from the alveoli diffuses into the blood in the capillaries while CO_2 diffuses from the capillaries into the alveoli to be **expired** (breathed out).

The amount of O_2 that can be carried dissolved in the blood plasma is not enough to meet the needs of the body. However, the ability of hemoglobin, a protein found in red blood cells, to carry O_2 increases the amount of O_2 that can be transported by the blood by 70 times. The ability of hemoglobin to carry CO_2 increases transport of CO_2 by 17 times.

Oxygen combined with hemoglobin is called **oxyhemoglobin**. Carbon dioxide combined with hemoglobin is called **carbaminohemoglobin**. **Association** (combining) and **disassociation** (release) of O_2 and CO_2 with hemoglobin depends on the **partial pressure** of each gas. (Partial pressure is the pressure exerted by one gas in a mixture of gases.) Oxygen associates with hemoglobin in the lungs where the partial pressure of oxygen (PO_2) is increased, and disassociates from hemoglobin at the tissues where the PO_2 is decreased. Carbon dioxide associates with hemoglobin at the tissues where the partial pressure of carbon dioxide (PCO_2) is increased, and disassociates from hemoglobin in the lungs where the PCO_2 is decreased.

RESPIRATORY SYSTEM DISORDERS

- *Upper respiratory infection (URI):* an infection of the nose, throat, larynx, or trachea such as caused by a cold virus.
- *Tonsillitis:* infection of the tonsils.
- *Asthma:* difficulty in breathing accompanied by wheezing caused by spasm or swelling of the bronchial tubes.
- *Bronchitis:* inflammation of the mucous membrane of the bronchial tubes.
- *Cystic fibrosis:* a genetic endocrine disease causing an excess production of mucus.
- *Emphysema:* chronic obstructive pulmonary disease.
- *Pleurisy:* inflammation of the pleural membrane.
- *Pneumonia:* inflammation of the lungs.
- *Pulmonary edema:* accumulation of fluid in the lungs.
- *Tuberculosis (TB):* infectious disease affecting the respiratory system caused by the bacteria *Mycobacterium tuberculosis.*
- *Respiratory distress syndrome (RDS):* severe impairment of respiratory function in a newborn due to a lack of a substance called *surfactant* in the infant's lungs.
- *Respiratory syncytial* (sin-si'shal) *virus:* a virus that is a major cause of respiratory distress in infants and children.
- *Rhinitis:* inflammation of the nasal mucous membranes.

DIAGNOSTIC TESTS

- Alkaline phosphatase
- Arterial blood gases
- Complete blood count
- Drug levels
- Electrolytes
- Microbiology cultures
- Pleuracentesis
- Skin tests

Circulatory System

The circulatory system consists of the cardiovascular system (heart, blood, and blood vessels) and the lymphatic system (lymph, lymph vessels, and nodes). The circulatory system is the means by which oxygen and food are carried to the cells of the body. It is also the means by which carbon dioxide and other wastes are carried away from the cells to the excretory organs: the kidneys, lungs, and skin. The circulatory system also aids in the coagulation process, assists in defending the body against disease, and plays an important role in the regulation of body temperature. The circulatory system is discussed in greater detail in Chapter 5.

Study & Review Questions

1. The transverse plane divides the body:
   a. diagonally into upper and lower portions
   b. horizontally into upper and lower portions
   c. vertically into front and back portions
   d. vertically into right and left portions

2. Proximal is defined as:
   a. away from the middle
   b. farthest from the center
   c. nearest to the point of attachment
   d. closest to the middle

3. The process by which the body maintains a state of equilibrium is:
   a. anabolism
   b. catabolism
   c. homeostasis
   d. venostasis

4. Which of the following is NOT a function of the skeletal system?
   a. protects internal organs
   b. provides a framework for shape and support
   c. produces red cells
   d. transports oxygen to the cells

5. The type of muscle that lines the walls of blood vessels is called:
   a. cardiac
   b. skeletal
   c. striated
   d. visceral

6. Which of the following is a test associated with the reproductive system?
   a. ABG
   b. BUN
   c. CK
   d. HCG

7. Which of the following is an accessory organ of the digestive system?
   a. heart
   b. lung
   c. liver
   d. ovary

8. Evaluation of the endocrine system involves:
   a. blood gas studies
   b. drug monitoring
   c. spinal fluid analysis
   d. hormone determinations

9. The spinal cord and brain are covered by protective membranes called:
   a. papillae
   b. meninges
   c. neurons
   d. viscera

10. The majority of gas exchange between blood and tissue takes place in the:
   a. arterioles
   b. pulmonary vein
   c. capillaries
   d. venules

Suggested Laboratory Activities

1. Demonstrate anatomic position and identify body surfaces, planes, and directional terms on a fellow student.

2. Identify body cavities and organs using anatomic models.

3. Label diagrams of the various body systems.

4. Create a chart of diseases and diagnostic tests associated with each body system.

5. Watch a film such as "The Human Body: Systems Working Together," (Coronet Film and Video, Northbrook, IL).

BIBLIOGRAPHY AND SUGGESTED READINGS

Byrne CJ, Saxton D: *Laboratory Tests: Implications for Nursing Care*. San Francisco: Addison-Wesley Publishing Company, 1986.

Fischbach F: *Laboratory Diagnostic Tests* (4th ed.). Philadelphia: JB Lippincott Company, 1992.

Marieb E: *Human Anatomy and Physiology*. New York: Benjamin/Cummings Publishing Co., Inc., 1989.

Memmler RL, Cohen BJ, Wood DL: *The Human Body in Health and Disease* (7th ed.). Philadelphia: JB Lippincott Company, 1992.

The Circulatory System

5

OBJECTIVES

On successful completion of this chapter, the reader should be able to:

1 Identify the layers and structures of the heart and the describe the function of each.

2 Describe the cardiac cycle, and how an ECG tracing relates to it; explain the origin of heart sounds and pulse rates.

3 Describe how to take blood pressure readings and what they represent.

4 Identify the two main divisions of the vascular system and trace the flow of blood throughout the system.

5 Identify the different types of blood vessels and describe the structure and function of each.

6 Name and locate the veins on which phlebotomy can be performed and describe the suitability of each.

7 List the major constituents of blood, differentiate between serum and plasma, and describe the function of each of the formed elements.

8 Define hemostasis and describe basic coagulation and fibrinolysis processes.

9 List the disorders of the circulatory and lymphatic systems.

10 Identify the structures and vessels and describe the function of the lymphatic system.

McCall: PHLEBOTOMY ESSENTIALS. © 1993
J. B. Lippincott Company.

THE HEART

The **heart** is the major structure of the circulatory system (Color Plate 1). It is the "pump" that circulates blood throughout the body. The heart is a four-chambered, hollow, muscular organ, slightly larger than a man's closed fist. It is located in the center of the thoracic cavity between the lungs with the apex (tip) pointing down and to the left of the body. The heart has three layers and is surrounded by a thin fluid-filled sac called the **pericardium** (per'i-kar'de-um).

Layers of the Heart

The three layers of the heart are the epicardium, the myocardium, and the endocardium. The **epicardium** (ep'i-kar'de-um) is the thin outer layer of the heart, continuous with the lining of the pericardium. The **myocardium** (mi-o-kar'de-um) is the thick, muscle layer of the heart. The **endocardium** (en'do-kar'de-um) is the thin membrane lining the heart. It is continuous with the lining of the blood vessels.

Heart Chambers

The heart has two sides, right and left, separated by a partition called the **septum**. Each side has two chambers; the upper chambers on each side are called **atria** (a'tre-a) and the lower chambers are called **ventricles** (ven'trik-ls). The atria are receiving chambers and the ventricles are pumping or delivering chambers.

The **right atrium** receives deoxygenated blood from the body via the **superior (upper)** and **inferior (lower) vena cavae** (ve'na ka'va). The **right ventricle** receives blood from the right atrium and pumps it to the lungs via the **pulmonary artery**.

The **left atrium** receives oxygenated blood from the lungs via the **pulmonary veins**. The **left ventricle** receives blood from the left atrium and pumps it into the **aorta** (a-or'ta). The walls of the left ventricle are nearly three times as thick as the right ventricle due to the force required to pump the blood into the arterial system.

Valves

Valves between the chambers of the heart prevent the backflow of blood, and thus keep it flowing in the right direction. The valves at the entrance to the ventricles are called **atrioventricular** (a'tre-o-ven-trik'u-lar) **valves**. The valves that exit the ventricles are called **semilunar** (sem'e-lu'nar) **valves** because they are crescent-shaped like the moon.

The **right atrioventricular valve** is called the **tricuspid** (tri-kus'pid) valve because it has three flaps or cusps. The **left atrioventricular valve** is called the **bicuspid** (bi-kus'pid) **valve** because it has two flaps. It is also called the **mitral** (mi'tral) **valve**.

Both of the atrioventricular valves are attached to the walls of the ventricles by thin threads of tissue called **chordae tendineae** (kor'de ten-din'e-e), which keep the valves from flipping back into the atria.

The **right semilunar valve** is called the **pulmonary** or **pulmonic** semilunar valve because blood passing through it goes into the pulmonary artery. The **left semilunar valve** is called the **aortic** semilunar valve because blood passing through it goes into the aorta.

Coronary Arteries

The heart does not receive nourishment or oxygen from the blood passing through it. The heart receives its own blood supply via the right and left **coronary arteries**, which are the first branches off of the aorta, just beyond the aortic semilunar valve. Obstruction of a coronary artery or one of its branches causes an insufficient supply of blood to the heart to meet oxygen needs and results in a condition called **myocardial ischemia** (is-kee'me-ah). Complete obstruction or prolonged ischemia leads to **myocardial** (mi'o-kar'de-al) **infarction** (MI) or "heart attack" due to necrosis (ne-kro'sis) or "death" of the surrounding tissue from lack of oxygen.

Cardiac Cycle

One complete contraction and subsequent relaxation of the heart is called a **cardiac cycle**. The contracting phase of the cardiac cycle is called **systole** (sis'to-le), which is followed by a relaxing phase called **diastole** (di-as'to-le).

Contraction is initiated by an electrical impulse generated from the **sinoatrial** (sin'o-a'tre-al) **node**, also called the pacemaker, located in the upper wall of the right atrium. The impulse causes both atria to contract simultaneously, pushing blood through the atrioventricular valves into the ventricles.

The impulse is then picked up by the **atrioventricular (AV) node**, located in the lower right atrium. As the atria relax, the pulse is relayed through the **AV bundle (bundle of His)** and along the **Purkinje** (pur-kin'jee) fibers throughout the ventricular muscle. This causes the ventricles to contract, forcing blood through the semilunar valves. Both atria and ventricles relax briefly before the entire cycle starts again. Each cycle lasts approximately 0.8 seconds. (See Figure 5-1 for diagram of the conduction system of the heart.)

Because the electrical impulses are detectable on the surface of the body, the cardiac cycle can be recorded by means of an **electrocardiogram (ECG or EKG)**. The ECG is an actual record of the electrical currents that correspond to each event in the heart muscle contraction. These contractions can be recorded as waves when electrodes (leads or

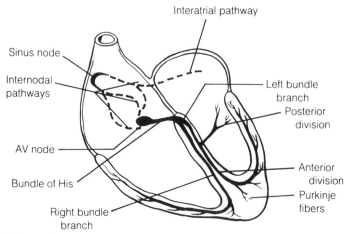

Figure 5–1 The electrical conduction system of the heart (Jones SA, Weigel A, White RD, McSwain NE, Breiter M).

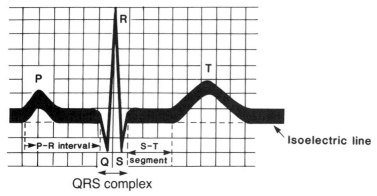

Figure 5–2 Normal ECG tracing showing one cardiac cycle (Jones SA, Weigel A, White RD, McSwain NE, Breiter M).

wires) are placed on the skin (Fig. 5-2). The P wave represents the activity of the atria and is usually the first wave seen. The QRS complex (a collection of three waves), along with the T wave, represents the activity of the ventricles. An ECG is useful in diagnosing tissue damage and abnormalities in heart rate.

Controlled exercise by means of the treadmill stress test is often used to uncover myocardial ischemia only exhibited when patients exert themselves. During this test, the patient walks on a treadmill while an ECG is continuously recorded. The patient's blood pressure and heart rate are also monitored. As the exercise rate is increased, the patient is closely observed and told to report any discomfort. The test is discontinued when the patient reports discomfort or when the maximum stress level is reached.

Origin of the Heart Sounds (Heart Beat)

As the ventricles contract, the atrioventricular valves close resulting in the first heart sound: a long, low-pitched sound commonly described as a "lubb." The second heart sound comes at the beginning of ventricular diastole and is due to the closing of the semilunar valves. It is shorter and sharper and described as a "dupp." Abnormal heart sounds, usually due to faulty valve action, are called **murmurs**.

Heart Rate and Cardiac Output

The number of heart beats per minute is called the **heart rate**. Normal adult heart rate is around 75 beats per minute. The volume of blood pumped by the heart in 1 minute is called the **cardiac output** and averages 5 liters per minute.

An irregularity in the heart rate, rhythm, or beat is called an **arrhythmia** (ah-rith'me-ah). A slow rate, less than 60 beats per minute, is called **bradycardia** (brad'e-kar'de-ah). A fast rate, over 100 beats per minute, is called **tachycardia** (tak'e-kar'de-ah). Extra beats before the normal beat are called **extrasystoles**. Rapid, uncoordinated contractions are called **fibrillations** and can result in lack of pumping action.

Pulse

The **pulse** is caused by a wave of increased pressure created as the ventricles contract and blood is forced out of the heart and through the arteries. In normal individuals, the **pulse rate** is the same as the heart rate. The pulse is most easily felt by compressing the radial artery on the thumb side of the wrist.

Blood Pressure

Blood pressure is a measure of the force (pressure) exerted by the blood on the walls of blood vessels. It is commonly measured in a large artery, such as the brachial artery in the upper arm. The pressure is measured using a **sphygmomanometer** (sfig'mo-mah-nom'e-ter), more commonly known as a blood pressure cuff. Blood pressure results are expressed in millimeters of mercury (mm Hg). Two components of the blood pressure are measured: the **systolic** (sis-tol'ik) and the **diastolic** (di-as-tol'ik).

Systolic pressure is the pressure in the arteries during contraction of the ventricles. It is the top number of a blood pressure reading and averages 120 mm Hg for adults.

Diastolic pressure is the pressure during relaxation of the ventricles. It is the lower reading and averages 80 mm Hg.

Taking a blood pressure reading involves placing a blood pressure cuff around the upper arm, and a stethoscope over the brachial artery. The cuff is inflated until the brachial artery is compressed and the blood flow is cut off. Then, the cuff is slowly deflated until the first sounds are heard with the stethoscope. The pressure reading at this time is equal to the systolic pressure. The cuff is then slowly deflated until a muffled sound is heard. The pressure at this time is equal to the diastolic pressure.

HEART DISORDERS

- *Angina pectoris* (an'-ji'na pek'to-ris): also called **ischemic heart disease**; pain on exertion caused by decreased blood flow to the myocardium from the coronary artery.
- *Aortic stenosis* (a-or'tik ste-no'sis): narrowing of the aorta or its opening.
- *Bacterial endocarditis* (en'do-kar-di'tis): an infection of the lining of the heart, most commonly caused by streptococci.
- *Congestive heart failure (CHF):* increased workload on the heart due to heart disease; causes impaired circulation to the lungs, which leads to fluid build-up in the lungs and other tissues.
- *Myocardial infarction (MI):* heart attack or death of heart muscle due to obstruction (occlusion) of the coronary artery.

DIAGNOSTIC TESTS

- Arterial blood gases
- AST (SGOT)
- Cholesterol
- CK (CPK)
- CK isoenzymes
- ECG
- LDH
- Potassium
- Triglycerides

THE VASCULAR SYSTEM

Blood circulates throughout the body within a closed system. There are two divisions to this system: the **pulmonary circulation** and the **systemic circulation**.

The **pulmonary circulation** carries blood from the heart to the lungs to remove carbon dioxide and pick up oxygen. It then returns the oxygenated blood to the heart to be pumped throughout the body.

The **systemic circulation** carries oxygenated blood from the heart, along with food from the digestive system, to all the cells of the body. The systemic circulation is also responsible for carrying carbon dioxide and other waste products of metabolism away from the cells for disposal.

Blood Vessels

Blood vessels are tubelike structures capable of expanding and contracting. Along with the heart, they form the closed system for the flow of blood.

TYPES OF BLOOD VESSELS

Arteries carry blood away from the heart (Fig. 5-3). They have thick walls because the blood is under pressure from the contraction of the ventricles. Except for the

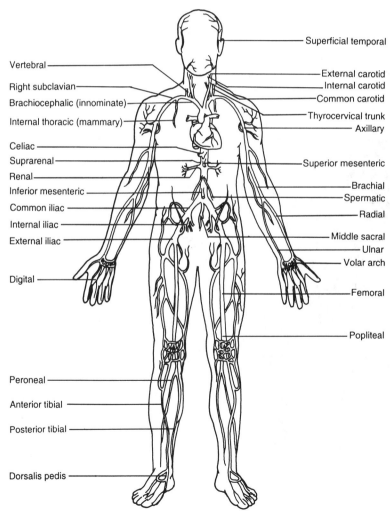

Figure 5–3   Principal arteries of the body (Rosdahl C).

pulmonary artery, which carries deoxygenated blood to the lungs, the arteries carry oxygenated blood. Because it is full of oxygen, normal arterial blood is bright cherry red in color. The smallest branches of arteries are called **arterioles** (ar-te're-olz). The largest artery in the body is the **aorta.** It is approximately 1 inch (2.5 cm) in diameter.

Veins return blood to the heart (Fig. 5-4). Veins carry deoxygenated blood, except for the pulmonary vein which carries oxygenated blood from the lungs back to the heart. Because venous blood is oxygen-poor, it is much darker in color than normal arterial blood. The walls of veins are thinner than arteries because the blood is under less pressure. Because the walls are thinner, veins collapse more easily than arteries. Blood is

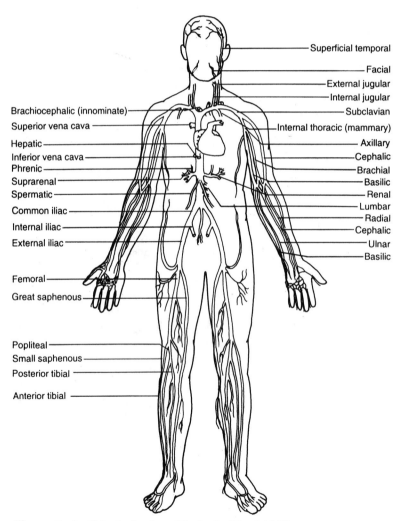

Figure 5-4   Principal veins of the body (Rosdahl C).

kept moving through veins primarily due to skeletal muscle movement. Most veins have **valves** to prevent the backflow of blood and keep it moving along. The smallest veins at the junction of the capillaries are called **venules** (ven'ulz). The largest vein in the body is the **vena cava.** The longest vein in the body is the **great saphenous** (sa-fe'nus) vein in the leg.

Capillaries are tiny vessels, one-cell thick, which connect the arterioles and venules and allow the exchange of oxygen and nutrients between the cells and the blood. Blood in the capillaries is a mixture of both venous and arterial blood.

BLOOD VESSEL STRUCTURE

Capillaries are composed of a single layer of endothelial cells. Arteries and veins are composed of three layers. Thickness of the layers varies with the size and type of blood vessel. (See Fig. 5-5 for a diagram of arteries, veins, and capillaries.)

The **tunica** (tu'ni-ka) **adventitia** (ad'ven-tish'e-a) is the outer layer. It is made up of connective tissue and is thicker in arteries than veins. The **tunica media** is the middle layer. It is made up of smooth muscle tissue; it is much thicker in arteries than veins. The **tunica intima** (in'ti-ma) is the inner layer or lining; it is made up of a single layer of endothelial cells. The internal space of a vessel through which the blood flows is called the **lumen** (lu'men).

The Flow of Blood

1. Blood returned to the heart via the superior and inferior (upper and lower) vena cavae enters the right atrium of the heart.
2. Contraction of the right atrium forces the blood through the tricuspid valve into the right ventricle.
3. Contraction of the right ventricle forces the blood through the pulmonary semilunar valve into the pulmonary artery.
4. The blood flows through the pulmonary artery to the lungs where the red blood cells release carbon dioxide and exchange it for oxygen.
5. Oxygen-rich blood flows back to the heart by way of the pulmonary veins and enters the left atrium.
6. Contraction of the left atrium forces the blood through the bicuspid valve into the left ventricle.
7. Contraction of the left ventricle forces the blood through the aortic semilunar valve into the aorta.
8. The blood travels throughout the body by way of the arteries, which branch into smaller and smaller arteries, the smallest of which are the arterioles.
9. The arterioles connect with the capillaries where oxygen, water, and nutrients from the blood diffuse through the capillary walls to the cells. At the same time, carbon dioxide and other end-products of metabolism enter the bloodstream.
10. The capillaries connect with the smallest branches of veins (venules).
11. The venules merge into larger and larger veins until the blood returns to the heart again by way of superior or inferior vena cava and the cycle starts again (Fig. 5-6 and Color Plate 3).

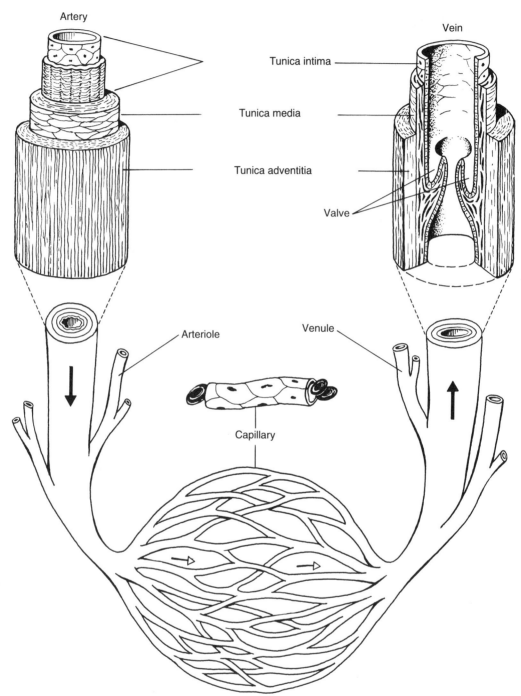

Figure 5–5   Artery, vein, and capillary structure.

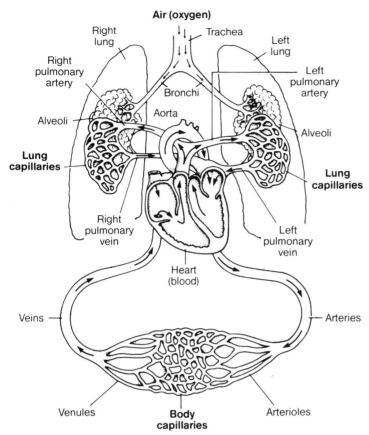

Figure 5–6   Representation of the vascular flow (National Tuberculosis and Respiratory Disease Association, New York, NY).

Vascular and Related Anatomy of the Arm and Leg

ANTECUBITAL FOSSA

The major veins for venipuncture are located in what is referred to as the **antecubital** (an'te-ku'bi-tal) **fossa**. This is the area of the arm that is anterior to (in front of) and below the bend of the elbow. Several major arm veins lie close to the surface in this area, making them easier to locate and penetrate with a needle. These veins are referred to as **antecubital veins** (Fig. 5-7A).

ANTECUBITAL VEINS SUBJECT TO VENIPUNCTURE

- *Median cubital:* the first-choice vein for venipuncture; it is usually large and well anchored so that it bruises less easily.
- *Cephalic:* the second-choice for venipuncture; it is often harder to palpate than the median cubital.

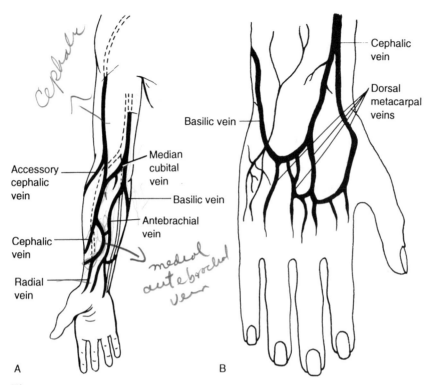

Figure 5–7 *A.* Major superficial arm veins subject to venipuncture; *B.* Hand veins subject to venipuncture (Timby BK, Lewis LW).

- *Basilic:* the third-choice vein for venipuncture. The basilic is generally easy to palpate but it is not as well anchored and rolls and bruises more easily. Venipuncture of this vein tends to be more painful to the patient. There is also the possibility of accidental puncture of the brachial artery, which lies close to the skin surface in this area.

OTHER ARM AND HAND VEINS SUBJECT TO VENIPUNCTURE

When antecubital veins are unsuitable or unavailable, other veins subject to venipuncture include veins of the forearm, the wrist, and the back of the hand (see Figure 5-7B).

LEG, ANKLE, AND FOOT VEINS SUBJECT TO VENIPUNCTURE

Leg, ankle, and foot veins (Fig. 5-8) should only be used for venipuncture when no other sites are available and with permission of the patient's physician. Puncture of the femoral vein is performed only by physicians or specially trained personnel.

ARTERIES SUBJECT TO PUNCTURE

Arterial puncture requires special training to perform, is more painful and hazardous to the patient, and is generally reserved for evaluating respiratory function. Ar-

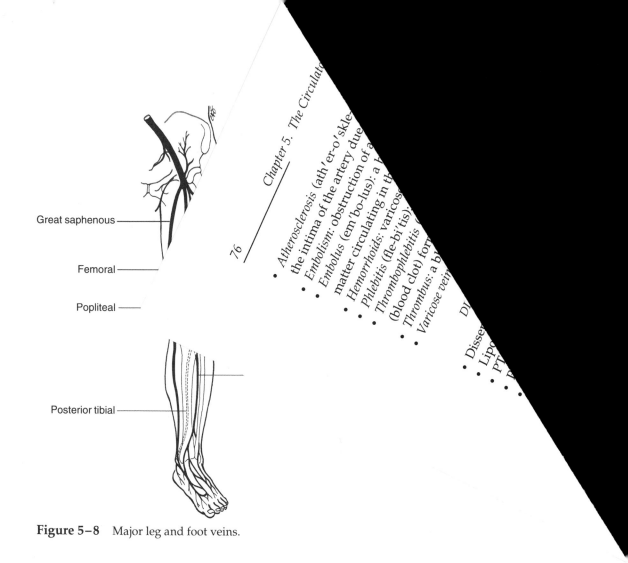

Great saphenous

Femoral

Popliteal

Posterior tibial

- Atherosclerosis (ath′er-o′skle
  the intima of the artery due
- Embolism: obstruction of a
- Embolus (em′bo-lus): a
  matter circulating in th
- Hemorrhoids: varicos
- Phlebitis (fle-bi′tis)
- Thrombophlebitis
  (blood clot) for
- Thrombus: a b
  Varicose vein

Figure 5–8 Major leg and foot veins.

teries of the arm subject to puncture are the **radial** and the **brachial arteries**. Puncture of the **femoral artery** of the leg may be performed during emergency situations or when no other arterial site is available. Puncture of the femoral artery is performed only by physicians and specially trained emergency room personnel. Arterial puncture is explained further in Chapter 13.

MEDIAN CUTANEOUS NERVE

Cutaneous nerves convey impulses for stimuli to the skin. The median cutaneous nerve is a major arm nerve that lies along the path of the brachial artery and in the vicinity of the basilic vein.

VASCULAR SYSTEM DISORDERS

- *Aneurysm* (an′u-rizm): a localized dilation or bulging in the wall of a blood vessel, usually an artery.
- *Arteriosclerosis* (ar-te′re-o-skle-ro′sis): thickening, hardening, and loss of elasticity of artery walls.

ro'sis): a form of arteriosclerosis involving changes in
to an accumulation of lipids, and so on.
blood vessel by an embolus.
lood clot, part of a blood clot, or other mass of undissolved
e blood stream.
veins in the rectal area.
inflammation of a vein.
throm'bo-fle-bi'tis): inflammation of a vein along with thrombus
mation.
ood clot in a blood vessel.
s (varices): swollen, knotted superficial veins.

AGNOSTIC TESTS

minated intravascular coagulation (DIC) screen
proteins

TT (APTT)
Triglycerides

THE BLOOD

Blood has been referred to as "the river of life." It flows throughout the circulatory system delivering nutrients, oxygen, and other substances to the cells, and transporting waste products away from the cells for elimination.

Blood is a mixture of fluid and cells that is about five times thicker than water, salty to the taste, and with a slightly alkaline *p*H of about 7.4 (*p*H is the degree of acidity or alkalinity on a scale of 1–14 with 7 being neutral). The fluid portion of the blood is called *plasma* and the cellular portion is referred to as the *formed elements* (Fig. 5-9). The average adult has about 5 liters (5.2 quarts) of blood, of which approximately 55% is plasma with the formed elements constituting the remaining 45%.

Plasma

Normal plasma is a clear, pale yellow fluid that is nearly 90% water (H_2O) and 10% solutes (dissolved substances). Composition of the solutes include the following:

- Proteins, such as **albumin,** which is manufactured by the liver and functions to help regulate osmotic pressure or the tendency of blood to attract water; **antibodies** which combat infection; and **fibrinogen** which is also manufactured by the liver and functions in the clotting process.
- Nutrients, which supply energy. Plasma nutrients include carbohydrates such as **glucose,** and **lipids (fats)** such as **triglycerides;** and **cholesterol.**
- Minerals, such as **sodium (Na), potassium (K), calcium (Ca),** and **magnesium (Mg).** Sodium helps maintain fluid balance, *p*H, and calcium and potassium balance necessary for normal heart action. Potassium is essential for normal muscle activity, and the conduction of nerve impulses. Calcium is needed for proper bone and teeth for-

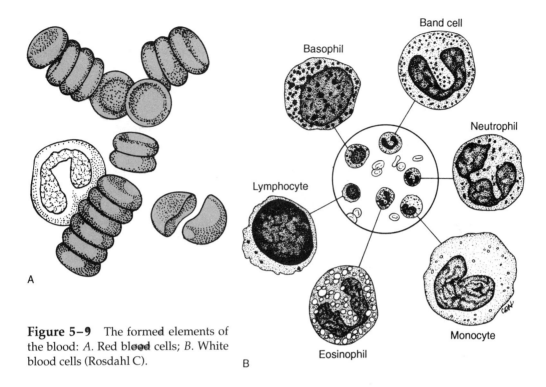

Figure 5-9 The formed elements of the blood: *A.* Red blood cells; *B.* White blood cells (Rosdahl C).

mation, nerve conduction, and muscle contraction; it is essential to the clotting process.

- Gases, such as oxygen (O_2), carbon dioxide (CO_2), and nitrogen (N).
- Other substances, such as vitamins, hormones, and waste products of metabolism such as blood urea nitrogen, creatinine, and uric acid.

Formed Elements

ERYTHROCYTES

Erythrocytes (e-rith'ro-sites), better known as red blood cells (RBCs), are the most numerous cells in the blood, averaging 4.5 to 5 million per cubic millimeter of blood. Their main function is to carry oxygen from the lungs to the cells. They also carry carbon dioxide from the cells back to the lungs to be exhaled. RBCs are produced in the bone marrow. They form with a nucleus, which they lose as they mature and enter the bloodstream. Immature RBCs in the bloodstream that contain nuclear remnants are called **reticulocytes** (re-tik'u-lo-sites). Mature RBCs have a life span of approximately 120 days after which they begin to disintegrate and are removed from the bloodstream by the spleen and liver. The main component of RBCs is **hemoglobin (Hgb or Hb)**, which enables them to transport oxygen and carbon dioxide, as well as gives them their red color. RBCs are described as anuclear (no nucleus), biconcave (indented from both sides) disks approximately 7 to 8 microns in diameter. RBCs function **intravascularly,** which means that they stay within the vascular system. An old term for RBCs is red corpuscles.

LEUKOCYTES

Leukocytes (loo'ko-sites) or white blood cells (WBCs) are cells containing a nucleus. The average adult has from 5,000 to 10,000 WBCs per cubic millimeter of blood. WBCs are formed in the bone marrow and lymphatic tissue. They function **extravascularly,** which means they have the ability to leave the bloodstream. They may appear in the bloodstream for only 6 to 8 hours while residing in the tissue for longer periods of time—days, months, or even years. The life span of WBCs varies with the type.

The main function of WBCs is to destroy pathogens. They accomplish this by a method called **phagocytosis** (fag'o-si-to'sis), in which the pathogen is surrounded and engulfed by the WBC. Some WBCs produce antibodies that destroy pathogens indirectly or release substances that attack foreign matter. An old term for WBCs is white corpuscles.

There are different types of WBCs, each identified by their size, shape of the nucleus, and whether there are granules present in the cytoplasm when the cells are stained with a special blood stain called **Wright's stain**. WBCs containing easily visible granules are called **granulocytes** (gran'u-lo-sites'). WBCs lacking easily visible granules are called **agranulocytes**.

Granulocytes.   Granulocytes can be differentiated by the color of their granules when stained with Wright's stain.

- *Neutrophils* (nu'tro-fils): Neutrophils are normally the most numerous of the WBCs, averaging 65% of the WBC total. The granules of neutrophils are fine in texture and stain lavender. Because a typical neutrophil is **polymorphonuclear (PMN)**, meaning its nucleus has several lobes or segments, neutrophils are sometimes referred to as PMNs, polys, or segs. Neutrophils are one of the main phagocytic cells. Bacterial infections are associated with the presence of increased neutrophils. The life span of neutrophils is from about 6 hours to a few days.
- *Eosinophils* (e'o-sin'o-fils): The granules of eosinophils (Eos) are beadlike and stain bright orange-red. The nucleus of an eosinophil has two lobes. Up to 3% of the WBCs in a normal adult are Eos. Eos ingest and detoxify foreign protein and help turn off immune reactions. Eos increase with allergies and parasitic infestations such as pinworms. The life span of an eosinophil is from 8 to 12 days.
- *Basophils* (ba'so-fils): Basophils (basos) are the least numerous of the WBCs, comprising less than 1% of the WBC population. The granules of basophils are large, stain dark blue, and often obscure the nucleus. Nuclei of basos are often in the shape of an S. Basos release histamine and heparin, which enhance the inflammatory response. Basos are thought to live several days.

Agranulocytes.   There are two types of agranulocytes: monocytes and lymphocytes. **Monocytes (monos)** are the largest of the WBCs. They comprise from 1% to 7%

of the WBC population. Monos have fine gray-blue cytoplasm and a large, dark-staining nucleus. Monos destroy pathogens by phagocytosis. They are sometimes referred to as macrophages after they leave the bloodstream. The life span of monos is several months.

Lymphocytes are the second most numerous of the WBCs. They comprise approximately 15% to 30% of the WBC population. A typical lymphocyte has a large round, dark purple nucleus that occupies the majority of the cell. The nucleus is surrounded by a thin rim of pale blue cytoplasm. The majority of lymphocytes stay in the lymph tissue, where they play an important role in immunity. Two main types of lymphocytes are T-lymphocytes, which directly attack infected cells; and B-lymphocytes, which give rise to plasma cells, which produce immunoglobulins (antibodies) that are released into the bloodstream where they circulate and attack foreign cells. The life span of lymphocytes varies from only a few hours to a number of years.

THROMBOCYTES

Thrombocytes (throm'bo-sits), better known as **platelets,** are the smallest of the formed elements. Platelets are actually parts of a large cell called a **megakaryocyte** (meg'a-kar'e-o-sit'), which is formed in the bone marrow. The number of platelets in the blood (platelet count) of the average adult is from 150,000 to 400,000 per cubic millimeter. Platelets are essential to **coagulation** (the blood clotting process) and are the first cell on the scene when an injury occurs. (See "Hemostasis," page 82.) The life span of platelets is around 10 days.

Blood Type

An individual's blood type (also called blood group) is inherited and is determined by the type of antigen present on his or her red blood cells. Some blood type antigens cause formation of antibodies to a different blood type. If a person receives a blood transfusion of the wrong type, the person's antibodies may react with the donor RBCs and cause them to **agglutinate** (a-gloo'ti-nat)—clump together—and **lyse** (lize)—be destroyed. Such a reaction, which can be fatal, is called a **transfusion reaction**. A person will not normally produce antibodies against his or her own RBC antigens. The most commonly used method of blood typing recognizes two blood group systems: the ABO system and the Rh factor system.

The ABO blood group system recognizes four blood types: A, B, AB, and O, based on the presence or absence of what are identified as the A and B antigens. Unique to the ABO system are the preformed antibodies present in the plasma of a person's blood that will react against RBCs carrying antigens that are not present on a person's own RBCs. These preformed antibodies are called **agglutinins**.

In the ABO system, type O is the most common blood type. Type AB is the least common. Table 5-1 shows the antigens and antibodies present in the four blood types.

Individuals with type AB blood were once referred to as **universal recipients** because they have neither A nor B antibody to the RBC antigens, and can "theoretically" receive any ABO type blood. In the same manner, type O individuals were once called **universal donors** because they have neither A nor B antigen on their RBCs and in an emergency their type can "theoretically" be given to anyone. However, type O blood *does* contain plasma antibodies to both A and B antigens and when given to an A or B

Table 5–1.
ABO Blood Group System

Blood Type	RBC Antigen	Plasma Antibodies (agglutinins)
A	A	Anti-B
B	B	Anti-A
AB	A and B	Neither Anti-A or Anti-B
O	Neither	Anti-A and Anti-B

type recipient can cause a mild transfusion reaction. To avoid reactions, patients are now given type-specific blood even in emergencies.

The Rh system is based on the presence or absence of an RBC antigen called the Rh factor. An individual whose RBCs have the Rh antigen is said to be positive for the Rh factor or **Rh positive (Rh+)**. An individual whose RBCs lack the Rh antigen is said to be **Rh negative (Rh−)**. It is important that a patient receive the correct Rh type blood, as well as the correct ABO type. Approximately 85% of the population is Rh+.

Unlike the ABO system, antibodies to the Rh factor (anti-Rh antibodies) are not preformed in the blood of Rh− individuals. However, an Rh− individual who receives Rh+ blood can become **sensitized**. This means that the individual may produce antibodies against the Rh factor. In addition, an Rh− woman, who is carrying an Rh+ fetus may become sensitized by the RBCs of the fetus, most commonly by leakage of the fetal cells into the mother's circulation during childbirth. This may lead to the destruction of the RBCs of a subsequent Rh+ fetus because Rh antibodies produced by the mother can cross the placenta into the fetal circulation. When this occurs, it is called **hemolytic disease of the newborn (HDN)**. A previously unsensitized Rh− mother can be given **Rh immunoglobulin** at certain times during her pregnancy, as well as immediately after the baby's birth. Rh immunoglobulin will destroy any Rh+ fetal cells that may have entered her bloodstream and prevent sensitization.

Other factors in an individual's blood can cause adverse reactions during a blood transfusion, even with the correct ABO and Rh type blood. For this reason, a compatibility test or **crossmatch** is performed using the patient's serum and cells, as well as the donor's serum and cells before a unit of blood is determined **compatible** for transfusion. Newly invented artificial blood, made by chemically altering donor blood, will soon be tested on humans. This blood was designed to be given to any blood type and poses no risk of transmitting disease.

Types of Blood Specimens

SERUM

Blood that has been removed from the body will coagulate or clot in about 20 to 30 minutes. The clot consists of the blood cells enmeshed in a fibrin network discussed below (see "Hemostasis"). The remaining fluid portion is called **serum** and can be separated from the clot by centrifugation (spinning the clotted blood at high RPMs in a machine called a centrifuge). Normal serum is clear, pale yellow and has the same composition as plasma **except** it *does not contain fibrinogen* because the fibrinogen was used in the formation of the clot. Many laboratory tests can be performed on serum.

PLASMA

To obtain plasma, a blood specimen must be prevented from clotting. This can be accomplished by the addition of a substance called an **anticoagulant**. Some anticoagulants prevent the blood from clotting by chemically binding calcium. Others prevent clotting by inhibiting the clotting factor **thrombin**.

The cells of a plasma sample can also be separated from the plasma by centrifugation. The resulting plasma is a clear, pale yellow fluid just like serum **except** it *contains fibrinogen*.

Some tests, such as certain coagulation tests can only be performed on plasma. Many chemistry tests can be performed on either serum or plasma. Stat chemistry tests (tests whose results are needed immediately) are often performed on plasma because the specimen can be centrifuged immediately instead of having to wait 20 to 30 minutes for the blood to clot.

WHOLE BLOOD

Some tests such as RBC, WBC, platelet counts, and other hematology tests need to be performed on blood that is in the same form as when it circulated in the bloodstream. It is important that the components of the blood *not* be allowed to separate. Such a specimen is called a *whole blood specimen*. To obtain a whole blood specimen, it is also necessary to add an anticoagulant to keep the blood from clotting. Because the components will separate if the specimen is allowed to stand undisturbed, the specimen must be mixed for a minimum of 2 minutes prior to performing the test. Because the anticoagulant may change the characteristics of the formed elements, blood smears for hematology studies must be made within 1 hour of collection.

BLOOD DISORDERS

- *Anemia:* an abnormal reduction in the number of RBCs in the circulating blood.
- *Leukemia:* an increase in WBCs characterized by the presence of a large number of abnormal forms.
- *Leukocytosis:* an abnormal increase in WBCs in the circulating blood.
- *Leukopenia:* an abnormal decrease of WBCs.
- *Polycythemia:* an abnormal increase in RBCs.
- *Thrombocytosis:* increased platelets.
- *Thrombocytopenia:* decreased platelets.

DIAGNOSTIC TESTS

- Bone marrow
- CBC
- Differential
- Eosinophil (Eo) count
- ESR
- Ferritin

- Hematocrit (Hct)
- Hemoglobin (Hb or Hgb)
- Indices (MCH, MCV, MCHC)
- Iron (Fe)
- Total iron binding capacity (TIBC)

HEMOSTASIS

Hemostasis (he'mo-sta'sis) is the process by which the body stops the leakage of blood from the vascular system after injury. It includes the process that leads to clot formation as well as clot dissolution. If an injury occurs to a blood vessel, the hemostatic process is set in motion to repair the injury. The process, also called the **coagulation** process, proceeds in four stages.

- Stage 1—**Vasoconstriction**: the damaged vessel constricts (narrows) to decrease the flow of blood to the injured area.
- Stage 2—**Platelet Plug Formation**: injury to the blood vessel exposes protein material in the basement membrane. Contact with this material causes the platelets to degranulate and stick to one another **(platelet aggregation)** and adhere to the injured area **(platelet adhesion)** forming a "platelet plug." Normal platelet plug formation depends on an adequate concentration of platelets in the blood (determined by a platelet count), normal functioning of platelets, and blood vessel integrity. A bleeding time test assesses platelet plug formation.

  Stages 1 and 2 are referred to as **primary hemostasis**. For some injuries, such as a needle puncture of a vein, primary hemostasis is all that is needed to heal the injury and the process proceeds no further. For larger injuries, the process continues to **secondary hemostasis** involving formation of a tougher "fibrin" clot formed of RBCs, platelets, and fibrin.
- Stage 3—**Fibrin Clot Formation**: fibrin clot formation involves the complex interaction of a series of coagulation **factors** designated by Roman numerals in the order of discovery. Once activated, each factor activates the next factor in sequence somewhat like a cascade. This **coagulation cascade** (Fig. 5-10) can be initiated by two separate pathways, the **intrinsic** and the **extrinsic**, both of which eventually join to form a common pathway that ends in the formation of a fibrin clot. Both pathways require the presence of calcium and phospholipid from the platelets.

  Intrinsic: The intrinsic pathway involves coagulation factors circulating within the bloodstream and is initiated with activation of factor XII. Functioning of the intrinsic pathway is measured by the activated partial thromboplastin test (APTT or PTT), which is also useful in monitoring heparin therapy.

  Extrinsic: The extrinsic pathway is initiated by the release of thromboplastin (factor III) from injured tissue and the activation of factor VII. The prothrombin test (PT) measures the functioning of the extrinsic pathway and is used to monitor coumarin therapy.

  Common pathway: Both pathways lead to the activation of factor X and the initiation of the factors of the common pathway. Ultimately prothrombin (factor II) is

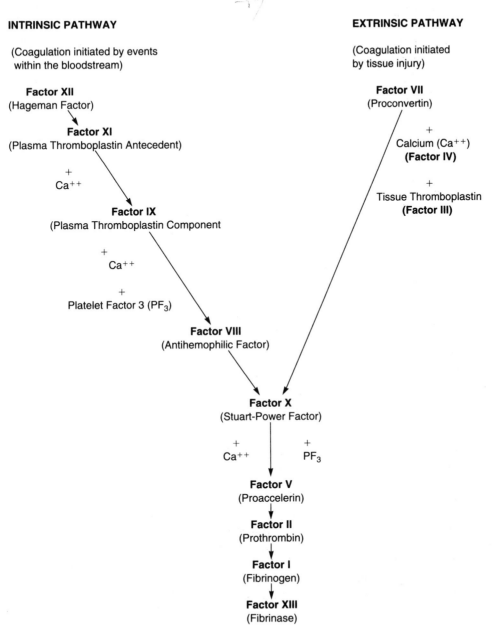

INTRINSIC PATHWAY

(Coagulation initiated by events
within the bloodstream)

Factor XII
(Hageman Factor)

Factor XI
(Plasma Thromboplastin Antecedent)

+
Ca^{++}

Factor IX
(Plasma Thromboplastin Component

+
Ca^{++}

+
Platelet Factor 3 (PF_3)

Factor VIII
(Antihemophilic Factor)

EXTRINSIC PATHWAY

(Coagulation initiated
by tissue injury)

Factor VII
(Proconvertin)

+
Calcium (Ca^{++})
(Factor IV)

+
Tissue Thromboplastin
(Factor III)

Factor X
(Stuart-Power Factor)

+   +
Ca^{++} PF_3

Factor V
(Proaccelerin)

Factor II
(Prothrombin)

Factor I
(Fibrinogen)

Factor XIII
(Fibrinase)

Figure 5–10   Simplified coagulation cascade.

converted into thrombin. Thrombin then splits fibrinogen (factor I) into the fibrin
necessary to form the fibrin clot also known as the **hemostatic plug**. The fibrin clot
is stabilized by factor XIII.

• Stage 4—**Fibrinolysis**: Fibrinolysis involves the ultimate removal or dissolution of the
fibrin clot once healing has occurred. This process is possible because activation of the

clotting process also releases substances that lead to the conversion of plasminogen to plasmin. Plasmin breaks the fibrin into small fragments called **fibrin degradation products (FDP)**, which are removed by reticuloendothelial cells (phagocytic cells).

The Role of the Liver in Hemostasis

The liver plays an important role in the hemostatic process. It is responsible for the synthesis (manufacture) of most of the coagulation factors. It also produces the bile salts necessary for the absorption of vitamin K, which is also necessary to the synthesis of the coagulation factors. When the liver is diseased, synthesis of coagulation factors is impaired and bleeding may result.

HEMOSTATIC DISORDERS

- *Hemophilia* (he′mo-fil′e-a): a hereditary condition characterized by increased coagulation time.
- *Thrombocytopenia* (throm′bo-si′to-pe′ne-a): an abnormal decrease in platelets.

DIAGNOSTIC TESTS

- Activated clotting time (ACT)
- Bleeding time (BT)
- Prothrombin time (PT)
- Partial thromboplastin time (PTT or APTT)
- Fibrin degradation products (FDP)

THE LYMPHATIC SYSTEM

The lymphatic system is made up of **lymphatic vessels, ducts, nodes** (masses of lymph tissue), and fluid called **lymph**. Lymph vessels spread throughout the entire body much like blood vessels. Lymph fluid is similar to plasma, but is 95% water.

Body cells are bathed in tissue fluid acquired from the bloodstream. Water, oxygen, and nutrients continually diffuse through the capillary walls into the tissue spaces. Much of the fluid diffuses back into the capillaries along with waste products of metabolism. Excess tissue fluid filters into **lymphatic capillaries**, where it is called **lymph**.

Lymphatic capillaries join with larger and larger lymphatic vessels until they empty into one of two terminal vessels: the **right lymphatic duct** or the **thoracic duct**. These ducts then empty into large veins in the upper body. Lymph moves through the vessels primarily by skeletal muscle contraction much like blood moves through the veins. Like veins, lymphatic vessels also have valves to keep the lymph flowing in the right direction.

Before reaching the ducts, the lymph passes through a series of structures called **lymph nodes**, which trap and destroy bacteria and foreign matter. The nodes also function in the production of lymphocytes. Lymph nodes are made of a special kind of tissue called **lymphoid tissue**. Lymphoid tissue has the ability to remove impurities and process lymphocytes. The tonsils, thymus, gastrointestinal tract and spleen also contain lymphoid tissue.

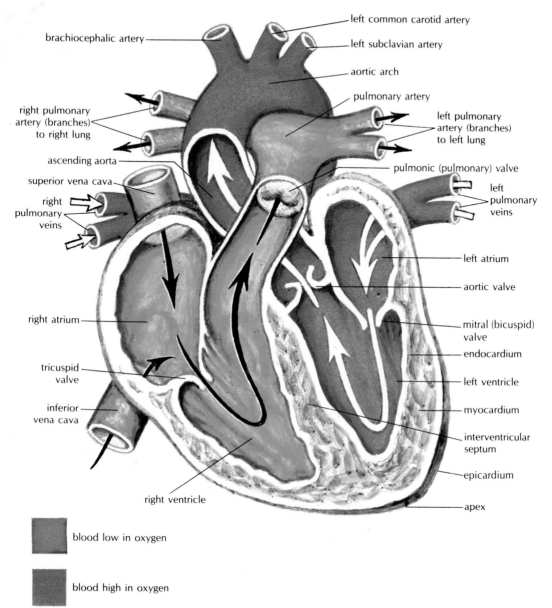

brachiocephalic artery

left common carotid artery

left subclavian artery

aortic arch

pulmonary artery

right pulmonary artery (branches) to right lung

left pulmonary artery (branches) to left lung

ascending aorta

pulmonic (pulmonary) valve

superior vena cava

left pulmonary veins

right pulmonary veins

left atrium

aortic valve

right atrium

mitral (bicuspid) valve

endocardium

tricuspid valve

left ventricle

inferior vena cava

myocardium

interventricular septum

epicardium

right ventricle

apex

blood low in oxygen

blood high in oxygen

Color Plate 1   Heart and great vessels.

HEMOGARD Closure	Conventional Stopper	Additive	Number of Inversions at Blood Collection (Invert gently, do not shake)	Laboratory Use
Gold		• Clot activator and gel for serum separation	5	SST Brand Tube for serum determinations in chemistry. Tube inversions ensure mixing of clot activator with blood and clotting within 30 minutes.
Light Green		• Lithium heparin and gel for plasma separation	8	PST Brand Tube for plasma determinations in chemistry. Tube inversions prevent clotting.
Red		• None	0	For serum determinations in chemistry, serology and blood banking.
Orange		• Thrombin	8	For stat serum determinations in chemistry. Tube inversions ensure complete clotting, usually in less than 5 minutes.
Royal Blue		• Sodium heparin • Na_2EDTA • None	8 8 0	For trace element, toxicology and nutrient determinations. Special stopper formulation offers the lowest verified levels of trace elements available (see package insert).
Green		• Sodium heparin • Lithium heparin • Ammonium heparin	8 8 8	For plasma determinations in chemistry. Tube inversions prevent clotting.

Stopper Color	Additive	Inversions	Use
Gray	• Potassium oxalate/ sodium fluoride • Sodium fluoride • Lithium iodoacetate • Lithium iodoacetate/ lithium heparin	8 8 8 8	*For glucose determinations. Glycolytic inhibitors stabilize glucose values for up to 24 hours at room temperature with iodoacetate, and for at least 3 days with fluoride. Tube inversions ensure proper mixing of additive and blood. Oxalate and heparin, anticoagulants, will give plasma samples. Without them, samples are serum.*
Brown	• Sodium heparin	8	*For lead determinations. This tube is certified to contain less than .01 µg/mL (ppm) lead. Tube inversions prevent clotting.*
Yellow	• Sodium polyanetholesulfonate (SPS)	8	*For blood culture specimen collections in microbiology. Tube inversions prevent clotting.*
Lavender	• Liquid K_3EDTA • Freeze-dried Na_2EDTA	8 8	*For whole blood hematology determinations. Tube inversions prevent clotting.*
Light Blue	• .105M sodium citrate (3.2%) • .129M sodium citrate (3.8%)	8 8	*For coagulation determinations on plasma specimens. Tube inversions prevent clotting. NOTE: Certain tests require chilled specimens. Follow recommended procedures for collection and transport of specimen.*

Color Plate 2 Common color-coded evacuated tube stoppers. (Courtesy Becton Dickinson, Franklin Lakes, NJ.)

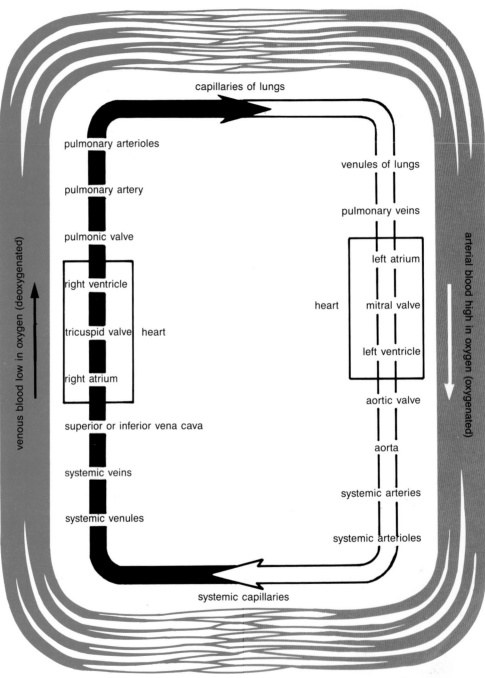

Color Plate 3   Blood vessels constitute a closed system for the flow of blood.

LYMPHATIC SYSTEM DISORDERS

- *Lymphangitis* (lim-fan-ji'tis): inflammation of the lymph vessels.
- *Lymphadenitis* (lim-fad'e-ni-tis): inflammation of lymph nodes. Inflamed lymph nodes may not be able to filter pathogens from the lymph before it returns to the blood-stream. This could lead to **septicemia** (sep-ti-se'me-ah).
- *Lymphadenopathy* (lim-fad'e-nop'ah-the): disease of the lymph nodes, often associated with enlargement such as seen in mononucleosis.
- *Splenomegaly* (splen'no-meg'ah-le): spleen enlargement.
- *Hodgkin's disease:* a chronic, malignant disorder, common in males, characterized by lymph node enlargement.
- *Lymphosarcoma* (lim-fo-sar-ko'mah): a malignant lymphoid tumor.
- *Lymphoma:* the term for any lymphoid tumor, benign or malignant.

DIAGNOSTIC TESTS

- Biopsy
- CBC
- Mononucleosis test (Monospot)
- Culture and sensitivity
- Bone marrow biopsy

Study & Review Questions

1. The thin membrane lining the heart which is continuous with the lining of the blood vessels is the:
   a. myocardium
   b. epicardium
   c. endocardium
   d. pericardium

2. The chamber of the heart that receives blood from the lungs is the:
   a. left atrium
   b. right atrium
   c. left ventricle
   d. right ventricle

3. The mitral valve in the heart is also called the:
   a. pulmonary semilunar valve
   b. tricuspid valve
   c. aortic valve
   d. bicuspid valve

4. The ECG shows P waves due to:
   a. atria contractions
   b. delayed contractions
   c. recovery of the electrical charge
   d. ventricle contraction

5. The relaxation phase of the heart is called the:
   a. cardiac cycle
   b. diastole
   c. pulse
   d. systole

6. A heart disorder that is characterized by fluid build-up in the lungs is called:
   a. aortic stenosis
   b. bacterial endocarditis
   c. congestive heart failure
   d. myocardial infarction

7. The internal space of a blood vessel is called the:
    a. atrium
    b. lumen
    c. septum
    d. valve

8. The longest vein in the body is:
    a. cephalic
    b. inferior vena cava
    c. pulmonary vein
    d. great saphenous

9. An individual's blood type—A, B, AB, or O—is determined by the presence or absence of _____ on the red blood cells.
    a. antigens
    b. chemicals
    c. clotting factors
    d. hormones

10. Which is the correct sequence of events following vessel injury?
    a. platelet aggregation, vasoconstriction, fibrin clot
    b. vasoconstriction, platelet aggregation, fibrin clot
    c. vasodilation, platelet adhesion, fibrin clot
    d. fibrinolysis, platelet adhesion, vasoconstriction

Suggested Laboratory Activities

1. Identify structures of the heart using an anatomic model.

2. Demonstrate how to take the blood pressure of a fellow student.

3. Locate and take the pulse at several locations on a fellow student.

4. Examine and compare tubes of whole blood, serum, and plasma.

5. Locate the major antecubital veins as well as other veins subject to venipuncture, on a fellow student.

6. Watch a film on the circulatory system.

7. Make a model of the extrinsic pathway of the coagulation cascade.

BIBLIOGRAPHY AND SUGGESTED READINGS

Corriveau D, Fritsma G: *Hemostasis and Thrombosis in the Clinical Laboratory.* Philadelphia: JB Lippincott Company, 1988.

Memmler RL, Cohen BJ, Wood DL: *The Human Body in Health and Disease* (7th ed.). Philadelphia: JB Lippincott Company, 1992.

Infection Control, Safety, and First Aid

6

KEY TERMS
biohazard
blood-borne pathogen standard
body substance isolation (BSI)
cardiopulmonary resuscitation (CPR)
Centers for Disease Control and Prevention (CDC)
electrical safety
engineering controls
fomites
infection
isolation procedures
material safety data sheets (MSDS)
microbes
nosocomial infection
occupational exposure
Occupational Safety and Health Administration (OSHA)
pathogen
personal protective equipment (PPE)
susceptible host
universal precautions
virulence

OBJECTIVES
On successful completion of this chapter, the reader should be able to:
1 Define infection and describe what is meant by the terms local, systemic, communicable, and nosocomial.
2 Identify the components of the chain of infection, give examples of each, and describe infection control procedures used to break the chain.
3 Define blood-borne pathogen, list examples, and describe the means of transmission of blood-borne pathogens in a health care setting.
4 Describe the universal precautions outlined by the CDC.
5 State safety rules that should be followed by the phlebotomist when working in the laboratory or in patient areas.
6 Identify guidelines to follow for electrical, chemical, and radiation safety in the health care setting.
7 Describe fire safety procedures, including the classes of fires and types of extinguishers recognized by the National Fire Protection Association (NFPA).
8 State first aid procedures for external hemorrhage and shock prevention.

McCall: PHLEBOTOMY ESSENTIALS. © 1993
J. B. Lippincott Company.

INFECTION CONTROL

Our environment is full of microscopic organisms referred to as **microbes**. Microbes include bacteria, fungi, protozoa, and viruses. The majority of microbes are **non-pathogenic**, meaning they do not cause disease under normal conditions. Microbes that are capable of causing disease (or **pathogenic**) are called **pathogens**. If a pathogen invades the body and the conditions are favorable for it to multiply and cause injurious effects or disease, the resulting condition is called an **infection**. Infection can be **local** (restricted to a small area of the body) or **systemic** (sis-tem'ik), in which the entire body is affected.

Communicable Infections

Some organisms cause infections that can be spread from person to person. These infections are called **communicable infections** and the diseases that result are called **communicable diseases**. A division of the U.S. Public Health Service called the **Centers for Disease Control and Prevention** (CDC) is charged with the investigation and control of various diseases, especially those that are communicable and have epidemic potential. The CDC recommends safety precautions to protect health care workers and others from infection.

Nosocomial Infections

Approximately 5% of patients in the United States contract some sort of infection *after* admission to a health care facility. Such infections are called **nosocomial infections**. Nosocomial infections can result from contact with infected personnel, other patients, visitors, or equipment. The most common nosocomial infection in the United States is urinary tract infection (UTI). A phlebotomist, whose duties require contact with many patients, must be fully aware of the infection process and take precautions to prevent the spread of infection.

The Chain of Infection

The process of infection requires the presence of three components, which make up what is referred to as the **chain of infection** (Fig. 6-1). These components or links in the chain of infection are a **source** (of microorganisms), a **means of transmission**, and a **susceptible host**. For an infection to occur, this chain must be complete. If the process of infection is stopped at any component or link in the chain, an infection is prevented. Whenever a pathogen successfully enters a susceptible host, thus completing the chain, the host becomes a new source of microorganisms and the process of infection continues.

Components of the Chain of Infection

SOURCE

Sources of infectious microorganisms can be infected humans or animals, or contaminated articles and equipment. Whether or not an inanimate source is capable of transmitting infection depends on the amount of contamination, the **viability** or ability of the organism to survive on the source, the **virulence** or degree to which an organism

Chain of Infection

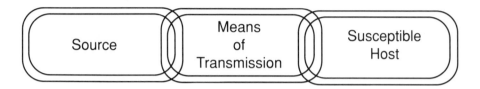

Breaking the Chain of Infection

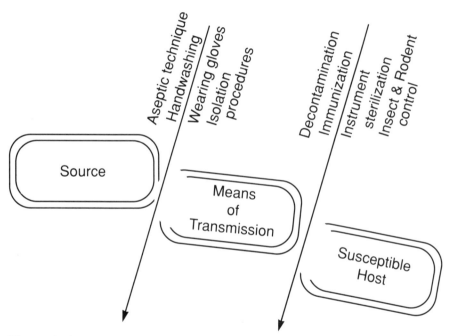

Figure 6–1   The chain of infection.

is capable of causing disease, and the amount of time elapsed between when the source was contaminated and when it was contacted.

For example, the virus that causes hepatitis B is much more virulent or capable of causing disease from a small amount of infective material than is the virus that causes acquired immunodeficiency syndrome (AIDS). It is also more viable, meaning it is capable of surviving on surfaces longer than the AIDS virus. However, if a long enough time elapses from the time of contamination until contact by a susceptible host, the microbe is no longer alive and it is not capable of transmitting disease.

MODES OF TRANSMISSION
There are four basic modes of transmission: contact, vehicle, vector, and airborne.

Contact transmission.   There are three types of contact transmission:

1. **Direct contact** involves direct, physical transfer of a pathogenic microbe to a susceptible host through close or intimate contact such as touching or kissing.
2. **Indirect contact** involves personal contact by a susceptible host with a contaminated inanimate object, such as bed linens, eating utensils, and clothing. Objects or substances that are capable of adhering to infectious material and transmitting infection are called **fomites** (fo'mi-tez). Fomites in the laboratory include telephones, computer terminals, and countertops.
3. **Droplet contact** involves the transfer of the infective microbe to the nose, mouth, or conjunctiva (mucous membrane of the eye) of a susceptible individual through sneezing, coughing, or talking by an infected person. This is considered "contact" transmission because droplets do not travel more than 3 feet.

Vehicle transmission.   Vehicle transmission involves the transmission of the infective microbe through contaminated food, water, or drugs. Examples of vehicle transmission are salmonella infection from handling contaminated chicken, and shigella infection from drinking contaminated water. The transmission of hepatitis and AIDS through blood transfusion is also considered vehicle transmission.

Vector transmission.   Vector transmission involves the transfer of the microbe by an insect, arthropod, or animal. An example of vector transmission is the transmission of malaria by a mosquito or the plague by rodent fleas.

Airborne transmission.   Airborne transmission involves droplet nuclei. Droplet nuclei are the residue of evaporated droplets generated by sneezing, coughing, or talking. Droplet nuclei can remain viable even though suspended in the air for a long time. Droplet nuclei can be inhaled by or deposited on a susceptible host.

SUSCEPTIBLE HOST
A **susceptible host** can be anyone. Susceptibility is affected by age, health, and the immune status of the individual. For example, newborns whose immune systems are not yet developed and old people whose immune systems are no longer functioning properly are more susceptible to infections. A healthy person who has received a vaccination against a disease-causing virus, as well as someone who has recovered from a particular virus, has developed antibodies against that virus and is **immune**, or unlikely to develop the disease and is therefore less susceptible.

Breaking the Chain of Infection
Breaking the chain of infection means stopping infections at the source, eliminating means of transmission, and reducing or eliminating susceptibility of potential hosts. A few of the ways to prevent transmission of organisms that are infectious or

capable of causing infection are proper handwashing; wearing gloves, gowns, or masks when indicated; isolation procedures; insect and rodent control; and the decontamination of surfaces and instruments. Susceptibility of potential hosts can be reduced through proper nutrition, reduction of stress, and immunization against common pathogens.

Infection Control Programs

Every health care institution must have an infection control program responsible for implementing procedures designed to break the chain of infection. Such procedures are aimed at protecting not only patients, but also employees, visitors, and others. An infection control program is also responsible for monitoring and collecting data on all infections occurring within the health care institution, and instituting special precautions in the event of outbreaks of particular infections. In addition, infection control programs screen employees for infectious diseases (*eg,* tuberculosis [TB] test), and provide vaccinations against hepatitis B, measles, and so on. Infection control programs follow regulations and guidelines established by the **Occupational Safety and Health Administration (OSHA)**, CDC, and the Joint Committee for Accrediting Healthcare Organizations (JCAHO), as well as other state and local regulatory agencies. Recent OSHA requirements concerning employee exposure to **blood-borne pathogens**, mandated by standard 1910.1030 in the code of federal regulations, supersede all other regulatory requirements.

Blood-borne Pathogens

Blood-borne pathogen is a term applied to any infectious microorganism present in blood and other body fluids and tissues. The term most commonly refers to hepatitis B virus (HBV) and human immunodeficiency virus (HIV). Other blood-borne pathogens include the microorganisms that cause syphilis, malaria, relapsing fever, and Creutzfeldt-Jakob disease. The main **parenteral** (any route other than the digestive tract) means of transmission of blood-borne pathogens in the health care setting are:

1. *Nonintact skin:* direct contact of pathogen-containing material with both visible and invisible preexisting cuts and scratches, (including those occurring with chapped hands), burns, lesions, and dermatitis.
2. *Percutaneous (through the skin):* direct inoculation of blood or other body fluids by accidental needlesticks and injuries from other sharp objects (sharps) such as broken glass, tubes, and so on. Transfusion of infected blood or blood products is also considered parenteral inoculation.
3. *Mucous membrane:* contact of the oral, nasal, or conjunctival mucosa by droplets, aerosols, or splashes of infectious material; or by touching the mouth, nose, or eyes with contaminated hands.

Universal Precautions

Because it is not always possible to know if a patient is infected with a blood-borne pathogen, such as HBV and HIV, the CDC introduced the concept of **universal precautions**. Under universal precautions, the blood and body fluids of *all* individuals are considered potentially infectious. Universal precautions is meant to be part of an overall infection control plan designed to prevent the spread of infection from other pathogens, in addition to blood-borne pathogens. Universal precautions include:

1. Using barrier protection to prevent skin and mucous membrane exposure when possible exposure to blood or body fluids is anticipated. Barriers include gowns, gloves, face masks, and shields. Barriers are also called personal protective equipment (PPE).
2. Wearing gloves when handling blood and body fluids.
3. Wearing gloves when performing vascular procedures, including all phlebotomy procedures.
4. Changing gloves between patients.
5. Wearing facial protection if splashing is possible.
6. Wearing aprons over gowns or lab coats if splashing is possible.
7. Washing hands after glove removal or when gloves are knowingly contaminated.
8. Following safe practices when handling sharp instruments, as well as prohibiting bending, breaking, or recapping of needles.

Isolation Procedures

One way an infection control program minimizes spread of infection is through the establishment of **isolation procedures**. Isolation procedures separate patients with certain transmissible infections or diseases from contact with other patients, as well as limit their contact with hospital personnel and visitors. Isolating a patient requires a doctor's order and is implemented either to prevent the spread of infection from a patient with a contagious disease or to protect a patient whose immune system is compromised. Patients are most commonly isolated in a private room. The type of isolation, including a description of the precautions necessary, is generally posted on the patient's door in the form of a color-coded card or sign. A cart containing all the supplies needed to enter the room and to care for the patient is placed outside the door.

Types of Isolation Systems

There are two basic types of isolation systems recommended by the CDC: the **category-specific** system and the **disease-specific** system. The diagnosis of, or suspicion of, a transmissible disease is necessary before implementation of either system. The CDC recommends that individual health care institutions modify one or the other of these systems to comply with universal precautions.

CATEGORY-SPECIFIC ISOLATION

There are seven categories in the category-specific system: strict, contact, respiratory, acid fast bacillus (AFB or tuberculosis), enteric, drainage/secretion, and blood/body fluid precautions. The blood/body fluid category has been replaced by universal precautions, which is followed for all categories. In addition, all categories require that articles leaving an isolated patient's room must be double-bagged and labeled "biohazard" prior to disposal or decontamination for reuse.

Strict isolation.   Strict isolation, also called complete isolation, is required for patients with highly contagious diseases such as chicken pox, bubonic plague, and diphtheria that can be spread by direct contact and through the air. Strict isolation requires the wearing of gowns, gloves, and masks by all persons entering the room.

Contact isolation. Contact isolation is indicated for highly transmissible diseases that are spread primarily by direct contact but do not warrant strict isolation. These infections include influenza (flu) and infections with antibiotic-resistant bacteria. Contact isolation requirements include gloves, gowns if soiling is likely, and masks if in close contact with the patient.

Respiratory isolation. Respiratory isolation is used for patients with infections that can be spread via droplets or through the air, such as whooping cough (pertussis), *Haemophilus* influenza, and meningococcal meningitis. Masks must be worn by those coming in close contact with the patient.

Acid-fast bacillus (AFB) isolation. AFB isolation is used for patients with active tuberculosis. Masks or particulate respirators, gowns, and gloves are indicated until there is clinical evidence that the infectiousness has substantially decreased and the patient is no longer coughing appreciably.

Drainage/secretion. Drainage/secretion isolation is often used for patients with skin infections, open wounds, or burns. It is sometimes used following surgery. Masks and gowns are indicated for procedures where splashing or soiling may occur.

Enteric isolation. Enteric isolation is used for patients with intestinal infections that can be transmitted by ingestion. Enteric infections include those caused by *Salmonella, Shigella, Campylobacter,* or other organisms causing diarrhea or dysentery. Masks and gowns are indicated for procedures where soiling or splashing may occur.

DISEASE-SPECIFIC ISOLATION

The disease-specific system recommends specific isolation procedures based on the mode of transmission for the most common diseases in the United States.

PROTECTIVE OR REVERSE ISOLATION

A special kind of isolation called **protective** or **reverse isolation** is used for patients who are highly susceptible to infections. In this instance, the protective measures are used to keep health care workers and others from transmitting infections to the patient rather than vice versa. Examples of patients requiring protective isolation include patients with suppressed immune systems such as transplant patients, patients with AIDS, some chemotherapy patients, and patients with extensive burns.

Body Substance Isolation

Because in some cases, transmission of infection can occur before a diagnosis is made, both the category-specific and the disease-specific systems are subject to error. In addition, the category-specific system covers many diseases and often results in overisolation and needless cost increases. For these reasons, a new system called **body substance isolation (BSI)** has gained acceptance.

Body substance isolation provides the equivalent of universal precautions for blood-borne pathogens while incorporating elements of disease-specific, as well as category-specific, precautions for all transmissible pathogens. Body substance isolation is fol-

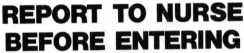

REPORT TO NURSE
BEFORE ENTERING

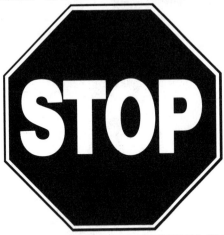

**FAVOR DE ANUNCIARSE A LA ENFERMERA DE PISO
ANTES DE ENTRAR AL CUARTO**

BRIGGS   L-9214   Des Moines, Iowa 50306   1-800-247-2343

Figure 6–2 Precaution "stop sign." (Adapted from Briggs Corp., Des Moines, IA.)

lowed for *every* patient without the need for suspicion or diagnosis of a transmissible disease. Body substance isolation goes beyond universal precautions by requiring the wearing of gloves when contacting *any* body substance. Special "stop signs" (Fig. 6-2) alert health care workers when additional precautions are needed such as for respiratory or strict isolation. Body substance isolation requires the following actions:

1. Wear gloves when in contact with blood, body fluids, secretions, mucous membranes, nonintact skin, and all moist substances from the body. Gloves *must* be changed between patients. To comply with OSHA regulations, wash hands as soon as gloves are removed or as soon as immediately feasible.
2. Perform handwashing before and after other contact with patients with ungloved hands.
3. Use additional barrier protection such as gowns and face masks when blood, body fluids, and secretions are apt to spill or splash onto the clothing of the health care worker.
4. Place all soiled articles into appropriate biohazard (see "Biological Hazards") containers or bags. If the container is contaminated on the outside, place it into a secondary container.
5. Dispose of needles and other sharp instruments in rigid puncture-resistant containers.
6. Use private rooms and additional precautions for certain airborne diseases, such as pulmonary tuberculosis, contagious diseases requiring strict isolation, and patients requiring reverse isolation.

7. Determine the immune status of health care workers and give necessary vaccinations if possible. Nonimmune workers should not enter rooms of patients with communicable diseases, such as measles and mumps. Immune workers (*ie*, workers who have had the disease or have been vaccinated against the disease) do not need extra precautions for those diseases.

8. Display body substance isolation precaution signs (Fig. 6-3) in every patient room. Place stop signs on the doors of patients requiring additional precautions indicating special precautions or directing those who enter the patient's room to first check with the patient's nurse.

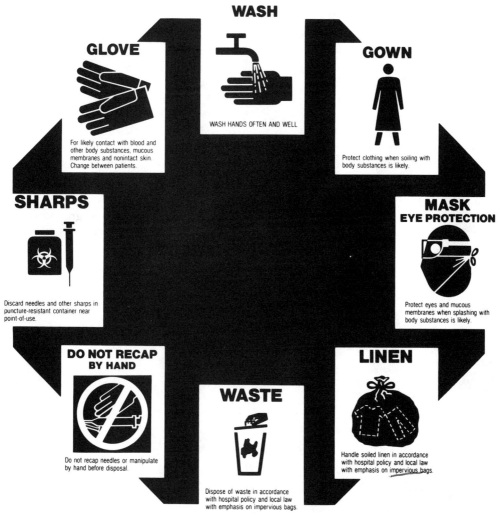

WASH
WASH HANDS OFTEN AND WELL

GLOVE
For likely contact with blood and other body substances, mucous membranes and nonintact skin. Change between patients.

GOWN
Protect clothing when soiling with body substances is likely.

SHARPS
Discard needles and other sharps in puncture-resistant container near point-of-use.

MASK EYE PROTECTION
Protect eyes and mucous membranes when splashing with body substances is likely.

DO NOT RECAP BY HAND
Do not recap needles or manipulate by hand before disposal.

WASTE
Dispose of waste in accordance with hospital policy and local law with emphasis on impervious bags.

LINEN
Handle soiled linen in accordance with hospital policy and local law with emphasis on impervious bags.

Figure 6–3   Body substance isolation sign. (Adapted from Briggs Corp., Des Moines, IA.)

Nursery Infection Control Technique

Because their immune systems are not yet fully developed, newborns are more susceptible to infections than healthy older children and adults. For this reason, special infection control techniques should be used by the phlebotomist, as well as all other personnel who enter the nursery. Most nurseries have a separate room just outside the nursery where handwashing and gowning is performed before entering. Typical proper nursery infection control techniques include:

1. Washing hands thoroughly with an antiseptic hand cleaner.
2. Putting on clean gloves, gown, and mask.
3. Leaving the blood collection tray in the wash room outside the nursery and taking into the nursery only those items necessary to perform the specimen collection.

Gowning

Sterile gowns are worn by health care workers to protect certain patients (*eg*, newborns) from contaminants on the health care worker's clothing. Gowns are also worn to protect health care workers from infectious materials encountered, for example, when entering strict isolation rooms. Gowns are most often made of disposable cloth or paper, have long sleeves with knit cuffs, and are generous in size to adequately cover clothing. Gowns usually fasten in the back. When putting on a gown, only inside surfaces of the gown should be touched. A properly worn gown has the sleeves pulled all the way to the wrist, the belt tied, and the gown overlapped and completely closed and securely fastened (Fig. 6-4). Gloves are pulled over the cuffs. A gown is removed from

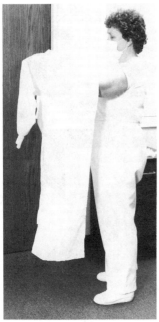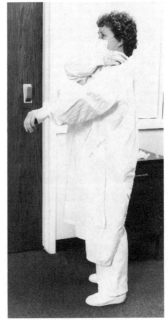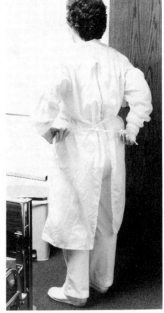

Figure 6–4   Proper gowning procedure (Craven RF, Hirnle CJ).

the inside by sliding the arms out of the sleeves. The gown is then held away from the body and folded so that the contaminated outer surface is to the inside.

Handwashing

The most important means of preventing and controlling the spread of infection is proper handwashing. Handwashing by the phlebotomist should be performed:

- Before and after each patient contact
- Between different procedures on the same patient
- Before putting on gloves and after taking them off
- Before leaving the laboratory
- Before going to lunch or break
- Before and after going to the bathroom
- Whenever hands become visibly or knowingly contaminated.

ROUTINE HANDWASHING PROCEDURE

1. Remove rings and watch.
2. Stand back so that you do not touch the sink.
3. Wet hands under warm, running water.
4. Apply soap and work up a lather. Rub your hands together to create friction, which loosens dead skin, dirt, and other debris. Scrub everywhere, including between the fingers and around the knuckles. Wash for at least 15 seconds. Debris under fingernails should be removed with an orange stick or similar device.
5. Rinse hands in a downward motion from wrists to fingertips.
6. Repeat steps 4 and 5.
7. Dry hands with a clean paper towel.
8. Turn the faucet off with another clean paper towel.

SAFETY

Providing quality care in an environment that is safe for employees, as well as patients, is a concern that is foremost in the minds of health care providers. Safe working conditions must be assured by employers as mandated by the Occupational Safety and Health Act of 1970 and enforced by the OSHA. Even so, there are biologic, electrical, radiation, and chemical hazards encountered in a health care setting, often on a daily basis. It is important for the phlebotomist to be aware of the existence of hazards and have knowledge of the safety precautions and rules necessary to eliminate or minimize them.

General Laboratory Safety Rules

1. *Never* eat, drink, smoke, or chew gum in the laboratory.
2. *Never* place food or beverages in a refrigerator used for storing reagents or specimens.
3. *Never* apply cosmetics in the laboratory or handle contact lenses.

4. *Never* wear long chains, large or dangling earrings, or loose bracelets.
5. *Always* wear a fully buttoned lab coat when engaged in lab activities. *Never* wear a lab coat to lunch, on break, or when leaving the lab to go home.
6. *Always* tie back hair that is longer than shoulder length.
7. *Always* keep fingernails short and well manicured. Do not wear nail polish or artificial nails.
8. *Always* wear a face shield when specimen processing or any activity that might generate splashes or aerosol of body fluids.
9. *Always* wear comfortable, sturdy shoes with nonslip soles. *Never* wear sandals, open-toed shoes, slippers, or high heels.
10. *Always* wear gloves for phlebotomy procedures.

Safety Rules When in Patient Rooms and Other Patient Areas

1. Handle all specimens following universal precautions guidelines.
2. Properly dispose of used and contaminated specimen collection supplies and return all other equipment to the specimen collection tray before leaving the patient's room. *Do not* recap needles.
3. Replace bedrails that were let down during patient procedures.
4. Do not touch electrical equipment in patient rooms, especially when in the process of drawing blood.
5. Report infiltrated intravenous (IV) lines or other IV problems to nursing.
6. Report unresponsive patients to nursing.
7. Watch out for and report food, liquid, and other items spilled or dropped on the floor to nursing or housekeeping.
8. Report unusual odors to nursing.
9. Be careful when entering and exiting patient rooms. Watch out for housekeeping equipment, dietary carts, housekeeping equipment, x-ray machines, and other equipment, which are often left in the halls outside patient rooms.
10. Avoid running. It is alarming to patients and visitors and may cause an accident.

Biological Hazards

A biological hazard or **biohazard** is any material or substance harmful to health. Biohazards are identified by a special symbol called a **biohazard symbol** (Fig. 6-5). Because the majority of laboratory specimens are blood and other body fluids and tissues with the potential to contain blood-borne pathogens and other infectious materials and

Figure 6–5   Biohazard symbol.

agents that could be harmful to health, they are considered biohazards. Common routes of entry for biohazards are

- Ingestion
- Skin contact
- Airborne

Proper handwashing, and following universal precautions, as well as proper isolation and body substance isolation procedures minimizes the risk posed by biohazards.

BLOOD-BORNE PATHOGEN STANDARD

OSHA has concluded that employees face a serious health risk as a result of **occupational exposure** to blood and other potentially infectious materials, including other body fluids and tissues because they may contain pathogenic microorganisms. For this reason, OSHA put into force the *Occupational Exposure to Blood-Borne Pathogens Standard*. Enforcement of this standard, which is mandated by federal law, is meant to minimize, if not eliminate, occupational exposure to the viruses that cause hepatitis B and AIDS (or HIV), as well as other blood-borne pathogens. This standard outlines the necessary engineering and work practice controls that OSHA believes will help minimize or eliminate exposure to employees. In addition, the standard requires the availability and use of PPE or personal protective equipment, special training, medical surveillance, and the availability of vaccination against HBV for all employees having contact with blood-borne pathogens.

EXPOSURE CONTROL PLAN

To comply with the OSHA standard, employers must have a written exposure control plan which includes:

1. An exposure determination: a list of all job classifications in which employees have or may have occupational exposure to blood-borne pathogens, as well as a list of tasks and procedures in which exposure may occur.
2. Methods of implementation and compliance:
   a. *A universal precautions statement:* requires all employees to observe universal precautions.
   b. *Engineering controls:* controls that isolate or remove the blood-borne pathogen hazard from the workplace. Examples are readily accessible handwashing facilities, sharps disposal containers, and self-sheathing needles.
   c. *Work practice controls:* practices that alter the manner in which a task is performed to reduce the likelihood of exposure. Examples of work practice controls are prohibiting needle bending, breaking, or recapping; requiring handwashing following glove removal; and prohibiting eating, drinking, smoking, or applying cosmetics in work areas of the laboratory.
   d. *Personal protective equipment (PPE):* PPE or barrier protection devices to minimize the risk of infection from blood-borne pathogens must be provided at no charge to all employees who have potential exposure. PPE includes gloves, gowns, lab coats, aprons, face shields, masks, and resuscitation mouthpieces. Laundry service for reusable protective outerwear such as gowns and lab coats must be provided by the employer.

    e. *Housekeeping schedule and methods:* Work surfaces must be cleaned at least once a day, as well as after any contact with blood or other potentially infectious material. A 10% solution of household bleach (5.25% sodium hypochlorite) is an acceptable disinfectant.

3. Hepatitis B vaccine and postexposure follow-up: hepatitis B vaccine series must be offered free of charge to all employees who have potential occupational exposure. Confidential medical evaluation and follow-up must be available immediately to employees with exposure incidents.

4. Communication of hazards to employees:
    a. *Warning labels and signs* must be affixed to containers of blood, contaminated waste containers, and other potentially infectious material. This includes refrigerators and freezers where infectious material may be stored. The labels should be predominantly fluorescent orange or orange-red, bearing the word *biohazard* and containing the biohazard symbol (see Figure 6-5). Red bags or containers may be substituted for labels.
    b. *Training and information* concerning blood-borne pathogens must be provided to employees at no cost and during working hours at the time of initial assignment to tasks involving occupational exposure. Employers should maintain an accessible copy of the *Blood-borne Pathogen Standard,* as well as an explanation of its contents. Annual training is to be provided within 1 year of initial training.

5. Record keeping:
    a. *Medical records:* Employers are required to maintain confidential medical records on each employee with occupational exposure. These records must include the employee's name, social security number, and HBV vaccination status.
    b. *Training records:* Employers are required to maintain records of training sessions that include the content, qualifications of persons conducting, and the names and titles of persons attending.

HEPATITIS B VIRUS (HBV)

Hepatitis B (formerly called serum hepatitis) is the most frequently occurring laboratory-associated infection, making it the major infectious occupational health hazard in the health care industry. The agent that causes hepatitis B, HBV, is a potentially life-threatening blood-borne pathogen that targets the liver. (Hepatitis means "inflammation of the liver.") HBV can survive for hours on work surfaces, telephones, and so on, and can be transmitted indirectly, *as well as* directly through needlesticks. In a nonmedical setting, it may be transmitted through sexual contact and sharing of dirty needles.

According to OSHA, every year approximately 8,700 health care workers contract hepatitis B and about 200 die as a result. Of those who recover, some become carriers with the ability to pass the disease on to others. Carriers are also at risk for developing cirrhosis of the liver and even liver cancer. Work practices to prevent HBV infection will also help protect against other types of hepatitis such as hepatitis A virus (HAV) or infectious hepatitis, as well as non-A, non-B hepatitis (hepatitis C), and Delta hepatitis.

HEPATITIS B VACCINATION

The best defense against HBV infection is vaccination, which consists of a series of three equal intramuscular injections of vaccine. The vaccine (*eg,* Recombivax B) is derived from yeast culture and poses no risk of transmitting HBV, HIV, or other blood-borne pathogens. Employers are required by OSHA to offer this vaccine free to employees. Employees who decline the vaccination must sign a declination form.

Hepatitis B vaccine protects against HBV, as well as Delta hepatitis, which can only be contracted concurrently with HBV infection.

HUMAN IMMUNODEFICIENCY VIRUS

Human immunodeficiency virus (HIV) is the virus responsible for causing AIDS. The virus attacks the body's immune or defense system, leaving the host susceptible to opportunistic infections. Because HIV is a blood-borne pathogen and because infection with HIV has a poor prognosis at best, it is of great concern to health care workers. Although the incidence of work-related infection with HIV is relatively low, studies by the CDC have shown that phlebotomy procedures are dangerous work-related activities, and are responsible for approximately 50% of the HIV exposures that have occurred so far in a health care setting. There is no vaccine to protect against HIV infection at this time.

PROCEDURE FOR NEEDLESTICKS AND OTHER EXPOSURES

OSHA requires employers to provide free medical evaluation and treatment to any employee in the event of an exposure incident. Initial response by the employee requires decontamination of a needlestick site with alcohol and flushing mucous membrane contact sites with water. The employee is to then report directly to a licensed health care provider for a medical evaluation and counseling, as well as any treatment required. Medical evaluation involves the following:

1. Testing the employees's blood for HIV in an accredited laboratory.
2. Testing the source patient for HIV and HBV, provided permission is granted by the patient.
3. If the source patient refuses testing, is HBV-positive, or in a high-risk category, the employee may be given immune globulin or HBV vaccination.
4. If the source patient is HIV-positive, the employee is counseled and evaluated for HIV infection at periodic intervals.
5. An exposed employee is counseled to be alert for acute viral symptoms (acute retroviral syndrome) within 12 weeks of exposure.

Electrical Safety

There are potential hazards, such as fire and electrical shock, associated with the use of electrical equipment. Knowledge of the proper use, maintenance, and servicing of electrical equipment (such as the centrifuge) can minimize hazards associated with their use.

Guidelines for electrical safety include:

1. Avoid extension cords.
2. *Do not* overload electrical circuits.
3. Inspect cords and plugs for breaks and fraying.
4. Unplug equipment when servicing, including when replacing a light bulb.
5. Unplug equipment that has had liquid spilled in it. Do not plug in again until the spill has been cleaned up and you are certain wiring is dry.

6. Unplug and do not use equipment that is malfunctioning.
7. Do not attempt to make repairs to equipment if you are not trained to do so.
8. Do not handle electrical equipment with wet hands or when standing on a wet floor.
9. Know the location of the circuit breaker box.
10. Do not touch electrical equipment in patient rooms, especially when in the process of drawing blood.

ACTIONS TO TAKE IF ELECTRICAL SHOCK OCCURS

1. Shut off the source of electricity.
2. If the source of electricity cannot be shut off, use nonconducting material (*eg,* hand inside a glass beaker) to remove the source of electricity from a victim.
3. Call for medical assistance.
4. Start cardiopulmonary resuscitation if indicated.
5. Keep the victim warm.

Fire Safety

All employees of any institution should be aware of procedures to follow in case of fire. They should know where fire extinguishers are located and be familiar with their use. They should also understand how to use fire blankets or heavy toweling to smother fires in clothing. In addition, they should be familiar with the location of emergency exits.

COMPONENTS OF FIRE

Three components, sometimes referred to as the fire triangle, are necessary for fire to occur. They are fuel, oxygen (or an oxidizing agent), and heat (or an ignition source).

CLASSES OF FIRE

Four classes of fire are recognized by the National Fire Protection Association (NFPA). Classification depends on the fuel source of the fire. The four classes are as follows:

1. *Class A fires* occur with ordinary combustible materials such as wood, papers, or clothing. Class A fires require water or water-based solutions to cool or quench the fire to extinguish it.
2. *Class B fires* occur with flammable liquids and vapors such as paint, oil, grease, or gasoline. Class B fires require blocking the source of oxygen or smothering the fuel to extinguish the fire.
3. *Class C fires* occur with electrical equipment and require nonconducting agents to extinguish them.
4. *Class D fires* occur with combustible or reactive metals such as sodium, potassium, magnesium, and lithium. Class D fires require dry powder agents or sand to extinguish. They are the most difficult fires to control and frequently lead to explosions.

FIRE EXTINGUISHERS

Fire extinguisher classes correspond with the class of fire.

Class A extinguishers use soda and acid or water to cool the fire. Class B extinguishers use foam, dry chemicals, or carbon dioxide to smother the fire.

Class C extinguishers use dry chemicals, carbon dioxide, or other nonconducting agents to smoother the fire. Class ABC (multipurpose) extinguishers use dry chemical reagents to smoother the fire. They can be used on Class A, B, and C fires and eliminate the confusion of having several different types of extinguishers. Multipurpose extinguishers are the type most frequently used in health care institutions.

Do's and Don'ts if a Fire Occurs

- *Do* pull the nearest fire alarm.
- *Do* call the fire department.
- *Do* attempt to extinguish a small fire.
- *Do* close all doors and windows if leaving the area.
- *Do* smother a clothing fire with a fire blanket or have the person roll on the floor in an attempt to smother the fire.
- *Do* crawl to the nearest exit if there is heavy smoke.
- *Don't* panic.
- *Don't* run.
- *Don't* use elevators.

The NFPA code word for action in the event of fire is RACE. R = *Rescue* individuals in danger. A = *Alarm:* sound the alarm. C = *Confine* the fire by closing all doors and windows. E = *Extinguish* the fire with the nearest suitable fire extinguisher.

Radiation Safety

The principles involved in radiation exposure are distance, time, and shielding. This means that the amount of radiation you are exposed to depends on how far you are from the source of radioactivity, how long you are exposed to it, and what protection you have from it. Exposure time is important because radiation effects are cumulative.

The phlebotomist may encounter radiation hazards when collecting specimens from patients who have been injected with radioactive dyes, when collecting specimens from patients in the radiology department, and when delivering specimens to radioimmunoassay departments of the laboratory. The phlebotomist should be aware of the institution's radiation safety procedures. In addition, the phlebotomist should recognize the symbol for radiation hazard (Fig. 6-6) and be cautious when entering areas displaying it. Because radiation is particularly hazardous to a fetus, pregnant employees should

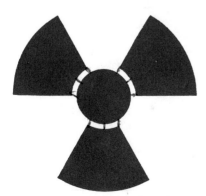

Figure 6–6   Radiation hazard symbol.

avoid areas displaying the radiation symbol and patients who have recently been injected with radioactive dyes.

Chemical Safety

The phlebotomist may come in contact with hazardous chemicals when using cleaning reagents, adding preservatives to 24-hour urine containers, or when delivering specimens to the laboratory. Inappropriate use of chemicals can have dangerous consequences. For example, mixing bleach with other cleaning compounds can release dangerous gases. In addition, many chemicals are acids, such as the HCl used as a urine preservative, or alkalis, which can cause severe burns. An important rule to remember when handling acids is to never add water to acid because a violent reaction could occur. Container labels contain important information as to the nature of the contents and should always be read carefully before use.

Table 6–1.
Placard Recognition Information

United Nations Hazard Class	Symbol	Background Color	Examples
Class 1 Explosives	Bursting ball	Orange	Fireworks Ammunition Dynamite

Class 2
Gases (compressed, liquified, or dissolved under pressure)
	Flammable
	Flame
	
	Nonflammable
	Cylinder
		Red
		
		Green
			Flammable:
			  butane
			  propane
			Nonflammable:
			  ammonia
			  chlorine

Class 3 Flammable liquids	Flame	Red	Brake fluid Camphor oil Glycol ethers Gasoline
Class 4 Flammable solids or substances	*Flammable Solid* Flame *Water-reactive Materials* Slashed W	Red and white vertical stripes Red and white vertical stripes with blue top quadrant	Lithium Magnesium Phosphorus Titanium

IDENTIFICATION OF CHEMICALS

Labeling of hazardous materials is required by the *OSHA Hazardous Communication (HazCom) Standard*. Labeling format may be different for each manufacturer; however, chemical manufacturers must comply with the labeling requirements set by the Manufacturers Chemical Association (MCA). Labels for hazardous chemicals must contain a statement of warning such as "danger" or "poison"; a statement of what the hazard is—toxic, flammable, or combustible, and precautions to eliminate risk; and first-aid measures in the event of a spill or other exposure.

Additional labels of precaution may include a Department of Transportation (DOT) symbol incorporating a United Nations' hazard classification number and symbol (Table 6-1). The Department of Transportation labeling system uses a diamond-shaped warning sign (Fig. 6-7) containing the name of the hazard and a symbol representing that hazard.

Table 6–1.
Placard Recognition Information (*Continued*)

United Nations Hazard Class	Symbol	Background Color	Examples
Class 5 Division 5.1: oxidizing substances Division 5.2: organic peroxides	Circle with flame	Yellow	Ammonium nitrate Benzoyl peroxide Calcium chlorite
Class 6 Poisonous and infectious substances	Skull with crossbones	White	Chemical mace Pesticides Cyanide AIDS specimens
Class 7 Radioactive materials	Propeller	Yellow over white	Cobalt 14 Plutonium Radioactive waste Uranium 235
Class 8 Corrosives	Test tube over hand Test tube over metal	White over black	Caustic potash Caustic soda Hydrochloric acid Sulfuric acid
Class 9 Miscellaneous dangerous substances	ORM-A ORM-B ORM-C ORM-D ORM-E	White	ORM-A: dry ice ORM-B: quick lime ORM-C: sawdust ORM-D: hair spray ORM-E: hazardous waste

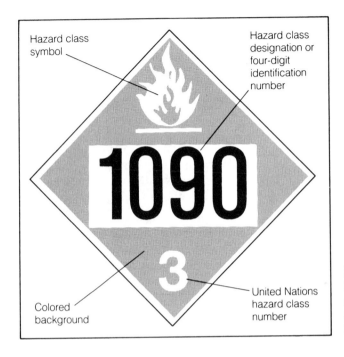

Figure 6–7 Example of DOT hazardous materials labels (flammable, poison, corrosive, etc.) (Jones SA, Weigel A, White RD, McSwain NE, Breiter M).

Another hazardous material rating system developed by the NFPA (Fig. 6-8) is often used to label areas where hazardous chemicals and other materials are stored in the event of a fire. This system uses a diamond-shaped symbol divided into four quadrants. Health hazards are indicated in a blue diamond on the left; the level of fire hazard is indicated in the upper quadrant in a red diamond; stability or reactivity hazards are indicated in a yellow diamond on the right; and other specific hazards are indicated in a white quadrant on the bottom.

In addition to requiring labeling, the *OSHA HAZCOM Standard* has become the "right-to-know" law. This standard requires manufacturers to supply Material Safety Data Sheets (MSDS) for their products. An MSDS contains general information and precautionary and emergency information for the product. All products with a hazardous warning on the label require an MSDS. This information helps ensure that products will be used safely and for their intended purpose.

SAFETY SHOWERS AND EYE WASH STATIONS

The phlebotomist should know the location of and be instructed in the use of safety showers and eye wash stations in the event of a chemical spill or splash to the eyes or other body part. The eyes or other body parts affected should be flushed with water for a minimum of 15 minutes, followed by a visit to the emergency room for evaluation.

CHEMICAL SPILLS

Chemical spills should be cleaned up using special clean-up kits containing absorbent and neutralizer materials.

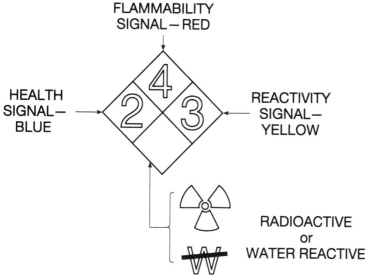

FLAMMABILITY
SIGNAL – RED

HEALTH
SIGNAL –
BLUE

REACTIVITY
SIGNAL –
YELLOW

RADIOACTIVE
or
WATER REACTIVE

Figure 6–8 National Fire Protection Association diagram (Jones SA, Weigel A, White RD, McSwain NE, Breiter M).

FIRST AID PROCEDURES

The ability to recognize and react quickly and skillfully to emergency situations may mean the difference between life and death for a victim.

External Hemorrhage

Control of hemorrhage (abnormal bleeding) from an obvious wound is most effectively accomplished by elevating the affected part above the level of the heart and applying direct pressure to the wound. However, do not attempt to elevate a broken extremity. Pressure should be applied using a clean cloth or compress. If the compress should become soaked with blood, a new compress should be placed over the original. The original compress should not be removed as removal may disrupt the clotting process.

If applying pressure over the site is ineffective in controlling bleeding, such as may be the case with a very large injury, apply strong finger pressure over the pressure point of the main artery supplying the area. *Avoid* use of a tourniquet to control bleeding. A tourniquet should only be used as a last resort to save a patient's life after all other means to control bleeding are unsuccessful, such as may occur with an avulsion (amputation) or a severely mangled or crushed body part.

Shock Prevention

A state of shock results when there is insufficient return of blood flow to the heart, resulting in inadequate supply of oxygen to all organs and tissues of the body. Numerous conditions including hemorrhage, heart attack, trauma, and drug reactions can lead to some degree of shock. Because shock can be a life-threatening situation, it is important that the symptoms be recognized and dealt with immediately.

COMMON SYMPTOMS OF SHOCK

- Pale, cold, clammy skin
- Rapid, weak pulse
- Increased, shallow breathing rate
- Expressionless face and staring eyes

FIRST AID FOR SHOCK

1. Maintain an open airway for the victim.
2. Call for assistance.
3. Keep the victim lying down with head lower than the rest of the body.
4. Attempt to control bleeding or other cause of shock if known.
5. Keep the victim warm. *Never* give fluids if patient has injuries likely to require surgery and anesthesia. *Never* give fluids if the patient is unconscious or semiconscious.

Cardiopulmonary resuscitation

Most health care institutions require their personnel to be certified in cardiopulmonary resuscitation (CPR). Cardiopulmonary resuscitation instruction generally includes instruction in recognizing and treating foreign body airway obstruction (choking) and rescue breathing. There are five different courses in CPR offered by the American Heart Association. The C course is required for health care personnel. Certification must be renewed every 2 years. Most phlebotomy programs require CPR certification as a prerequisite/corequisite or include it as part of the course.

Study & Review Questions

1. Which of the following situations involves a nosocomial infection?
   a. a patient admitted to the hospital with a severe urinary tract infection
   b. an employee who contracts HBV infection from a needlestick
   c. a patient in ICU whose surgical wound is infected
   d. a baby in the nursery with congenital herpes

2. Reverse isolation may be used for:
   a. a pediatric patient with measles
   b. an adult patient with the flu
   c. a patient with a urinary tract infection
   d. a patient with severe burns

3. Under BSI procedures, a stop sign on a patient's door means:
   a. no visitors allowed
   b. check with the nurse for special precautions before entering
   c. do not enter without a mask
   d. knock before entering

4. The single most important means of preventing the spread of infection is:
   a. proper handwashing
   b. wearing a mask
   c. wearing gloves
   d. nosocomial infections cannot be prevented

5. Safe working conditions for employees are mandated by:
   a. CDC
   b. OSHA
   c. CAP
   d. ASCP

6. The most frequently occurring lab acquired infection is:
   a. HBV infection
   b. HIV infection
   c. syphilis
   d. tuberculosis

7. Electrical safety involves:
   a. distance, time, and shielding
   b. knowing where the fire extinguishers are
   c. knowing the circuit breaker box locations
   d. none of the above

8. In the event of a chemical splash in the eye, the first thing the victim should do is:
   a. go to the emergency room
   b. call the paramedics
   c. wipe the eye with a tissue
   d. immediately flush the eye with water for 15 minutes

Suggested Laboratory Activities

1. Practice proper handwashing procedures.

2. Practice the proper way to put on and remove gloves.

3. Touch your hand to a blood agar plate after touching various surfaces or before and after handwashing. Incubate the plates overnight and observe growth of microorganisms.

4. Examine safety equipment such as face shields, goggles, and splash guards.

5. Determine the location of fire extinguishers and other safety equipment in your laboratory, as well as other areas of your facility.

6. Write an exposure control plan for the student laboratory.

BIBLIOGRAPHY AND SUGGESTED READINGS

Davis B, Bishop ML, Mass D: *Clinical Laboratory Science: Strategies for Practice.* Philadelphia: JB Lippincott Company, 1989.

Grime D, Grime R, Hamelink M: *Infectious Diseases.* St. Louis: Mosby Clinical Nursing Series, 1991.

National Committee for Clinical Laboratory Standards, M29-T2: *Protection of Laboratory Workers from Infectious Disease Transmitted by Blood, Body Fluids and Tissue* (2nd ed.). Villanova, PA: NCCLS Tentative Guideline, September 1992.

Nursing Photobook. *Controlling Infections* (Skill Book Series). Springhouse, PA: Intermed Communciations, 1982.

OSHA Compliance Encyclopedia, vol. III. Madison, CT: Business and Legal Reports, revision July 1992.

Blood Collection Equipment and Supplies

7

OBJECTIVES

On successful completion of this chapter, the reader should be able to:

1   List the equipment and supplies needed to collect blood by venipuncture and skin puncture.
2   Identify types of additives used in blood collection, how they work, and the color coding associated with each type.
3   Contrast antiseptics and disinfectants.
4   Explain the purpose of using a tourniquet for venipuncture and name, as well as describe, the various types.
5   List order of draw for the evacuated tube system and the syringe system.
6   Describe evacuated tube system and syringe parts and needles; define lumen, bevel, and gauge.

KEY TERMS

additives
antiseptics
bevel
Caraway tubes
disinfectants
evacuated tubes
gauge
lancet
lumen
microcollection containers
microhematocrit tubes
Natelson tubes
sweeps
winged infusion set

McCall: PHLEBOTOMY ESSENTIALS. © 1993
J. B. Lippincott Company.

GENERAL BLOOD DRAWING EQUIPMENT

The primary duty of the phlebotomist is to collect blood specimens for laboratory analysis. This chapter will discuss the equipment and supplies needed to facilitate this process.

Blood Drawing Station

A blood drawing station is a special area of the laboratory equipped for performing phlebotomy procedures on patients, primarily outpatients. (Outpatients are non-hospitalized patients who have been sent by their doctors to the laboratory to have blood tests performed.)

A blood drawing station includes, at the minimum, a table for supplies and a chair or bed for the patient. The table should be a convenient height for the phlebotomist to work from, with enough space to hold supplies for numerous phlebotomy procedures. The chair should be comfortable for the patient and have an adjustable armrest to achieve proper arm positioning. There should be a safety device to lock the armrest in place to prevent the patient from falling out should he or she become faint.

There should be a bed or reclining chair available for patients with a history of fainting, persons donating blood, and other special situations. A reclining chair does not require a locking armrest. A bed or padded table is also needed for performing heelsticks or other procedures on infants and small children.

Carts and Trays

The use of carts and trays make blood drawing equipment portable. This is especially important in a hospital setting and other instances where the patient cannot come to the laboratory.

Carts are made of stainless steel or strong synthetic material. They have swivel wheels, which glide the carts smoothly and quietly down hospital hallways and in and out of elevators. They also have several shelves to carry adequate supplies for obtaining blood specimens from many patients. Carts are generally used for early morning phlebotomy rounds when many patients need laboratory work and for scheduled "**sweeps**" (rounds that occur at regular intervals throughout the day). Because carts can present a risk of transmitting nosocomial infections, they are not normally brought into patients' rooms. Instead, they are parked outside in the hallway. To have extra supplies, as well as a container for needle disposal at the bedside as required by the Occupational Safety and Health Administration (OSHA), a tray of supplies to be taken into the room is often carried on the cart.

Trays (Fig. 7–1) are designed to be easily carried by the phlebotomist and to contain enough equipment for numerous blood draws. They are convenient for "stat" or emergency situations or when relatively few patients need blood work. Trays are often part of the equipment on a phlebotomy cart. Making certain that carts and trays are adequately stocked is an important duty of the phlebotomist.

Gloves

"Universal precautions" guidelines by the Centers for Disease Control and Prevention (CDC) and regulations by OSHA require the wearing of gloves when perform-

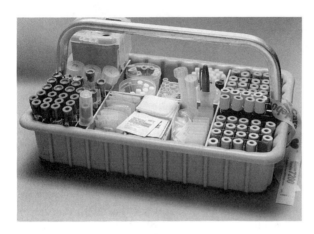

Figure 7–1   One type of blood collection tray.

ing phlebotomy procedures (see Chapter 6). A new pair of gloves must be used for each patient and removed when the procedure is completed. Nonsterile, disposable latex, vinyl, or polyethylene examination gloves are acceptable. A good fit is essential. Cotton gloves to wear under latex or plastic gloves are available for persons who develop dermatitis from wearing gloves.

Antiseptics and Disinfectants

Antiseptics are substances or solutions used to prevent **sepsis** or a disease state resulting from the presence of microorganisms or their toxic products in the bloodstream. Antiseptics are bacteriostatic, that is, they prevent or inhibit the growth of bacteria. They are safe for use on human skin and are used to clean the skin prior to venipuncture or skin puncture.

The most common antiseptic used for routine blood collection is 70% isopropyl alcohol (isopropanol) in the form of individually wrapped prep pads. Other antiseptics include povidone iodine in several forms, including swab sticks and sponge pads for blood culture collection, and prep pads for blood gas collection. Preparations of 0.5% chlorhexidene gluconate can be used for those allergic to iodine.

Disinfectants are bactericidal (*ie,* they kill bacteria). They are used on surfaces and instruments. They are not safe for use on human skin. Household bleach (5.25% sodium hypochlorite) in a 1:10 solution is a disinfectant that can kill the viruses that cause AIDS and hepatitis. It is commonly used to wipe surfaces and clean up blood spills.

Sterile Gauze Pads

Sterile 2 × 2 gauze pads folded in fourths are used to hold pressure over the site following venipuncture or skin puncture. Cotton or rayon balls may be used, however, they have a tendency to stick to the site and reinitiate bleeding on removal.

Bandages

Adhesive bandages are used to cover the site once the bleeding has ceased. Paper, cloth, or knitted tape over a folded gauze square can also be used, especially for patients who are allergic to adhesive bandages. Two-inch-wide roll gauze or self-

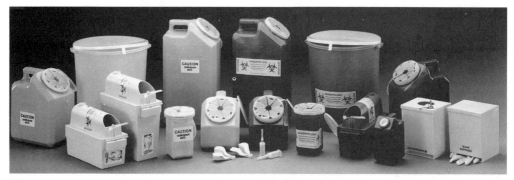

Figure 7–2   Several styles of sharps containers. (Courtesy of PRO TEC Containers, Inc., Irvine, CA)

adhesive gauze such as Coban (a special type of gauze that sticks to itself but not the skin) is occasionally used over a gauze pad or cotton ball to form a pressure bandage following arterial puncture or for patients with bleeding problems. Bandages should not be used on infants under 2 years of age because of the danger of aspiration and suffocation.

Needle and Sharps Disposal Containers

Used needles, lancets, and other sharp objects must be disposed of immediately in special containers usually referred to as "sharps" containers (Fig. 7–2). A variety of styles and sizes are available from manufacturers. They are usually red or bright orange for easy identification and also are marked "biohazard." Containers must be rigid, puncture-resistant, leak-proof, disposable, and easily sealed when full. Those selected for phlebotomy use should contain a device to aid in removing needles from evacuated tube adapters. Needles are *not* to be recapped, cut, bent, or broken prior to disposal.

Slides

Precleaned 5 × 75 mm (1 × 3 inch) glass microscope slides are used to make blood films for hematology determinations. Slides are available either plain or with a frosted area at one end where the patient's name or other information can be written in pencil.

VENIPUNCTURE EQUIPMENT

In addition to the aforementioned supplies and equipment, venipuncture procedures require the use of the following special equipment.

Tourniquets

A *tourniquet* (Fig. 7–3) is applied to a patient's arm prior to venipuncture. It should be applied tightly enough to slow the venous flow without affecting the arterial flow. This allows more blood to flow into the area than out, which causes the veins to

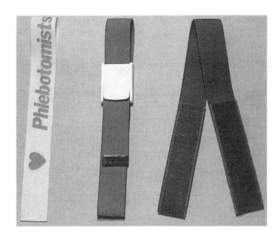

Figure 7–3 Several types of tourniquets (left to right): latex strap, Seraket®, and velcro closure.

enlarge, making them easier to find and penetrate with a needle. Tourniquets are available in adult and pediatric sizes.

The most commonly used tourniquet is a flat strip of stretchable latex, 15 to 18 inches long. A length of latex Penrose drain tubing serves the same purpose. Latex does not readily support bacterial growth and, if soiled, can easily be wiped clean with disinfectant. Inexpensive disposable latex tourniquets are available.

A blood pressure cuff may be used in place of a tourniquet by those familiar with its operation. The patient's blood pressure is taken and the pressure is then maintained below the patient's diastolic pressure.

Velcro-closure tourniquets are also available. They usually are made of elastic material with a long band of Velcro to allow a wide range of adjustment capability. A disadvantage of Velcro tourniquets is that they may not fit around the arms of extremely obese patients.

Another type of tourniquet, called a Seraket tourniquet is made of cloth webbing and has a buckle closure. This type stays on the patient's arm when released and can be tightened again if necessary. A disadvantage of this type, as with the Velcro tourniquet and blood pressure cuff, is that it is not easily cleaned if soiled with blood or otherwise contaminated.

Needles

Blood-drawing needles are sterile, disposable, and for single use only. They are silicon-coated, which enables them to penetrate the skin smoothly. The end of the needle that is inserted into the vein is called the **bevel** because it is cut on a slant or "beveled" to allow the needle to penetrate the vein easily and prevent coring (removal of a portion of the skin or vein). The long, cylindrical portion is called the **shaft**, and the end that connects to the blood-drawing apparatus is referred to as the **hub**.

The **gauge** of a needle indicates the size of the needle and refers to the diameter of the **lumen** (internal space) or "bore" of the needle. Like wire or nail gauges, the larger the gauge number, the smaller the actual diameter of the needle. Gauge selection depends on the size and condition of the vein.

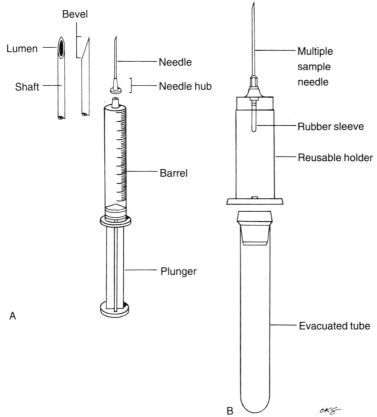

Figure 7-4 *A.* Syringe components; *B.* Components of the evacuated tube collection system.

Evacuated Tube System

The most commonly employed system for collecting blood samples is the *evacuated tube system* (Fig. 7-4). It is a closed system in which the patient's blood goes directly from the vein into a stoppered tube without being exposed to the air. The evacuated tube system allows numerous tubes to be collected using a single venipuncture. Evacuated tube collection systems are available from several manufacturers. Mixing components from different manufacturers may lead to problems, such as needles coming unscrewed and tubes popping off during venipuncture procedures. To avoid problems and ensure proper needle fit and smooth removal of tubes, it is necessary for all components of the system to be from the same manufacturer.

COMPONENTS OF THE SYSTEM

Needles. Needles used with the evacuated tube system are threaded in the middle and have a beveled point on each end. One end is used to pierce the skin and enter the vein; the other end penetrates the rubber stopper of a collection tube. The threaded portion allows easy and secure attachment to a tube holder. The end of the needle that penetrates the vein is longer and has a longer bevel. The end of the needle that penetrates the stopper of the collecting tube has a rubber sleeve, which covers it when the tube is removed. This feature prevents leakage of blood when changing tubes during a multiple-tube draw, as well as when the tube is removed prior to withdrawing the needle from the vein. Because multiple tubes can be drawn with evacuated tube system needles, they are called **multiple-sample needles.**

Evacuated tube system needles come in two lengths: 1 inch and 1½ inches. Length selection depends primarily on user preference and also the depth of the vein. Many phlebotomists prefer to use the 1-inch needle in routine situations because it is less intimidating to the patient. It is also less intimidating to a phlebotomy student using it. However, some phlebotomists feel that the 1½-inch needle allows for easier placement of the anchoring thumb.

Evacuated tube system needles are available in sizes from 20 to 22 gauge, with 21-gauge needles most commonly used for routine venipuncture.

Needles come enclosed in sealed twist-apart shields to ensure sterility; they should not be used if the seal is broken. The shields are color-coded by the manufacturer according to gauge for easy identification.

Holders.   The needle and tube **holder,** sometimes referred to as an **adapter,** is a clear plastic cylinder with a small opening at one end to receive the threaded needle. There is a large opening at the other end to receive the evacuated blood drawing tube. There are flanges (extensions) on the sides of the tube end of the holder to aid in tube placement and removal.

Holders come in at least two sizes: one for regular-diameter tubes and a smaller one for small-diameter tubes used for pediatric patients or difficult draws. It is important to use the proper holder for the size of the tube. Some manufacturers supply adapter inserts so that both large and small tubes may be used with the regular-sized holder.

Special holders designed to reduce the risk of accidental needle sticks are also available. One such holder is the Safety-lok needle holder from Becton Dickinson Vacutainer Systems (Franklin Lakes, NJ). This single-use holder has a protective shield that the user can slide over the needle and lock in place after the needle is withdrawn from the vein, ensuring immediate protection from accidental needle puncture. However, using the holder requires a large needle disposal container to accommodate its bulk and creates much more waste than a needle by itself.

A similar holder that shields the needle prior to disposal is the SAF-T-CLIK tube holder manufactured by Ryan Medical, Inc., Brentwood, TN.

A needle disposal system from Becton Dickinson Vacutainer Systems (Franklin Lakes, NJ) features a reusable holder combined with a needle disposal container. The holder combines a safe, one-handed resheathing process and a locking needle enclosure. This devices enables the phlebotomist to retract the used needle and safely resheath it while retracted. At this point, the entire unit with the needle locked inside may be discarded, or the needle may be safely removed from the holder using the special needle disposal container. The needle may also be retracted and removed without resheathing.

Another holder designed with safety in mind is the PRO-JECT Safety Needle Holder by PRO-TEC, Irvine, CA. This holder has a special release mechanism that allows the user to release the needle into the needle container without unscrewing it from the holder. This prevents injuries associated with needle disposal caused by the needle slipping out of the holder while being unscrewed, or the needle being stuck in the holder with the rubber guard end pointed up. It will not, however, protect the user from injuries associated with dropping the needle before disposal.

Evacuated tubes. **Evacuated tubes** are used with both the evacuated tube system and the syringe method of obtaining blood specimens. With the evacuated tube system, the blood is collected directly into the tube during the venipuncture procedure. With the syringe method, the blood from the syringe must be transferred into the tubes after collection.

Evacuated tubes fill with blood automatically because of the vacuum that exists inside the tube. The amount of vacuum is premeasured so that the tube will draw a precise amount of blood. A tube that has lost its vacuum will not fill with blood. Tube vacuum is guaranteed by the manufacturer until the expiration date; however, premature loss of vacuum can occur from opening the tube, dropping the tube, advancing the tube too far onto the needle holder, or pulling the needle bevel partway out of the skin during venipuncture.

Evacuated tubes come in various sizes from 2 to 15 ml. The size is selected according to the age of the patient, the amount of blood needed for the test, and the size and condition of the patient's vein. Some evacuated tubes, especially those for serum determinations, are coated on the inside with silicon to help prevent destruction of red blood cells and to keep the blood from sticking to the sides of the tube. Evacuated tubes may or may not contain an additive. Blood collected in tubes without additives will clot and yield serum on centrifugation. Tubes that contain additives may or may not clot, depending on the type of additive they contain (Table 7–1.)

TUBE ADDITIVES

An **additive** is any substance placed in a tube other than the coating of the tube or tube stopper (closure). Additives have specific functions. The most common additives are categorized below.

Anticoagulants. An anticoagulant is a substance that prevents the blood from coagulating or clotting. Tubes containing anticoagulants yield whole blood specimens which may be separated by centrifugation to yield plasma. The most common anticoagulants include:

• *EDTA.* Ethylenediaminetetraacetic acid in a tripotassium (K_3) or disodium (Na_2) base. EDTA prevents coagulation by finding calcium in the form of a potassium or sodium salt. EDTA is the anticoagulant of choice for whole blood hematology studies.

• *Heparin.* There are three heparin formulations: ammonium, lithium, and sodium heparin. Heparin prevents coagulation by inhibiting the clotting component thrombin. Heparin is the anticoagulant of choice for plasma chemistry determinations and is often used for "stat" chemistry determinations to save the time required for a serum specimen to clot.

Table 7–1.
Specimen Type and Collection Tubes

Specimen Type	Color Code	Additive	Type of Additive	Department
Clotted Blood				
Serum	Red	None		Chemistry
				Serology
		Sterile		Blood bank
	Red / yellow	Glass particles	Clot activator	Chemistry
	Black / yellow	Thrombin		Chemistry
	Red / gray	Thixotropic gel	Clot activator	Chemistry
	Rose	Thixotropic gel	Clot activator	Chemistry
	Navy	None		Special chemistry
Whole Blood				
Plasma	Light blue	Sodium citrate	Anticoagulant	Coagulation
	Gray	Sodium fluoride	Anticoagulant	Chemistry
	Green	Lithium heparin	Anticoagulant	Chemistry
		Sodium heparin	Anticoagulant	
	Navy	Sodium heparin	Anticoagulant	Special chemistry
		Ethylenediamine-tetraacetate (EDTA)	Anticoagulant	Special chemistry
Whole Blood	Lavender	EDTA	Anticoagulant	Hematology
	Green	Sodium heparin	Anticoagulant	Hematology
	Yellow	Sodium polyanethole sulfonate (SPS)	Anticoagulant	Microbiology
		Acid Citrate Dextrose (ACD)	Cell preservative	Blood bank

• *Sodium citrate.*   Prevents coagulation by binding calcium. Sodium citrate is the anticoagulant of choice for coagulation studies performed on plasma.

• *Potassium or ammonium oxalate.*   Prevents coagulation by binding calcium. Oxalate along with an antiglycolytic agent (see below) is often used to collect plasma specimens for glucose testing.

Antiglycolytic agent.   An antiglycolytic agent is a substance that inhibits metabolism of glucose by the cells of the blood. The most common antiglycolytic agents are sodium fluoride and iodoacetic acid.

Clot activators.   Clot activators are substances that initiate or enhance coagulation. They include substances that provide increased surface for platelet activation, such as glass or silica particles and inert clays like siliceous earth and celite, as well as the clotting components thromboplastin and thrombin.

Thixotropic gel separator. A thixotropic gel separator is an inert (non-reacting) synthetic substance that forms a physical barrier between the cellular portion of a specimen and the serum or plasma portion after the specimen has been centrifuged.

TUBE STOPPERS

Tube stoppers (Color Plate 2) are made of rubber and are color-coded to indicate the presence and type of additive or the absence of additive. Stopper colors may vary slightly by manufacturers. The most common tube stopper colors and additives, if applicable, are as follows:

Red: no additive
Red/gray: gel separator and glass or silica particles
Green/gray: gel separator and heparin
Green: heparin
Royal blue: may be non-additive (red label) or contain EDTA (lavender label) or heparin (green label). Stopper indicates that the tube is designed to be as free of trace elements as possible.
Lavender: EDTA, the additive of choice for hematology studies
Light blue: sodium citrate, the additive of choice for coagulation studies
Gray: potassium oxalate and sodium fluoride, prevents coagulation and glycolysis. Used for glucose and alcohol (ethanol) determinations.

New Becton Dickinson Hemogard Closure tubes (see Color Plate 2) have a rubber stopper covered by a plastic shield. The plastic shield is designed to protect lab personnel from blood remaining on the stopper after the tube is removed from the needle, as well as when the stopper is removed from the tube. The rigidity of the plastic also prevents a "thumb roll" technique and subsequent aerosol (misting) of contents when removing the stopper from the tube. The color coding of Hemogard stoppers varies slightly from that of regular stoppers.

Order of draw

EVACUATED TUBE METHOD

When using the evacuated tube system, and when multiple tubes are to be drawn, the following "order of draw" is recommended to avoid contamination of non-additive tubes by additive tubes, as well as cross-contamination between different types of additive tubes: *yellow*

1. Blood culture tubes (and other tests requiring sterile specimens)
2. Red stopper or red/gray stopper: nonadditive and gel separator, respectively
3. Light blue stopper: sodium citrate, or other citrate-containing tubes or tubes for coagulation studies (*Note:* if a light blue-stoppered tube is the first or only tube to be drawn, a 5-ml red stopper tube should be drawn first and discarded to eliminate contamination from tissue thromboplastin picked up during needle penetration.)
4. Green or green/gray stopper: heparin
5. Lavender stopper: EDTA (K_3 or Na_2)
6. Gray stopper: oxalate/fluoride

SYRINGE METHOD

With the exception of tubes for sterile specimens which are collected first in either method, the order of filling evacuated tubes with blood obtained by syringe differs from the evacuated tube order of draw. It is assumed that the blood that enters the syringe last is the freshest and will be the first blood out of the syringe in the transfer process. Because the clotting process is activated the minute the blood starts to fill the syringe, it is important to transfer the blood quickly and to fill anticoagulant tubes before serum tubes. The suggested syringe order of draw for the most common tubes is as follows:

1. Blood culture (or other tube requiring sterile specimens)
2. Light blue: sodium citrate (or other citrate-containing tubes)
3. Lavender: EDTA
4. Green: heparin
5. Gray: oxalate/fluoride
6. Red or red and gray: serum tubes

Syringe System

Although the evacuated tube system is the preferred method of blood collection, the syringe system is sometimes used for patients with difficult veins. The syringe system consists of a hypodermic needle attached to a sterile, disposable plastic syringe.

Syringe needles are sterile, prepackaged, designed for single use, and come in a wide range of gauges for many different uses. Only those gauges appropriate for phlebotomy procedures should be used, generally 21 to 23 gauge for blood drawing and 18 gauge for transferring specimens into evacuated tubes. Syringe needles also come in different lengths, with 1-inch and 1½-inch lengths most commonly used for blood drawing.

Syringes come in various sizes, with 2 to 10 ml most commonly used for phlebotomy procedures. Syringes have two parts, a **barrel** with graduated markings in either milliliters (ml) or cubic centimeters (cc), and a **plunger** which fits in the barrel of the syringe. When drawing blood with a syringe, the plunger is slowly retracted by the phlebotomist, allowing the barrel to fill with blood. Blood specimens collected by syringe must be transferred to evacuated tubes following proper order of draw.

Winged Infusion Set

A winged infusion set (butterfly) (Fig. 7–5) consists of a ½- to ¾-inch stainless steel needle connected to a 5- to 12-inch length of tubing. It is called a butterfly because of its wing-shaped plastic extensions that are used for gripping the needle.

Butterflies generally come with attachments that allow them to be used with syringes. There are, however, butterflies that come with a special multiple sample luer adapter, which allows them to be used with an evacuated tube system. Special multiple sample luer adapters are also available to convert a syringe attachment butterfly for use with the evacuated tube system.

The butterfly needle is an indispensable tool for collecting blood from small or difficult veins, such as hand veins or veins of elderly or pediatric patients. It allows much more flexibility and precision than a needle and syringe. Butterfly needles come in vari-

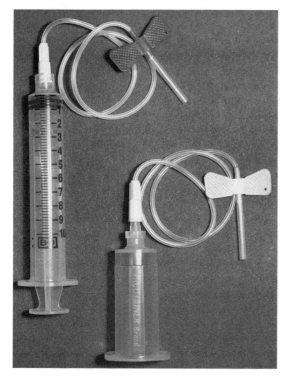

Hemody zing .

Figure 7-5 Winged infusion sets: (left) attached to a syringe; (right) attached to evacuated tube holder by means of a luer adapter.

ous sizes with a 23 gauge being the one most commonly used in difficult phlebotomy situations. Using a needle with a smaller bore than a 23 gauge increases the chance of hemolyzing the specimen.

Several types of "high risk" butterfly needles are now on the market. These needles contain a shield, which covers the needle on withdrawal from the patient's vein, reducing the possibility of accidental needle sticks. Examples are the Shamrock (Ryan Medical Inc., Brentwood, TN) and Angel Wing Safety Needle System (MBO Laboratories, North Chelmsford, MA).

SKIN PUNCTURE EQUIPMENT

In addition to the general blood drawing equipment, the following equipment is needed for skin puncture, which is also referred to as microcollection or capillary collection:

Lancets

A **lancet** (Fig. 7-6) is a sterile, single-use, disposable, sharp-pointed instrument used to pierce the skin to obtain droplets of blood used for testing. Only lancets specifically designed for skin puncture should be used. To avoid penetrating bone, depth of puncture must be controlled. A number of companies manufacture special skin puncture devices which control the depth of puncture. Examples are the Microtainer Brand

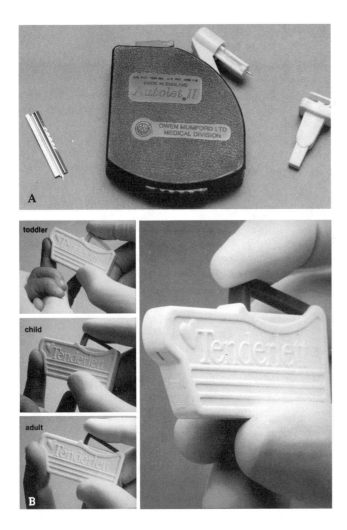

Figure 7-6 Several types of skin puncture lancets. *A.* Metal lancet; Autolet (Ulster Scientific Inc., New Paltz, NY); Safety Flow Lancet (Becton Dickinson, Franklin Lakes, NJ). *B.* Tenderlett Toddler, Junior, and Adult lancet devices (International Technidyne Corp., Edison, NJ).

Safety Flow Lancet (Becton Dickinson, Franklin Lakes, NJ) in sizes for heelstick and finger stick; and the Tenderfoot for neonates (newborns), Tenderlett Toddler, and Tenderlett Jr. for children (International Technidyne Corp., Edison, NJ). Also available are the Autolet II and Autolet Lite Clinisafe (Ulster Scientific, Inc., New Paltz, NY) spring-activated, reusable puncture devices that both feature a removable, single-use lancet and platform. The platform, which is positioned over the site prior to puncture, controls the depth of puncture and is available in three color-coded depths: white (1.8 mm), yellow (2.4 mm), and orange (3.0 mm). The Autolet Lite Clinisafe has a safety mechanism which prevents reuse of the device without replacing the lancet and platform unless the lancet and platform are replaced.

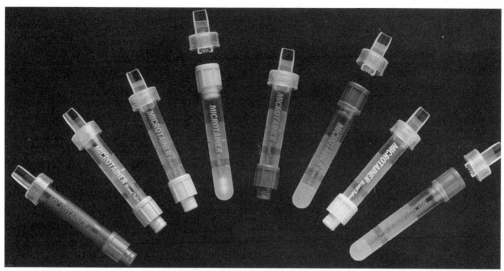

Figure 7–7   Microtainers. (Courtesy of Becton Dickinson and Co., Franklin Lakes, NJ)

Collection Devices

MICROCOLLECTION CONTAINERS

A number of companies manufacture special **microcollection containers** (Fig. 7–7) to be used for obtaining blood from skin punctures. These tubes are made of plastic and have color-coded stoppers, which indicate the presence or absence of an additive, as well as the type of additive if present. Color-coding corresponds to that of blood collection tubes used in venipuncture. Examples of microcollection tubes include the Microtainers and Microvettes by Becton Dickinson (Franklin Lakes, NJ), Capiject tubes by Terumo TMG, and Samplette capillary blood collectors (Sherwood Medical, St. Louis, MO).

MICROHEMATOCRIT TUBES

Disposable, narrow-bore glass or plastic capillary tubes designed to hold 50 to 75 microliters of blood are primarily used for hematocrit (packed cell volume) determinations on micro samples. They fill with blood by capillary action. They are designed to be used with special centrifuges. **Microhematocrit tubes** (Fig. 7–8) are also used to collect other micro specimens. Microhematocrit tubes come coated with ammonium heparin for hematocrit determinations, other hematology tests, and tests requiring plasma, or plain for collection of serum specimens. Ammonium heparin-coated tubes have a red band at one end of the tube; plain tubes have a blue band. Special plain capillary tubes are available for capillary coagulation tests.

Special microhematocrit tubes designed to be used exclusively with special centrifuges from Statspin Technologies, require as little as 9 microliters of blood and are gaining popularity for use in screening programs and pediatric clinics.

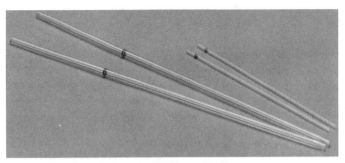

Figure 7–8   Microcollection tubes: Natelson tubes on the left and microhematocrit tubes on the right.

CARAWAY TUBES AND NATELSON TUBES

Caraway and Natelson tubes are disposable, glass microcollection tubes (see Figure 7–8). They can be used for most tests that can be performed on skin puncture blood. They are tapered at one end and come with or without an anticoagulant. Anticoagulated tubes for plasma determinations come with a yellow circular band at the nontapered end and generally contain lithium heparin. Nonanticoagulated tubes have a blue band. Caraway tubes are 75 mm in length and have a capacity of approximately 350 microliters. Natelson tubes are 147 mm in length and have a capacity of approximately 250 microliters.

CAPILLARY BLOOD GAS COLLECTION EQUIPMENT

Capillary blood gas collection tubes are used to collect skin puncture blood gas specimens (Fig. 7–9). Tubes vary according to volume requirements for different testing methods and instrumentation. Tubes 100 mm in length with a capacity of 100 microliters are most common. A color-coded band identifies the type of anticoagulant coating the inside of the tube, usually green for sodium heparin.

Stirrers.   Metal *stirrers* (often referred to as "fleas") are inserted into the tube after collection of a capillary blood gas specimen to aid in mixing the anticoagulant.

Magnet.   A *magnet* is required to aid in mixing capillary blood gas specimens after collection. The magnet often has a hole in the center so that it can be slipped over the capillary tube. It then is moved back and forth along the tube length, pulling the metal stirrer with it and mixing the anticoagulant into the blood specimen.

CLAY

Plastic or *clay* sealants are commonly used to seal one end of microhematocrit tubes, as well as tubes for chemistry determinations. Both ends of capillary blood gas tubes need to be sealed.

PLASTIC CAPS

Plastic end caps or closures are available in place of clay to seal microcollection tubes. Capillary blood gas collection tubes often come with their own caps.

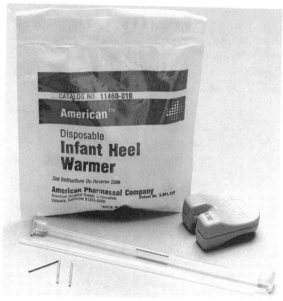

Figure 7-9   Capillary blood gas equipment.

MICROPIPET DILUTION SYSTEMS

A *micropipet dilution system* (Fig. 7–10) serves as both a collection device and a dilution unit for the blood sample. Components of this disposable system are a sealed plastic reservoir, which contains a premeasured amount of reagent; a detachable glass self-filling capillary pipet; and a pipet shield, which also serves as a device to puncture the reservoir covering or diaphragm, prior to adding the sample.

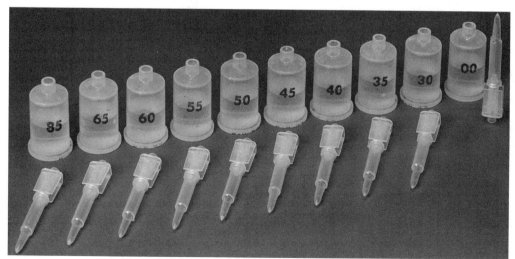

Figure 7-10   Unopette system (Courtesy of Becton Dickinson and Co., Franklin Lakes, NJ)

WARMING DEVICES

Warming the area prior to skin puncture can increase the blood flow as much as seven times. This is especially important when performing heelsticks on newborns. Several *heelwarming devices* are commercially available (see Figure 7–9). To avoid burning the patient, these devices provide a uniform temperature that does not exceed 42°C. A towel or diaper wet with warm tap water can also be used to wrap the hand or foot prior to skin puncture. However, care must be taken not to use water so hot it scalds the patient.

Study & Review Questions

1. Containers used for disposing needles and other sharp objects must be all of the following EXCEPT:
   a. clearly marked "biohazard"
   b. disposable
   c. puncture-resistant
   d. recyclable

2. The most common antiseptic for routine blood collection is:
   a. antibacterial soap and water
   b. povidone iodine
   c. 70% isopropyl alcohol
   d. 5.25% sodium hypochlorite

3. Needles are color-coded according to their:
   a. brand
   b. gauge
   c. length
   d. expiration date

4. The needle gauge with the smallest diameter is:
   a. 19
   b. 20
   c. 21
   d. 23

5. In the recommended order of draw for the evacuated tube method, which tube should be filled last?
   a. red top
   b. lavender top
   c. light blue top
   d. blood culture

6. The color-coded tube that is most often associated with hematology tests is:
   a. green
   b. light blue
   c. lavender
   d. red

7. Which of the following is NOT skin puncture equipment?
   a. Autolet
   b. Safety flow lancet
   c. Shamrock butterfly
   d. Tenderfoot

8. A microcollection tube that has a green cap contains which additive?
   a. EDTA
   b. citrate
   c. oxalate
   d. heparin

Suggested Laboratory Activities

1. Identify, handle, and describe the use of various blood collection equipment. Practice equipment assembly, if applicable.

2. Properly stock a laboratory blood collection tray.

3. Make 8 × 10 cards with different collection tubes attached and write a thought-provoking question on each concerning its use.

4. Arrange blood collecting tubes in the proper order of draw for both the evacuated tube and the syringe methods.

BIBLIOGRAPHY AND SUGGESTED READINGS

National Committee for Clinical Laboratory Standards, H3-A3: *Procedures for the Collection of Diagnostic Blood Specimens by Venipuncture* (3rd ed.). Villanova, PA: NCCLS, July 1991.

National Committee for Clinical Laboratory Standards, H4-A3: *Procedures for the Collection of Diagnostic Blood Specimens by Skin Puncture* (3rd ed.). Villanova, PA: NCCLS, July 1991.

National Committee for Clinical Laboratory Standards, H14-A2: *Devices for Collection of Skin Puncture Blood Specimens* (2nd ed.). Villanova, PA: NCCLS, July 1990.

National Committee for Clinical Laboratory Standards, M29-T2: *Protection of Laboratory Workers from Infectious Disease Transmitted by Blood, Body Fluids and Tissue* (2nd ed.). Villanova, PA: NCCLS Tentative Guideline, September 1992.

Factors to Consider Prior to Blood Collection

8

OBJECTIVES
On successful completion of this chapter, the reader should be able to:

1 Define basal state and list factors influencing this state.
2 List and define test status designations and describe the procedure to follow for each.
3 List factors to consider in site selection; describe causes for concern and procedures to follow when encountering each.
4 List complications associated with blood collection and describe how they may affect the patient or the integrity of the specimen.
5 Describe how to avoid complications, as well as how to handle those that occur.

KEY TERMS
basal state
cannula
diurnal variation
edema
fistula (shunt)
hematoma
hemoconcentration
hemolysis
heparin lock
indwelling lines
lipemic
patency
petechiae
STAT (stat)
syncope
venous stasis

PHYSIOLOGIC FACTORS

Basal State

Because constituents of the blood are affected by diet, exercise, and other factors, the ideal time for collecting blood specimens is early in the morning while the body is still at rest and **fasting**, or approximately 12 hours after the last intake of food. This condition is known as **basal state**. **Reference (normal)** values for lab tests on hospital patients are usually established using basal state specimens. Outpatient specimens are not basal state specimens and may have slightly different normal values.

Factors Influencing Basal State

AGE

Values for numerous blood components vary considerably with the age of the patient. For example, red blood cell (RBC) and white blood cell (WBC) values are higher in newborns than adults.

Some physiologic functions decrease with age in adults. For example, creatinine clearance, a kidney function test, is directly related to the patient's age, which must be used in calculating test results. *higher in ~ old pts. people elderly*

ALTITUDE

Decreased oxygen content of the air at higher altitudes causes the body to produce more RBCs to fulfill the body's oxygen requirements. The higher the altitude, the greater the increase. Red blood cell counts and related determinations such as hemoglobin (Hgb) and hematocrit (Hct) will have higher normal ranges at higher elevations.

DEHYDRATION

Dehydration (a decrease in total body fluid) that occurs with persistent vomiting or diarrhea, for example, causes **hemoconcentration**, which can falsely increase some blood components such as RBCs, enzymes, iron (Fe), calcium (Ca), and sodium (Na). In addition, it is often much more difficult to obtain a blood specimen from a dehydrated patient.

DIURNAL (DAILY) VARIATIONS

Many blood constituents show diurnal variation or normal fluctuations throughout the day. White blood counts, eosinophil counts, and iron levels are lower in the morning than in the afternoon. Cortisol levels are highest in the morning.

DIET

Blood composition is significantly altered by ingestion of food. Glucose levels increase dramatically with the ingestion of sugar-laden substances but should return to normal within 2 hours.

Ingestion of fatty substances, such as those found in many fast food items, butter, and cheese, increases lipid content in the blood for anywhere from 1 to 10 hours or more, causing the serum or plasma to appear **lipemic** (or cloudy). Some chemistry determinations cannot be performed on lipemic specimens because the cloudiness interferes with testing procedure.

Excessive fluid intake may cause decreased hemoglobin levels and alter electrolyte balance. Consumption of caffeine has been demonstrated to affect cortisol levels.

Most dietary influences on blood and urine specimens can be eliminated by requesting a fasting specimen.

DRUGS

Many drugs alter physiologic functions. In most instances, the altering effect is desired. In some individuals, however, there are also unwanted physiologic effects called "side effects" or sensitivities. As an example, thiazide diuretics often cause increased calcium levels and may cause low potassium levels. To check for side effects, it is not uncommon for doctors to monitor levels of certain blood components while a person is receiving drug therapy.

Chemotherapeutic drugs often cause a decrease in blood cells, especially WBCs and platelets. Numerous drugs are toxic to the liver, causing an increase in liver enzymes such as PT (ALT), alkaline phosphatase, and lactate dehydrogenase (LDH). Steroids and diuretics can cause pancreatitis and an increase in serum amylase and lipase values.

Drugs may also interfere with test performance in the laboratory, causing false increases or decreases in test results. Many lab test procedures are based on fluorescent, chromogenic (color-producing), peroxide-generating or reagent-binding reactions. A drug may compete with the test reagents for the substance being tested, causing a false-negative or falsely low result, or the drug may enhance the reaction, causing a false-positive or falsely high result.

According to the **College of American Pathologists (CAP)**, drugs known to interfere with blood tests should be stopped or avoided 4 to 24 hours prior to obtaining the blood sample for testing. Drugs known to interfere with urine testing should be avoided for 48 to 72 hours prior to urine sample collection.

It is up to the physician to recognize or eliminate drug interferences; however, it is helpful to the technician or technologist performing the test in the laboratory if the phlebotomist notes on the lab slip if he or she observes medication being administered just prior to blood collection.

ENVIRONMENT

Environmental factors such as temperature and humidity are known to affect test values. Environmental factors associated with geographic location are accounted for when establishing normal or reference values. Temperature and humidity in the laboratory are closely monitored to insure proper functioning of equipment and to maintain specimen integrity.

EXERCISE

Muscular activity, however moderate, will elevate the blood levels of a number of blood components, such as lactic acid, creatinine, protein, and certain enzymes. Levels of these substances return to normal soon after the activity is stopped, with the exception of enzymes such as creatine phosphokinase (CPK) and lactate dehydrogenase (LDH), which may remain elevated 24 hours or more.

POSITION

The position of a patient both before and during venipuncture influences blood composition. Going from a supine to standing position causes the water or plasma portion of the blood to filter into the tissues. This causes a decrease in plasma volume and an increase in nonfilterable elements or substances such as proteins, iron, calcium, and blood cells that cannot easily pass through the walls of the blood vessels. As an example, the RBC count on a patient who has been standing for approximately 15 minutes will be higher than the basal state RBC on the same patient.

PREGNANCY

Pregnancy causes physiologic changes in many body systems. As a result of these changes, a number of laboratory test results will differ from regular normal values and must be compared to normal ranges established for pregnant populations. For example, body fluid increases, which are normal during pregnancy, have a diluting effect on the red blood cells, leading to lower RBC counts.

GENDER

A patient's gender or sex has a determining effect on the concentration of numerous blood components. Most differences are apparent only after sexual maturity. These differences are reflected in separate normals for male and female patients. For example, RBC, hemoglobin, and hematocrit normals are higher in males.

STRESS

Emotional stress in the form of fear or anxiety has been shown to cause short-lived elevations in WBC counts, decreases in serum iron, and increased adrenal hormone values. For example, studies performed on crying infants demonstrated marked increases in WBC counts. Counts returned to normal within 1 hour after crying stopped. For this reason, complete blood count or WBC specimens should not be obtained unless the infant has been sleeping or resting quietly for approximately 1 hour.

A new field called **psychoneuroimmunology (PNI)** deals with the study of interactions between the brain, the endocrine system, and the immune system. Studies in this field have demonstrated that receptors on the cell membrane of WBCs can sense stress in a person and react by stimulating an increase in cell numbers.

TEST STATUS

Some tests require specimens collected at specific times or under specific conditions. Certain test requests take priority over others. The "status" of the test request should be clearly noted on the test request form. It is up to the phlebotomist to assess each test request and determine the priority and conditions involved in obtaining the specimen. Test status designations, priorities, and response times are determined by individual laboratories and may differ somewhat from one lab to another. The following are common test status designations in order of priority.

STAT (stat)

Stat comes from the Latin word "statim," meaning immediately. Stat blood tests should only be ordered on patients whose condition is or has become critical and test results are urgently needed to respond to the situation. Stat requests should not only be drawn expediently but should be processed and results reported immediately. The phlebotomist who draws and delivers a stat specimen to the lab should alert lab personnel to its presence.

Medical Emergency (Med Emerg)

Due to misuse of the term "stat," such as using the designation for requesting tests when there is not a medical emergency, some institutions have started using the designation "Med Emerg" to identify specimens that are needed in critical or "life-or-death" situations. This designation replaces "stat"; consequently, the same procedure is followed.

Timed Specimens

Some tests are requested to be collected at a particular time. It is important that the specimen be collected as near to the time requested as possible with the actual time of collection recorded on the request form and on the specimen container.

Commonly ordered timed tests include 2-hour postprandial glucose levels, glucose tolerance tests, cortisol levels, cardiac enzymes, and specimens for therapeutic drug monitoring peaks and troughs.

ASAP

ASAP stands for "as soon as possible." This means test results are needed soon for the doctor to respond to a serious situation, but the patient's condition is not critical.

Fasting

Some tests such as glucose, cholesterol, and triglycerides require that the patient abstain from eating or drinking (except water) for approximately 12 hours prior to collection of the specimen. It is up to the phlebotomist to ascertain if the patient is fasting. If the test has been ordered fasting and the phlebotomist determines that the patient has eaten, the phlebotomist must check with the patient's nurse (or the phlebotomy supervisor in the case of outpatients) to see if the test should still be performed. If the test is still wanted, the phlebotomist should draw the specimen and write "nonfasting" on the lab slip.

Pre-op

"Pre-op" means before an operation or surgery. Pre-op tests are needed to determine if the patient's condition is suitable for surgery. Examples of such tests may include complete blood count, partial thromboplastin time, or bleeding time tests.

Routine

Routine tests are those tests commonly ordered by the physician in the course of establishing a diagnosis or monitoring a patient's progress. Specimens should be collected in a timely fashion; however, there is no urgency involved. Most routine tests are ordered for early morning rounds. Routine tests ordered after morning rounds are collected during the next scheduled rounds or sweeps.

Routine Admission

Routine admission tests are required of all patients by the health care facility on admission. For example, many hospitals require all patients to have a complete blood count (CBC), chemistry profile, and urinalysis (UA) on admission. However, as consumers become more responsible for the cost of their health care, hospitals are moving away from batteries of admission tests toward more individualized (discrete) tests for each patient.

FACTORS TO CONSIDER IN SITE SELECTION

Scars and Burns

When selecting sites for phlebotomy tests, avoid tatooed, burned, or scarred areas of the skin. Veins are difficult to palpate and penetrate in scarred areas. Healed burn sites with extensive scarring often have impaired circulation and may yield erroneous test results. Newly burned areas are painful and also are susceptible to infection.

Mastectomy *never Draw blood from the one of the side of the mastectomy*

The patient's physician should be consulted before drawing blood from an arm on the same side as a recent mastectomy (breast removal). Due to lymphostasis (a stoppage of lymph flow) caused by lymph node removal, blood specimens obtained from the arm on the same side as a mastectomy may yield erroneous test results. These patients are also more susceptible to infection. In addition, application of a tourniquet to that arm may cause injury.

Hematoma

A venipuncture should not be made in the area of a **hematoma**. A hematoma is a swelling or mass of blood (usually clotted) caused by blood leaking from a blood vessel during or following venipuncture. **Venous stasis**, a slowdown of blood flow to the area due to obstruction by the hematoma, may lead to inaccurate test results. The area may also be painful to the patient. If there is no alternative site, it is acceptable to perform the venipuncture distal to the hematoma.

Edema

Edema is an abnormal accumulation of fluid in the tissues that causes swelling. Edema impairs circulation and may disrupt the exchange of nutrients and oxygen between the blood and tissues. Consequently, drawing blood specimens from edematous areas may result in inaccurate test results. Edematous tissue may also be fragile and easily injured by tourniquet and antiseptic application. Choose another site if possible.

Obesity

Veins on obese patients may be deep and difficult to find. The cephalic vein is often the vein of choice and can be located more easily by rotating the antecubital fossa inward.

Damaged Veins

Some patient's veins feel hard and cordlike and lack resiliency. These veins are said to be hardened or sclerosed. This may be due to inflammation, disease, or irritation from chemotherapeutic drugs. Sometimes it is due to the scarring caused by numerous venipunctures, as in the case of regular blood donors and people with chronic illnesses. Damaged veins are difficult to penetrate, often yield erroneous test results due to impaired blood flow, and should be avoided. Draw below the damaged area or choose another site.

Intravenous Therapy

Blood specimens should not be drawn from an arm with an intravenous (IV). Drawing a specimen from an arm with an IV may result in the dilution of the blood with the IV fluid, causing erroneous results, especially if the specimen is drawn above the IV. However, if no other site is available, the specimen may be collected *below* the IV (*never above*) using the following procedure:

1. Have the nurse turn off the IV for a minimum of 2 minutes prior to collection.
2. Apply the tourniquet distal to the IV.
3. Perform the venipuncture in a different vein than the one with the IV.
4. Collect a 5-ml tube of blood (10 ml for coagulation tests) and discard before collecting test specimens.
5. Have the nurse restart the IV.
6. State on the requisition form that the specimen was collected from an arm with an IV. It is also helpful to indicate the type of IV fluid.

Vascular Access Devices

A **vascular access device (VAD)**, also called an **indwelling line**, consists of tubing inserted into a main vein or artery. It is used primarily for administering fluids and medications, monitoring pressures, and drawing blood.

The most common type of VAD is a **central venous catheter (CVC)**, also called a **central venous line (CVL)**.

A CVC (Fig. 8-1) is inserted into a large vein such as the subclavian and advanced into the superior vena cava, proximal to the right atrium. The exit end is surgically tunneled under the skin to a site several inches away in the chest. Several inches of tubing protrude from the exit site, which is normally covered with a transparent dressing.

Another type of VAD, an **implanted port** is a small chamber that is attached to an indwelling line. The chamber is surgically implanted under the skin. The device is located by palpating the skin. Access is gained by inserting a needle through the skin into the self-sealing septum (wall) of the chamber. The site is not normally covered with a bandage when not in use.

The latest VAD, a **peripherally inserted central catheter (PICC)** is inserted into the peripheral venous system and threaded into the central venous system. It does not require surgical insertion. PICCs are commonly placed in either the basilic or cephalic vein with the exit in the vicinity of the elbow. Because a PICC tends to collapse on aspiration, drawing blood from a PICC is not recommended.

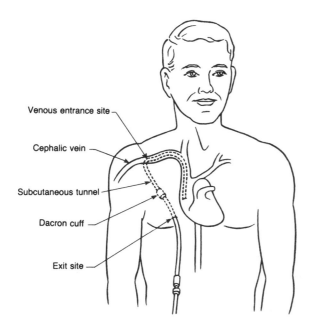

Venous entrance site

Cephalic vein

Subcutaneous tunnel

Dacron cuff

Exit site

Figure 8–1   Central venous catheter (CVC) (Metheny NM).

VADs that are to be used for blood drawing should only be accessed by specially trained personnel. However, the phlebotomist may be asked to assist in delivering the specimen to the appropriate tubes. Because lines are routinely flushed with heparin, a minimum of 5 ml of blood must be discarded before the test specimen is collected. Because of possible interference due to heparin, line draws are not recommended for co-agulation specimens. However, some hospital policies allow the sample to be drawn after clearing 10 ml of fluid.

Heparin Lock

A **heparin lock** is a special winged needle set that can be left in a patient's vein for up to 48 hours. It is used to administer medication and draw blood. It is periodically flushed with heparin to keep it from clotting; therefore, a 5 ml discard tube should be drawn prior to specimen collection. Drawing coagulation test specimens from heparin locks is not recommended. Only specially trained personnel should draw blood from a heparin lock.

Cannula

A **cannula** (Fig. 8-2) is a temporary surgical connection between an artery and a vein used for dialysis and blood drawing. Tubing of the cannula extends to the outside surface of the arm and has a rubber diaphragm cap through which a needle may be inserted to draw blood. A discard tube must be drawn prior to specimen tubes. Drawing blood from a cannula should be done only by specially trained personnel with the permission of the patient's physician.

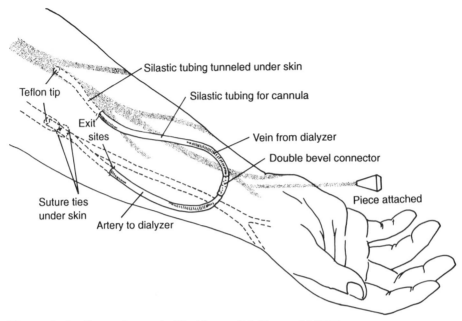

Figure 8–2   External cannula (Slockbower JM, Blumenfeld TA).

Fistula (shunt)

A **fistula** is created by a surgical procedure, which fuses a vein and artery together permanently. It is used for dialysis and should not be used for phlebotomy procedures. Specimens should be drawn from the other arm.

COMPLICATIONS ASSOCIATED WITH BLOOD COLLECTION

The phlebotomist must be aware of complications associated with blood collection procedures. Complications may affect the patient, the integrity of the specimen, or both. Some complications are unavoidable; others can be avoided by employing proper collection technique, or can be minimized by the alert response of a knowledgeable phlebotomist.

Complications Affecting the Patient

ALLERGIES TO ANTISEPTICS AND ADHESIVES

Occasionally, a patient is allergic to the antiseptic used in skin preparation prior to venipuncture or skin puncture. In this case, an alternate antiseptic should be used.

Some patients are allergic to the glue used in adhesive bandages. Usually paper tape over a folded gauze square can be used instead. If the patient is also allergic to paper tape, the area can be wrapped with gauze and fastened with paper tape over the gauze.

SEIZURES

In the rare event that a patient should have a seizure while the phlebotomist is drawing a blood specimen, it is important to remove the needle as quickly as possible. Try to hold pressure over the site without completely restricting the patient's movement. Do not try to put anything into the patient's mouth.

EXCESSIVE BLEEDING

Normally a patient will stop bleeding from the venipuncture site within a few minutes. Some patients, particularly those on anticoagulant therapy, may take longer to stop bleeding. Pressure must be maintained over the site until the bleeding stops. If the bleeding continues after 5 minutes, notify the nurse. Do not leave until bleeding has stopped or the nurse takes charge of the situation.

FAINTING (SYNCOPE)

Some patients become faint at the thought or sight of their blood being drawn, especially if they are ill. A patient who feels faint or has a history of syncope should be asked to lie down for the procedure. If a patient starts to faint during venipuncture:

1. Remove the tourniquet.
2. Withdraw the needle as quickly as possible.
3. Talk to the patient to divert attention away from the procedure as well as to help keep him or her alert.
4. Have the patient lower his or her head and breathe deeply, while physically supporting the patient to prevent injury in case of collapse.
5. Loosen a tight collar or tie if possible.
6. Apply a cold compress or washcloth to the forehead and back of the neck.
7. Use an ammonia inhalant to bring the patient around if necessary.
8. Alert the pathologist if the patient does not respond.

Once the patient has recovered, he or she must remain in the area for at least 15 minutes. The patient should be instructed *not* to operate a vehicle for at least 30 minutes. It is important for the phlebotomist to document the incident (following hospital policy) in case of future litigation.

HEMATOMA

A **hematoma** or bruise is caused by blood leaking into the tissues around the venipuncture site. It is identified by swelling at or near the venipuncture site. A hematoma can be painful to the patient, as well as unsightly.

A hematoma may form if:

1. The vein is too small for the needle size.
2. The needle penetrates all the way through the vein.
3. The needle is only partly inserted into the vein.
4. The needle is removed while the tourniquet is still on.
5. Pressure is not adequately applied following venipuncture.

If a hematoma should start to form while the phlebotomist is attempting to draw a specimen, the phlebotomist should immediately release the tourniquet, withdraw the needle, and hold pressure over the site.

INFECTION

Infection at the site following venipuncture is not unheard of, but is rare. Using proper aseptic technique and reminding the patient to keep the bandage on for at least 15 minutes should minimize the risk of infection.

NAUSEA

A patient who becomes nauseous should be reassured and made comfortable. Ask the patient to breathe slowly and deeply. Apply a cold, wet washcloth to the patient's forehead. If the patient is an inpatient, ask for assistance from the nurse before proceeding with the specimen collection.

PAIN

A small amount of pain is associated with routine venipuncture and skin puncture. Putting the patient at ease prior to blood collection helps relax the patient and seems to make the procedure less painful. Warning the patient prior to needle insertion will avoid a startle reflex by the patient.

A stinging sensation on venipuncture can be avoided by allowing the alcohol to dry completely prior to needle penetration.

Excessive, deep, or blind probing with the needle can be very painful to the patient and should be avoided.

PETECHIAE

Petechiae are small, nonraised red spots which appear on the patient's skin when a tourniquet is applied. This may be due to a defect of the capillary walls or as a result of platelet defects. It is *not* an indication that the phlebotomist has used incorrect procedure. However, it is an indication that the venipuncture site may bleed excessively.

REFLUX OF ANTICOAGULANT

In rare instances, it is possible for blood to backflow (reflux) into the patient's veins from the collection tube during the venipuncture procedure. Some patients have had adverse reactions to tube additives, particularly EDTA, due to reflux. Reflux can occur when the contents of the collection tube are in contact with the tube stopper while the specimen is being drawn. To prevent reflux reactions, keep the patient's arm in a downward position so that the collection tube remains below the venipuncture site and fills from the bottom up. Raising the head of the bed, extending the patient's arm over the side of the bed, or supporting the arm with a rolled towel will help achieve proper positioning. Back-and-forth movement of the contents of the tube should also be avoided until the tube is removed from the evacuated tube holder.

VEIN COLLAPSE

Too much vacuum for the size of the vein can cause the vein to collapse. This can result from using an evacuated tube that is too large or from pulling too forcefully on the plunger of a syringe when drawing blood from a small or fragile vein.

VEIN DAMAGE

Properly performed, an occasional venipuncture will not impair the **patency** (state of being freely open) of a patient's veins. Numerous venipunctures in the same area over an extended period of time, however, will eventually cause a buildup of scar tissue and increase the difficulty of performing subsequent venipuncture. Blind probing and improper technique when redirecting the needle can also damage veins and impair patency.

NERVE DAMAGE

Excessive or blind probing while performing a venipuncture can lead to injury of a main nerve (such as the median cutaneous nerve), causing permanent damage and the possibility of a lawsuit.

INADVERTENT ARTERIAL PUNCTURE

If accidental puncture of an artery is suspected during a venipuncture procedure, it is important to hold pressure over the site for a full 5 minutes. A phlebotomist can usually recognize arterial blood by its bright red color or by the fact that it spurts into the tube. If an arterial specimen is submitted to the lab for testing, it should be labeled as arterial because some lab values are different for arterial specimens.

Collection Techniques Affecting Specimen Integrity

Sometimes the character or integrity of a specimen can be compromised by the methods (techniques) used in collection. That the integrity of a specimen has been compromised is not always discernible by the phlebotomist or other laboratory personnel. However, a poor quality specimen will generally yield poor quality results and affect the care of the patient. Obviously, this is to be avoided. It is important for the phlebotomist to be aware of the following "pitfalls" of collection.

HEMOCONCENTRATION/VENOUS STASIS

Prolonged application of the tourniquet causes stagnation of the normal blood flow (venous stasis). When venous stasis occurs, the plasma portion of the blood filters into the tissues, causing hemoconcentration or an increase in nonfilterable blood components such as RBCs, enzymes, iron, and calcium.

Hemoconcentration can also be caused by vigorous hand pumping, probing, long-term IV therapy, and sclerosed or occluded veins.

HEMOLYSIS

Hemolysis results from the destruction of RBCs and the liberation of hemoglobin into the fluid portion of the specimen. Hemolysis of a specimen causes the serum or plasma to be pink (slight hemolysis) to red (gross hemolysis) in color. Severe hemolysis will affect certain tests, such as enzymes and potassium, and the specimen may have to be redrawn.

Hemolysis can be caused by:

1. Mixing additive tubes too vigorously or using rough handling during transport.
2. Drawing blood from a vein that has a hematoma.
3. Pulling back the plunger on a syringe too quickly.
4. Using a needle with too small of a bore for venipuncture.
5. Using too large a tube when using a small diameter butterfly needle.
6. Frothing of the blood caused by improper fit of the needle on a syringe.

7. Forcing the blood from a syringe into an evacuated tube.
8. Not wiping away the first drop of blood (which may contain alcohol residue) from a skin puncture.
9. Excessively squeezing the site when obtaining a skin puncture specimen.

PARTIALLY FILLED TUBES

Filling additive tubes until the vacuum is exhausted is important for proper ratio of additive to blood. Improper ratios can cause erroneous test results. A proper ratio of anticoagulant to blood is especially important for coagulation studies because of the critical ratio of anticoagulant to blood. Partially filled tubes for coagulation tests are unacceptable.

Unintentional partially filled tubes may result from loss of vacuum and may indicate that a tube is cracked. Cracked tubes present a safety hazard because they may leak or break with further handling. Never use a tube that is cracked or has been dropped; discard it instead.

SPECIMEN CONTAMINATION

Microbial contamination of a specimen for blood cultures can result from improper antiseptic application to the site or collection container, or from touching the site after it has been prepped.

Antiseptic contamination of a specimen can result from use of the wrong antiseptic in collection, such as the use of povidone iodine for skin puncture. Contamination of a skin puncture specimen with povidone iodine can result in an increase in potassium, phosphate, and uric acid.

Antiseptic contamination of blood culture specimens can occur if the antiseptic is not allowed to dry prior to inserting the needle into the vein or into the culture bottles. Inhibiting effects of antiseptics can cause false-negative blood culture results. Powder from gloves can contaminate skin puncture specimens and blood films on slides.

Study & Review Questions

1. Values for this test are normally highest in the morning:
   a. cortisol
   b. white blood count
   c. iron (Fe)
   d. eosinophil count

2. What tests may be affected most if the patient is not fasting?
   a. CBC and protime
   b. glucose and triglycerides
   c. RA and cardiac enzymes
   d. blood culture and thyroid profile

3. Drugs known to interfere with urine tests should be stopped:
   a. 4 to 24 hours prior to the test
   b. 24 to 36 hours prior to the test
   c. 48 to 72 hours prior to the test
   d. not at all; drugs do not interfere with urine tests

4. Veins that feel hard and cordlike when palpated are called:
   a. collapsed veins
   b. fistulas
   c. sclerosed veins
   d. young venules

5. A hematoma may result from all of the following EXCEPT:
   a. the needle bevel is only partly inserted into the vein
   b. not enough pressure is applied to the site following venipuncture
   c. the tourniquet is released before needle withdrawal
   d. the needle has penetrated all the way through the vein

6. Small red spots that appear on a patient's arm when the tourniquet is applied are called:
   a. edema
   b. hematoma
   c. hemolysis
   d. petechiae

7. When fingers and hands of the patient are swollen with excess fluids, the condition is called:
   a. atherosclerosis
   b. edema
   c. hemoconcentrated
   d. hypertensive

8. A fistula is
   a. always a congenital problem
   b. part of the dialysis machine
   c. a good source of arterial blood
   d. the fusion of a vein and artery

Suggested Laboratory Activities

1. Prioritize a list of tests with special timing or circumstances involved.

2. Change specimen integrity by improper handling and evaluate results.

3. Collect a specimen from a student who has just eaten and check for lipemia.

4. Ask a lab to evaluate specimens taken before and after a change in basal state, *ie*, draw a CK before and after jogging.

BIBLIOGRAPHY AND SUGGESTED READINGS

Bishop ML, Duben-Engelkirk JL, Fody EP: *Clinical Chemistry: Principles, Procedures, Correlations* (2nd ed.). Philadelphia: JB Lippincott Company, 1992.

Byrne CJ, Saxton D: *Laboratory Tests: Implications for Nursing Care.* San Francisco: Addison-Wesley Publishing Company, 1986.

National Committee for Clinical Laboratory Standards, H3-A3: *Procedures for the Collection of Diagnostic Blood Specimens by Venipuncture* (3rd ed.). Villanova, PA: NCCLS, July 1991.

National Committee for Clinical Laboratory Standards, H4-A3: *Procedures for the Collection of Diagnostic Blood Specimens by Skin Puncture* (3rd ed.). Villanova, PA: NCCLS, July 1991.

National Committee for Clinical Laboratory Standards, H21-A: *Collections, Transport and Preparation of Blood for Coagulation Testing and Performance of Coagulation Assays.* Villanova, PA: NCCLS, December 1986.

Specimen Collection Preparation

9

OBJECTIVES
On successful completion of this chapter, the reader should be able to:

1   Describe the process involved in requesting a test and the types of requisitions that might be used.
2   List information needed on the test requisition.
3   Describe the way to approach a patient and how to handle special situations associated with patient contact.
4   Explain the importance of proper patient identification, and describe what information is verified, how to handle discrepancies, and what to do if a patient's identification band is missing.
5   Describe proper bedside manner; explain its importance.
6   Describe how to prepare patients for testing; answer inquiries concerning tests.
7   Describe how to handle difficult patients and what to do if a patient objects to the test.
8   Describe how to verify diet information and what to do when diet requirements have not been followed.

KEY TERMS
bedside manner
ID band
ID card
medical record number
patient identification
test requisition

McCall: PHLEBOTOMY ESSENTIALS. © 1993
J. B. Lippincott Company.

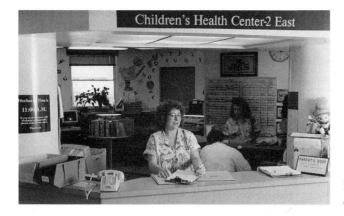

Figure 9–1 Health unit clerk at nurses station.

INITIATION OF THE TEST REQUEST

Hospital laboratories generally perform tests on inpatients, as well as outpatients from doctor's offices, clinics, and so forth. The following procedures refer to inpatient test collection. Outpatient procedures are the same, if applicable, unless otherwise indicated.

The test collection process begins when the physician orders or "requests" a test to be performed on a patient. All laboratory testing must be requested by a physician and results reported to a physician.

In a hospital setting, a **health unit coordinator** (Fig. 9-1), also known as a **health unit clerk** or **secretary**, fills out the paper work or enters the order in the computer under the direction of the patient's nurse.

In an outpatient setting, the doctor's office may call and inform the lab of the order, or the patient may arrive at the lab with order in hand from the doctor's office.

Test Requisitions

The form on which the test is ordered and sent to the lab is called the **test requisition**. The requisition may be a computer-generated form or a manual form.

Computer requisitions (Fig. 9-2) usually contain the actual labels that are to be placed on the specimens once they have been collected. There are a several different types of

```
          OP     1400  W642     07/22 W642      1400 07/22 W642       07/22 W642      1400 07/22
H#356421         07/22 H#356421       H#356421        43Y M H#356421        H#356421       43Y M
DOE , JOHN             DOE , JOHN     DOE , JOHN            DOE , JOHN      DOE , JOHN
S                     W642     07/22  1 BLUE              W642     07/22   1 BLUE
                W642  H#356421        PT-S                H#356421         PT-S
          1     BLUE  DOE , JOHN                OP        DOE , JOHN                       OP
          1400  W642      07/22 W642      1400 07/22 W642       07/22 W642      1400 07/22
                07/22 H#356421       H#356421        43Y M H#356421        H#356421       43Y M
                      DOE , JOHN     DOE , JOHN            DOE , JOHN      DOE , JOHN
S                     W642     07/22  1 RED               W642     07/22   1 RED
                W642  H#356421        GLUC-S              H#356421         GLUC-S
          1     RED   DOE , JOHN                OP        DOE , JOHN                       OP

COLLECTION REPORT COMPLETED
```

Figure 9–2 Computer requisition (Sunquest System, courtesy J. C. Lincoln Hospital, Phoenix, AZ.)

computer requisitions. Besides the pertinent patient identification information, many also indicate the type of tube needed for the specimen, as well as other patient information such as "potential bleeder" or "no venipuncture right arm."

Manual requisitions (Fig. 9-3) come in many different styles and types. Some laboratories require separate requisitions for each department. There are often different colors

JOHN C. LINCOLN HOSPITAL & HEALTH CENTER
250 E. DUNLAP AVENUE, PHOENIX, AZ 85020-2871

EMERGICENTER LAB ORDERS

☐ **PARADISE VALLEY EMERGICENTER** CLARK D. K. LAMBE, M.D., PATHOLOGIST
4232 E. CACTUS ROAD, PHOENIX, AZ 85032

☐ **LINCOLN METRO EMERGICENTER** ROBERT P. REISMAN, M.D., PATHOLOGIST
3131 W. PEORIA AVENUE, PHOENIX, AZ 85021

ORDERING PHYSICIAN:

X	TESTS AVAILABLE
	COLLECTION FEE
	ARTERIAL BLOOD GASES
	CBC
	HGB & HCT
	WBC
	DIFFERENTIAL
	SED RATE
	PLATELET COUNT
	RETICULOCYTE COUNT
	PROTIME
	PTT
	BLEEDING TIME
	PREGNANCY TEST - SERUM
	LYTES (Na, K, Cl, CO2)
	POTASSIUM
	CHEM 7 (LYTES, BUN, GLUC., CREAT.)
	GLUCOSE
	BUN AND CREATININE
	AMYLASE
	CPK
	SGOT
	LDH
	TOTAL PROTEIN
	ALKALINE PHOSPHATASE
	TOTAL BILIRUBIN
	SGPT
	MONOTEST
	THEOPHYLLINE
	SERUM ACETONE
	TRICHOMONAS / YEAST
	URINALYSIS

BACTERIOLOGY

	GRAM STAIN (PRELIMINARY)
SPECIMEN SOURCE	
TRICHOMONAS / YEAST PREP	
SPECIMEN SOURCE	
COMMENTS / REMARKS	

BLOOD GASES

	PATIENT	NORMAL
☐ ARTERIAL BLOOD		
☐ VENOUS BLOOD		
☐ ARTERIALIZED CAPILLARY		
☐ ROOM AIR		
☐ RECEIVING O2		
pH		7.38 - 7.42
PA O2		RA 76 - 96 mmHg / O2 Rx 76 - 550
SAT		94 - 99%
PA CO2		38 - 42 mmHg
BASE EXCESS / DEFICIT		0±2.5
ACTUAL BICARB		22 - 26 mEq / L
TOTAL CO2		23 - 27 mEq / L

SEROLOGY

		NORMAL
MONOTEST		NEG.

URINALYSIS

COLOR:		
CHARACTER:		

CHEMICAL SCREEN	PATIENT	EXPECTED
SPECIFIC GRAVITY		1.016 - 1.022
pH		5 - 9
PROTEIN		NEG
GLUCOSE		NEG
KETONES		NEG
BILIRUBIN		NEG
OCCULT BLOOD		NEG
UROBILINOGEN		0.1 - 1.0 mg / dl
LEUKOCYTE ESTERASE		
NITRITE		
CASTS / TYPE		/ LPF
WBC'S		/ HPF
RBC'S		/ HPF
EPITHELIAL'S		/ HPF
MUCUS		
AMORPHOUS		
BACTERIA		
YEAST		
CRYSTALS		
OTHER		

CHEMISTRY

TEST	PATIENT	NORMAL
GLUCOSE		65 - 110 mg/dl
BUN		7 - 18 mg/dl
CREATININE		0.5 - 1.1 mg/dl
SODIUM		137 - 145 mEq/L
POTASSIUM		3.6 - 5.0 mEq/L
CHLORIDE		98 - 107 mEq/L
CO2		22 - 31 mMole/L
AMYLASE		30 - 110 IU/L
CPK		30 - 170 IU/L
LDH		313 - 618 U/L
SGOT		5 - 40 IU/L
TOTAL PROTEIN		6.3 - 8.2 g/dl
ALKALINE PHOSPHATASE		38 - 126 U/L
TOTAL BILIRUBIN		0 - 1.4 mg/dl
SGPT		7 - 56 IU/L
THEOPHYLLINE		10 - 20 ug/ml
SERUM ACETONE		NEG.
PREGNANCY TEST (SERUM)		

COAGULATION		**NORMAL**
PROTIME		11.0 - 13.0 sec.
PTT		23.0 - 34.0 sec.
BLEEDING TIME		2.5 - 9.5 min.

HEMATOLOGY

PATIENT	NORMAL		DIFFERENTIAL
	WBC X10³	M = 7.8±3 / F = 7.8±3	SEGS 45 - 65 / BANDS 0 -5
	RBC X10⁶	M = 5.4±0.7 / F = 4.8±0.6	LYMPHS 25 - 45 / ATY. LYMPHS O
	HGB GM	M = 16.0±2 / F = 14.0±2	MONOS 3 - 7 / EOS 1- 5
	HCT %	M = 47±5 / F = 42±5	BASO 0 -1 / METAS 0
	MCV U³	M = 87 ± 7 / F = 90 ± 9	MYELOS 0 / NRBC 0/100 WBC
	MCH UUG	M = 29±2 / F = 29±2	PLATELETS APPEAR ☐NOR ☐INC ☐ DEC
	MCHC %	M = 34±2 / F = 34±2	HYPOCHROMIA / POLYCHROMASIA
SED. RATE		M = 0 - 15 / F = 0 - 20	ANISOCYTOSIS / POIKILOCYTOSIS
PLATE-LETS		3±1.5 / 100,000	OVALOCYTE / SPHEROCYTES
RETICS %		0.5 - 1.5	TARGET CELLS / SCHISTOCYTES
REVIEWED BY:			DATE

TECHNOLOGIST: DATE: COLLECTED BY:

Figure 9–3 Manual requisition. (Courtesy of John C. Lincoln Hospital, Phoenix, AZ.)

for each department so that they can be easily distinguished. Many institutions use one large form with separate sections for the different departments. Some requisitions are a three-part form that serves as a request, a report, and a billing form. When a manual requisition is used, the phlebotomist is responsible for labeling the specimen tube with the required patient information.

Whatever the system used, it is essential for the phlebotomist to become familiar with the various forms to be able to quickly and accurately interpret them.

Information Needed on the Requisition

- Ordering physician's name
- Patient's name
- Patient's medical record number
- Patient's date of birth
- Room number and bed (if inpatient)
- Type of test to be performed
- Date test is to be performed
- Test status (timed, fasting, priority, and so on)
- Billing information (if outpatient)

Receipt of Test Requisition by the Lab

Computer requisitions are usually printed out at the phlebotomist station in the laboratory. Manual requisitions are sent by courier or pneumatic tube system or are collected during sweeps by a member of the phlebotomy team. Someone is then in charge of sorting the requisitions by date, time, and priority of collection, as well as location of the patient.

Preparing to Collect Requested Specimens

When it is time to collect the specimens, the phlebotomist checks the requisitions to see that all of the needed equipment is on the blood-collecting tray or cart. The phlebotomist then proceeds to the first patient.

PATIENT CONTACT

Entering the Patient's Room

Doors to patient's rooms are usually open. If the door to the room is closed, the phlebotomist should knock lightly and open the door slowly, and say something like "good morning," before proceeding into the room. Even if the door is open, its a good idea to knock lightly to make occupants aware that you are about to enter. Curtains are often pulled when nurses are working with patients or when patients are using bedpans or urinals. Making your presence known to patients before proceeding or opening the curtain may avoid embarrassing them.

Identifying Yourself

Identify yourself to the patient by stating your name, that you are from the lab, and why you are there (*ie*, "Good morning. My name is Mr. Smith, I'm from the lab, and

I'm here to collect a blood specimen ordered by your doctor."). If you are a student, communicate this information to the patient as well. This is a part of informed consent and patient rights. The patient has a right to refuse to have blood drawn by a student.

Handling Special Situations

IF THE PATIENT IS ASLEEP

If the patient is asleep, as is often the case on early morning rounds, wake him or her gently. Try not to startle the patient. (Startling can cause a change in test results.) Nudge the bed rather than the patient. Speak softly but distinctly, and avoid turning on bright overhead lighting, at least until the patient's eyes have adjusted to being open. *Never* attempt to collect a blood specimen from a sleeping patient. Such an attempt may startle the patient and cause injury to the patient or the phlebotomist.

IF THE PATIENT IS UNCONSCIOUS

If the patient is unconscious, as is often encountered in intensive care units, continue to speak to the patient. Identify yourself and inform the patient of your intent just as you would an alert patient. Unconscious patients can often hear what is going on around them even though they are unresponsive. They may also be able to feel pain and may move when you insert the needle to draw the specimen. It may, therefore, be necessary to have someone assist you in holding an unconscious patient's arm.

IF A DOCTOR OR CLERGYMAN IS WITH THE PATIENT

If the patient's doctor or a clergyman is with the patient, don't interrupt. The patient's time with the doctor or clergy is private and limited. Proceed to the next patient and come back to that patient later. If the request is for a stat or timed specimen, excuse yourself, explain why you are there, and ask permission to proceed.

IF THE PATIENT IS NOT IN THE ROOM

If the patient is not in the room, check at the nurses' station to find out where the patient is. If the patient has been taken to another department such as x-ray, you may still be able to collect the specimen from the patient in the waiting area of that department before procedures have begun.

Every attempt should be made to find the patient, especially if the test is timed. However, if the patient cannot be located, is unavailable, or you are unable to obtain the specimen for any other reason, it is the policy of most laboratories for you to fill out a form stating that you were unable to obtain the specimen at the requested time and the reason why. The original copy of this form is left at the nurses' station and a copy goes back to the lab.

Handling Family and Visitors

Often there are family members or visitors in the room when you arrive to collect a specimen. It is best to ask them to step outside the room until you are finished. Most will prefer to do so. Occasionally, a family member, especially a spouse, is willing to assist you if needed. It is acceptable to let a family member help by steadying the arm or holding pressure over the site while you label tubes.

PATIENT IDENTIFICATION

Importance of Proper Identification

The most important step in specimen collection is patient identification. Obtaining a specimen from the wrong patient can have serious, even fatal, consequences, as in the case of specimens for type and crossmatch prior to blood transfusion. Misidentification of a patient can be grounds for dismissal of the person responsible and could even lead to a malpractice lawsuit against that person.

Determining the Patient's Name and Date of Birth

When identifying a patient, ask the patient to state his or her name and date of birth. For example, *never* say, "Are you Mrs. Smith?" A person who is very ill, hard of hearing, or on heavy medication may say "yes" to anything. Using a "memory jogger" such as having a patient spell an unusual name or commenting in some positive way about a name, will help you remember that you verified it.

Checking the Patient's Identification Bracelet

If the patient's response matches the information on the requisition, proceed to check the patient's **identification** (ID) bracelet (Fig. 9-4) (also called ID **band** or *arm band*).

All hospital patients are required to wear an ID band, usually on the wrist. The ID band lists the patient's name and hospital ID number or **medical record number**. Additional information includes the patient's birthdate, room number and bed designation, and physician's name (Fig. 9-5).

It is important that the information on the ID band match the information on the requisition *exactly*. It is not unusual to have patients with the same or similar names in the hospital at the same time. (Examples are patients with common last names, fathers and sons, multiple-birth babies, and relatives involved in tissue transplant procedures.) There have even been instances where two patients shared the same name and birthdate. Two patients will *not*, however, have the same hospital or medical record number, although they may be similar.

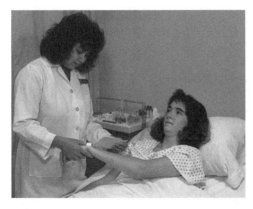

Figure 9–4   Phlebotomist at bedside checking patient identification band.

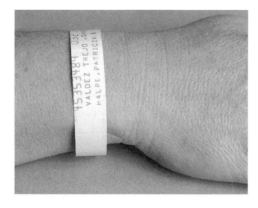

Figure 9–5   Typical identification bracelet.

How to Handle ID Discrepancies

If any discrepancy between the information on the ID band and the information on the requisition is noted, the specimen should not be obtained until the discrepancy is addressed and the patient's identity is verified.

If the ID Band is Missing

If there is no ID band on the patient's wrist, check to see if it is on an ankle. Intravenous (IV) lines in patient's arms often infiltrate the surrounding tissues and cause swelling that necessitates removal of the ID band. When this occurs, especially on a patient with IVs in both arms, nursing personnel will often place the ID band around the ankle.

In some instances, harried personnel remove ID bands from IV-infiltrated arms or during other procedures on patients, and place them on the night table by the patient's bed. An ID band on a night table could belong to a patient who previously occupied that bed. It is also not unusual for a new patient to occupy a bed before the nursing staff has a chance to attach his or her ID band. For this reason, identification should *never* be verified from an ID band that is *not* attached to the patient. In such instances, as well as when no ID band can be found, it is necessary to ask the patient's nurse to make positive identification and attach an ID band before the specimen is drawn. In an emergency situation where there is no time to wait for attachment of the ID band, the name of the nurse making the ID verification should be written on the requisition.

Emergency Room Identification Procedures

It is not uncommon for an emergency room to receive an unconscious patient with no identification. Specimens should not be collected without some way to positively connect the specimen with the patient. In many institutions, the phlebotomist will attach a special three-part ID band, such as a Typenex Blood Recipient ID band (Fenwal Laboratories, a division of Travenol Laboratories, Deerfield, IL) to an unidentified emergency room patient's wrist. The same number is on all three parts. The first part becomes the patient's ID band. The second part is attached to the specimen. The third part is used if the patient needs a transfusion, and is attached to the unit of blood.

Identification of Infants and Young Children

Infants can be identified by the ID band that is usually located on the ankle. The phlebotomist should be very careful when identifying as-yet-unnamed newborn infants. They are commonly identified, for example, as baby boy Jones, and so on. Be especially careful when identifying twins or other multiple-birth babies. They are commonly identified as Jones, twin A or B. *Never* rely on the name card on the infant's bed for identification purposes. Always check the ID band.

The identification of young children can be confirmed by a parent or relative. Identity of young children missing ID bands should be confirmed by the patient's nurse, and an ID bracelet attached the same as for adults.

Identification of Outpatients

Outpatients do not normally have ID bands. However, they may have an **ID card**. Some clinics give their patients ID cards from which specimen labels can be imprinted using an address-o-graph machine.

Outpatients often arrive with the order from their doctor in hand. The receptionist will verify the identity of the patient and fill out the proper lab requisition or generate one via computer. Some labs supply the doctors that use their services with the proper lab forms so that the patient arrives with the lab requisition already filled out.

Even if the patient has been properly identified by the receptionist, the phlebotomist must verify the patient's ID once the patient is actually called into the blood drawing area from the waiting room. Simply calling a person's name and having someone respond is not verification enough. Anxious or hard of hearing patients may think that they heard their name called, when in effect the phlebotomist called a similar name. There could also be two patients in the waiting area with the same name. The phlebotomist should ask an outpatient his or her name and date of birth in the same manner described for inpatients.

PREPARING THE PATIENT FOR TESTING

Bedside Manner

Gaining the patient's trust and confidence and putting the patient at ease are important aspects of **bedside manner**. The phlebotomist who has a professional appearance and who behaves in a professional manner will more easily gain a patient's trust. A confident phlebotomist will convey that confidence to the patient.

A cheerful and pleasant manner and an exchange of small talk with the patient will help to put a patient at ease, as well as divert attention from any discomfort associated with the procedure.

Handling Difficult Patients

A phlebotomist's cheerful and pleasant manner may not be echoed by the patient. Hospitalization is usually a stressful situation for a patient. A patient may be lonely, scared, fearful, or just plain disagreeable, and may react in a negative manner toward the phlebotomist. The phlebotomist should remain calm and professional and treat the patient in a caring manner under any circumstances.

Explaining the Procedure

Most patients have had a blood test before. To them the phlebotomist's statement of intent to perform a blood test is usually sufficient for them to understand what is about to occur. To a patient who has never had a blood test, a more detailed explanation may be necessary. Special procedures may require additional information.

If a patient does not speak or understand English, the phlebotomist may have to use sign language or other nonverbal means to demonstrate what is to occur. If this fails, an interpreter must be located. Speaking slowly and distinctly, using sign language, or writing down information may be necessary for patients with hearing problems.

In any event, as part of "informed consent" the phlebotomist must always inform the patient of the procedure and determine that the patient understands what is about to take place before proceeding.

Handling Patient Inquiry About Tests

Some hospitals will allow the phlebotomist to tell the patient the name of the test or tests to be performed. Others prefer that all inquiries be directed to the patient's physician. Because a particular test may be ordered to rule out a number of different problems, an attempt by the phlebotomist to explain the purpose of a test could be very misleading and unduly alarming to the patient. The phlebotomist usually handles such inquiries by stating that the doctor has ordered the tests as part of the patient's care and that the doctor will be happy to explain the tests to him or her if asked.

In cases where bedside testing is being performed (such as glucose monitoring), and the patient is already aware of the type of test being performed and asks about results, the phlebotomist should check with the patient's nurse to see if it is acceptable to tell the patient the results.

If the Patient Objects to the Procedure

Most patients understand that blood tests are needed in the course of their treatment. Occasionally a patient will object to the procedure. Reminding the patient that the test was ordered by the doctor as part of their care will sometimes convince the patient to cooperate. If not, often the patient's nurse may be able to convince the patient to cooperate. It is not up to the phlebotomist to attempt to badger the patient into cooperating, nor should a conscious, mentally alert adult patient be restrained to obtain a specimen. REMEMBER, the patient has the right to refuse to have the test done.

When it has been determined that a patient truly refuses to cooperate, the phlebotomist should write on the requisition that the patient has refused to have blood drawn. The phlebotomist should also notify the patient's nurse and the phlebotomy supervisor that the specimen was not obtained due to patient refusal. Some health care organizations have a special form for this purpose.

Verifying Diet Restrictions

Once the patient has been properly identified and has consented to the procedure, the phlebotomist should verify that the patient has followed any special diet instructions or restrictions. The most common diet requirement is for the patient to fast for a certain period of time, commonly overnight or "nothing past midnight."

If the phlebotomist determines that the patient did not fast or otherwise follow diet instructions, the nursing staff should be informed so that a determination can be made regarding whether to proceed with the test. In the event that the phlebotomist is told to proceed to collect the specimen, the phlebotomist should write "nonfasting" on the specimen requisition and the specimen label.

Proceeding With Specimen Collection

Once the patient has been properly identified and informed, diet restrictions have been met, and the patient has consented to the procedure, the phlebotomist can proceed to collect the test specimen. See Chapter 10 for routine venipuncture procedure.

Study and Review Questions

1. Which of the following is not normally required on a specimen label?
   a. room number and bed
   b. patient's first and last name
   c. date and time
   d. initials of the phlebotomist

2. Information you as a phlebotomist would normally share with the patient before collecting a specimen includes all of the following EXCEPT:
   a. your name
   b. why you are there
   c. if you are a student
   d. why the test was ordered

3. The most important step in specimen collection is:
   a. entering the patient's room correctly
   b. handling visitors
   c. identifying the patient
   d. identifying yourself

4. Information on the patient's armband should include all of the following EXCEPT:
   a. patient diagnosis
   b. medical record number
   c. patient's name
   d. physician's name

5. If a patient adamantly refuses to have blood drawn, the phlebotomist should:
   a. convince the patient to cooperate.
   b. notify the nurse and make a note on the requisition or fill out a patient refusal form.
   c. restrain the patient and proceed with the collection.
   d. write a note to the physician explaining what happened.

6. You are sent to draw a specimen on an inpatient. The patient is not wearing an ID band. What do you do?
   a. Ask the patient's name and proceed to collect the specimen.
   b. Refuse to draw the specimen and return to the lab.
   c. Have the patient's nurse put an ID band on the patient before drawing the specimen.
   d. Identify the patient by the name card on the door.

Suggested Laboratory Activities

1. Compare a manual requisition with a computer-generated requisition.

2. Fill in the required information on several types of lab requisitions.

3. Practice reading physician lab orders on patient charts.

4. Practice proper bedside manner by role-playing with another student.

5. Compare identification on sample requisitions with information on ID bands worn by students since the first day of lab.

BIBLIOGRAPHY AND SUGGESTED READINGS

Bishop ML, Duben-Engelkirk JL, Fody EP: *Clinical Chemistry: Principles, Procedures, Correlations* (2nd ed.). Philadelphia: JB Lippincott Company, 1992.

National Committee for Clinical Laboratory Standards, H3-A3: *Procedures for the Collection of Diagnostic Blood Specimens by Venipuncture* (3rd ed.). Villanova, PA: NCCLS, July 1991.

National Committee for Clinical Laboratory Standards, H4-A3: *Procedures for the Collection of Diagnostic Blood Specimens by Skin Puncture* (3rd ed.). Villanova, PA: NCCLS, July 1991.

Venipuncture Procedures

10

OBJECTIVES

On successful completion of this chapter, the reader should be able to:

1 List equipment and supplies needed for routine venipuncture.
2 Describe preliminary procedures in the venipuncture collection.
3 Identify potential sites for venipuncture collection and describe the steps in preparing the puncture site.
4 List the steps in the venipuncture procedure in order.
5 List necessary information found on specimen tube labels.
6 Describe the follow-up steps after a specimen has been collected.
7 List reasons for failure to obtain blood.
8 Describe collection procedure when using a butterfly and syringe and how to dispense blood into tubes following collection.

KEY TERMS

collapsed vein
concentric circles
luer adapter
needle sheath
palpate
pediatric tubes
pumping
reflux
resheathing
sclerosed

McCall: PHLEBOTOMY ESSENTIALS. © 1993
J. B. Lippincott Company.

ROUTINE VENIPUNCTURE PROCEDURE

Most tests require collection of a blood specimen by venipuncture. Performance of a venipuncture is often referred to as "drawing blood." A routine venipuncture involves the following steps (*Note:* The following steps were written using guidelines established by the National Committee for Clinical Laboratory Standards [see Chapter 2]. In a clinical setting there may be some variation in methods due to individual technique and special circumstances.)

Prepare Necessary Paperwork
Refer to Chapter 9 for guidelines.

Identify Patient
See Chapter 9 for proper procedure.

Verify Diet Restrictions
See Chapter 9.

Assemble Equipment and Supplies
A routine venipuncture requires the following equipment and supplies (Fig. 10-1):

1. Gloves
2. Tourniquet
3. 70% isopropanol (alcohol) prep pads or preferred antiseptic for the test (*eg*, povidone iodine for blood cultures and blood alcohol); alternate antiseptic such as green soap or soap and water for a patient allergic to the preferred antiseptic
4. Gauze pads or cotton balls

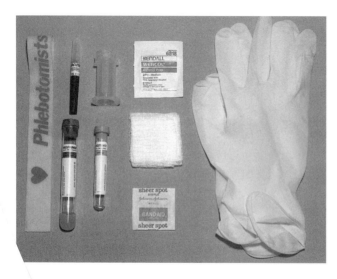

Figure 10-1 Routine venipuncture equipment.

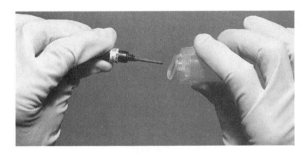

Figure 10–2 Needle and holder assembly.

5. Needle and evacuated tube holder (assembled) (Fig. 10-2)
6. Appropriate tubes for the tests, arranged in proper order of draw with the first tube inserted into the evacuated tube holder (expiration dates on the tubes must be checked to make certain that they have not expired)
7. Needle disposal container
8. Adhesive bandage or other bandaging materials
9. Permanent marker or pen

Wash Hands and Put on Gloves

Proper handwashing followed by glove application is an important part of the venipuncture procedure. Hands may be washed in a downward motion, scrubbing from wrists to fingertips, which prevents backflow of contaminated water and soap. A circular scrubbing motion using plenty of friction will help dislodge surface debris and bacteria. It is important to pay particular attention to areas between the fingers and around the nails. Hands should be rinsed from wrists to fingertips also and dried with a clean paper towel. Once the hands have been dried, the water can be shut off using a clean, dry paper towel. The phlebotomist then puts on a clean pair of gloves.

Reassure Patient

Reassuring the patient is a part of bedside manner discussed in Chapter 9. If the patient is worried about the amount of pain associated with the procedure, be honest and tell him or her that there will be a small amount of discomfort but that it will be of short duration. *Never* tell a patient that it won't hurt. Even children expect to be told the truth.

Explain to the patient the importance of holding the arm very still. A child's cooperation can be gained by having him or her take an active part in the process, such as holding the gauze pad. Rewards such as stickers, character badges, or "smiley face" bandages will help leave the child with a positive memory of the procedure.

Position Patient

A patient should be either seated or lying down while having blood drawn. A patient should *never* be standing or seated at a high stool.

SEATED PATIENT

Outpatients are most commonly seated in a special blood drawing chair (Fig. 10-3). When seated, a patient's arm should be supported firmly on a slanted armrest

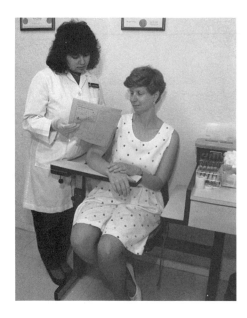

Figure 10–3 Phlebotomist explains procedure to outpatient seated in blood-drawing chair.

and extended downward in a straight line from the shoulder to the wrist. The arm should *not* be bent at the elbow.

SUPINE PATIENT

Inpatients normally have blood drawn while in a supine position. An outpatient in a weakened condition or one who has fainted previously when having a blood test should also have blood drawn lying down. As with the seated patient, the arm should be extended in a straight line from shoulder to wrist and not bent at the elbow. In proper position, the hand should be lower than the elbow. A pillow or a rolled towel may be used to support and position the arm if necessary.

OTHER CONSIDERATIONS

Bedrails may be let down, being careful not to catch intravenous lines, catheter bags and tubing, or other patient apparatus.

Bedrails *must* be raised again when the phlebotomist is finished. If the phlebotomist lowers a bedrail and forgets to replace it when finished, and a patient subsequently falls out of bed and is injured, the phlebotomist can be held liable. Many phlebotomists have learned to collect specimens with bedrails in place so as not to forget to put them back up.

A patient should not be eating, drinking, or chewing gum, or have a thermometer, toothpick, or any other foreign object in the mouth when having blood drawn. Objects in the mouth can cause choking. A bite reflex could break a thermometer and injure a patient.

Apply Tourniquet

A tourniquet is applied to increase pressure in the veins and aid in vein selection (Fig. 10-4*A*). If a patient has prominent veins, tourniquet application can wait until after cleansing, just prior to needle insertion.

(text continues on page 160)

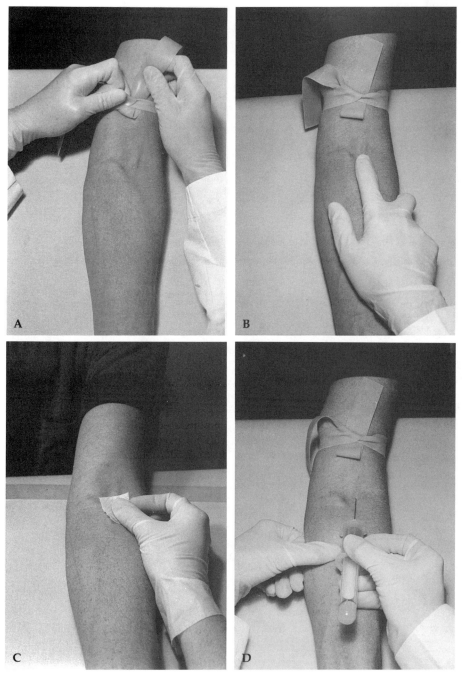

Figure 10–4   *A.* Appyling the tourniquet; *B.* selecting the site; *C.* cleaning the site (note: the tourniquet has been removed for this procedure); *D.* entering the vein, notice the thumb drawing the skin taut (note: the tourniquet has been retied).

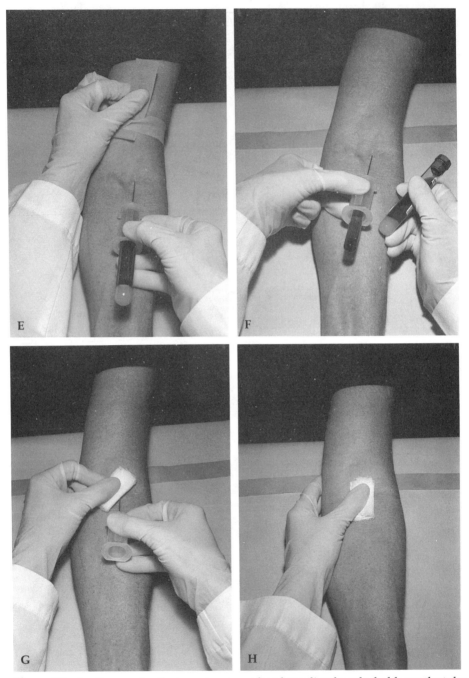

Figure 10–4   *E.* removing the tourniquet: one hand steadies the tube holder as the tube fills with blood, the other pulls the tucked under end of the tourniquet to release it from the patient's arm; *F.* filling a second tube while mixing the first; *G.* placing the gauze; *H.* phlebotomist holding pressure.

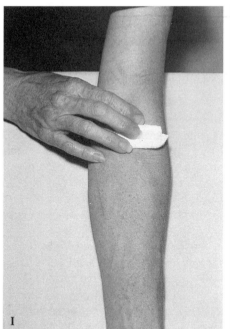

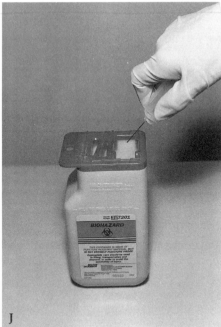

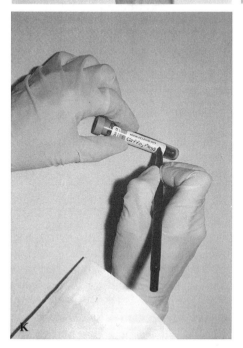

Figure 10-4 *I.* patient holding pressure; *J.* disposing of the needle; and *K.* labeling a blood specimen tube.

The tourniquet is applied 3 to 4 inches above the intended venipuncture site. If a patient has sensitive skin, the tourniquet may be applied over a sleeve, or a dry washcloth or gauze wrapped around the arm.

- *Do not* apply a tourniquet over an open sore. Use another site.
- *Do not* apply a tourniquet to an arm on the side of a mastectomy without the permission of the patient's physician.

A latex strip tourniquet is applied by positioning it around the arm while grasping the ends and applying a small amount of tension. While continuing to maintain tension, the left end is crossed over the right end and both ends are grasped between the thumb and forefinger of the left hand, close to the patient's arm. While the two ends are still grasped securely, the left end is tucked under the right end using either the left middle finger or right index finger. The result should be a loop with the end of the tourniquet pointing toward the shoulder. A slight tug on this end of the tourniquet should easily release it from the patient's arm.

The tourniquet should feel slightly tight to the patient. It should not be rolled or twisted and it should not be so tight that it pinches or hurts. It should not be so tight that the arm turns red or purple.

A tourniquet that is tied too tightly may prevent arterial blood flow into the area and result in failure to obtain blood. A tourniquet that is too loose will be ineffective. To minimize the effects of stasis and hemoconcentration, the tourniquet should *never* be left in place longer than 1 minute (see NCCLS Document H3-A3; National Committee for Clinical Laboratory Standards, 771 E. Lancaster Ave., Villanova, PA 19085).

Select Venipuncture Site

Venipuncture is most commonly performed in the antecubital area of the arm where the median cubital, cephalic, and basilic veins lie fairly close to the surface. This area should be examined first. A patient will generally have the most prominent veins in the dominant arm.

Having the patient make a fist will help make the veins more prominent. Vigorous **pumping** (opening and closing) of the fist should be avoided as it may cause erroneous results in a number of tests due to hemoconcentration.

Use the tip of the index finger to **palpate** (feel) the vein (see Figure 10-4B). Palpating will help to determine the size, depth, and direction of the vein. Select a vein that is large and well-anchored (does not move to the side or roll easily).

If you have trouble feeling a vein, close your eyes while feeling. (Closing your eyes enhances your sense of touch.) A vein has a bounce or resilience to it. An artery will pulsate. To avoid inadvertently puncturing an artery, *do not* select a vein that overlies or is close to an artery. In addition, *do not* select a vein that feels hard and cordlike or lacks resiliency; such veins are said to be **sclerosed**. Sclerosed veins are hard to penetrate, roll easily, and may not have adequate blood flow to yield a representative blood sample. A **thrombosed** vein (a vein containing a thrombus, or clot), will also feel hard and should not be used for venipuncture.

Once you have selected a vein, try to mentally visualize the location of the vein. It often helps to note the position of the vein in reference to a mole, hair, or skin crease to make relocation easier after cleansing the site.

If no suitable antecubital vein can be found, check the other arm. When no suitable antecubital vein can be found in either arm, check for wrist or hand veins. If a suitable vein still cannot be found, wrap a warm, wet towel around the arm or hand for a few minutes. Warming the site will increase blood flow and help to make veins more prominent.

Ankle veins should only be used as a last resort and after checking with the patient's doctor. Blood flow to the extremities, especially in bedridden patients and patients with coagulation problems, is not representative of the general circulation and may yield erroneous results. Ankle vein puncture of a patient with coagulation problems may have dangerous consequences, such as thrombus (blood clot) formation and impaired circulation.

Release Tourniquet

If the tourniquet was applied during vein selection, it should be released during the cleansing process (see NCCLS document H3-A3).

Cleanse the Site

Cleansing the venipuncture site with an antiseptic helps prevent microbial contamination of the patient and the specimen (see Figure 10-4C). However, it will *not* sterilize the site. The recommended antiseptic is 70% isopropyl alcohol. Most health care institutions use a commercially prepared, sterile prepackaged alcohol pad referred to as an *alcohol prep pad.*

Clean the site using a circular motion, starting at the center of the site and moving outward in ever widening **concentric circles**. Use sufficient pressure to remove surface dirt and debris. If the site is especially dirty, clean it again with a second alcohol prep pad.

Allow the area to dry for 30 seconds to 1 minute. The evaporation and drying process helps to destroy microbes.

Penetrating the site with a needle while the alcohol is wet may cause hemolysis of the specimen, as well as a burning sensation to the patient.

- *Do not* contaminate the site by drying the alcohol with unsterile gauze.
- *Do not* blow on the site. Blowing on the site or fanning it with your hand may introduce airborne contaminants.
- *Do not* touch the site after cleaning. If it is necessary to repalpate the vein, the site must be cleaned again unless the gloved finger used to palpate has first been cleaned in the same manner as the arm.

Verify Equipment and Tube Selection

Check to see that the correct tubes and other equipment have been selected for the tests ordered. Make certain that the needle is securely fastened to the evacuated tube holder and the first tube is properly seated in the holder.

- *Do not* push the tube past the guideline on the holder or loss of vacuum may result.
- *Do not* remove the **needle sheath** (cover) until just prior to needle insertion.
- Place blood drawing equipment within easy reach. Make certain that extra equipment or the blood collecting tray, as well as the sharps container are also within easy reach.
- *Do not* place equipment on the patient's bed.

Reapply Tourniquet

Reapply the tourniquet, being careful not to touch the cleansed area. Have the patient make a fist if necessary.

Pick Up Blood Drawing Equipment and Remove Needle Sheath

Hold the blood-drawing apparatus in your dominant hand with the thumb on top of the evacuated tube holder and the fingers underneath. (Some phlebotomists like to position the index finger near the hub of the needle during vein entry; however, the finger *must not* touch the needle.) Verify that the tube is positioned in the evacuated tube holder. A properly positioned tube is pushed onto the needle just far enough to hold the tube and keep it from falling out of the holder, but not far enough to release the vacuum of the tube. (Most tube holders contain a guideline beyond which the tube should not be pushed.)

Remove the needle cover. Visually inspect the needle tip for obstructions, imperfections, or barbs. Do not let the needle touch anything prior to venipuncture. If it does, it must be removed and replaced with a new needle.

Anchor the Vein

Grasp the patient's arm with your nondominant hand, using your thumb to pull the skin taut 1 to 2 inches below the intended venipuncture site. This anchors the vein and helps keep it from moving or rolling to the side on needle entry. The fingers of the same hand can be used to support the back of the arm in the area of the elbow. This helps keep the patient from pulling away as the needle enters the vein.

For safety reasons, using the index finger and the thumb for anchoring the vein (two-finger technique) is no longer recommended.

Insert the Needle into the Vein

Line the needle up with the vein with the bevel of the needle facing up and pointing in the same direction as the venous flow. Warn the patient by saying something like, "There is going to be a little poke now." Insert the needle into the skin at a 15- to 30-degree angle, using one smooth motion to penetrate first the skin and then the vein (see Figure 10-4D). When the needle enters the vein, you will feel a slight "give" or decrease in resistance.

At this point, some phlebotomists switch to holding the blood-drawing apparatus in their nondominant hand so that tube changes can be made with their dominant hand. This is accomplished by gently slipping the fingers of the opposite hand under the holder and placing the thumb atop the holder as the other hand lets go. Another method is to grasp the holder between the thumb and index finger, with the hand resting on the patient's arm over (but not touching) the needle. Other phlebotomists, particularly those who are left-handed, do not change hands but continue to steady the holder in the same hand and change tubes with the opposite.

Whatever the method, it is important to hold the blood-drawing apparatus steady so there is minimal needle movement.

Fill the Tubes

As soon as you sense that the needle is in the vein, push the tube to the end of the holder, using your thumb to push the tube while your index and middle fingers grasp the flange of the tube holder. Blood should begin to flow freely into the evacuated tube. If not, exert constant forward pressure on the end of the tube in case the rubber needle sleeve has pushed the tube off of the needle.

As soon as blood flows into the tube, *release the tourniquet* and have the patient release his or her fist (see Figure 10-4*E*). Blood should continue to flow and multiple tubes can still be collected. *DO NOT* leave the tourniquet on for more than 1 minute. *Exception:* On patients with fragile veins that might collapse, or in other difficult draw situations where release of the tourniquet might cause stoppage of blood flow, the tourniquet is sometimes left on until the last tube is filled. Three or four tubes can usually be filled in under 1 minute if the tourniquet was applied just prior to needle insertion.

Steady the needle in the vein. Try not to pull up or press down on the needle while it is in the vein. Both actions can be painful to the patient and may enlarge the hole in the vein, resulting in leakage of blood and hematoma formation.

Try to maintain the arm and the tube in a downward position so that blood fills the tube from the bottom up and does not touch the needle. This will help to prevent reflux (flow of blood from the tube back into the vein), as well as carry-over of additives to other tubes by means of blood left on the needle as tubes are changed.

To ensure a proper ratio of additive to blood, let the tube fill until the vacuum is exhausted and blood ceases to flow. Tubes will not fill completely. Remove the tube, using a twisting and pulling motion while bracing the thumb against the flange of the holder.

If the tube contains an additive, mix it immediately by gently inverting it five to ten times before putting it down (see Figure 10-4*F*). Vigorous mixing or shaking the tube can cause hemolysis. Lack of or inadequate mixing can lead to clot formation. Non-additive tubes do not require mixing.

If other tubes are to be drawn, place them into the holder and push them all the way onto the needle. Steady the tube holder so that the needle does not pull out or penetrate through the vein as tubes are placed and removed. Be certain to follow the proper order of draw (see Chapter 7).

Withdraw the Needle

After the last tube has been filled, removed from the holder, and mixed (if necessary), fold a clean gauze square in half or in fourths and place it directly over the needle without pressing down (see Figure 10-4*G*). (Applying pressure to the needle during removal is painful and the needle may slit the vein and the skin as it is withdrawn.) Withdraw the needle in one smooth motion, and immediately apply pressure to the site with the gauze pad for 3 to 5 minutes, or until the bleeding has stopped (see Figure 10-4*H*). Failure to apply pressure will result in leakage of blood and hematoma formation. It is acceptable to have the patient hold pressure while you proceed to label tubes, provided the patient is fully alert (see Figure 10-4*I*). *Do not bend the arm up.* Keep it extended or raised.

A clean cotton ball may be used over the site instead of gauze; however, cotton balls tend to stick to the site and reinitiate bleeding when removed.

Dispose of the Needle

Dispose of the needle immediately by placing it in the proper slot of a biohazard sharps container and turning it clockwise until it unscrews from the evacuated tube holder (see Figure 10-4*J*). If the needle remains in the slot of the sharps container with the rubber guard sticking up out of the container, use the tube holder to push it to the side and into the container. *Do not* attempt to loosen it with your fingers.

If the needle refuses to separate from the holder, throw the entire unit away.

If using a PRO-JECT Safety Needle Holder (PRO-TEC, Irvine, CA), hold the needle over the opening of the sharps container and press the release mechanism. The needle should drop into the container.

Do not cut, bend, break, or recap needles. *Do not* stick the needle into the patient's mattress. If you find yourself in a situation where a sharps container is not readily accessible, a *one-handed* **resheathing** technique or a resheathing device may be used according to the national standards outlined in NCCLS document M29-T2.

Label the Tubes

Specimen tube labels (see Figure 10-4*K*) should contain the following information as a minimum:

- Patient's name
- Hospital number (if applicable) or date of birth
- Time of collection
- Date
- Phlebotomist's initials

Compare the information on the label with the patient's identification band and the requisition before leaving the patient.

- *Do not* label tubes prior to venipuncture.
- *Do not* leave the room before labeling the tubes.
- *Do not* dismiss an outpatient before labeling is completed.
- *Do not* label tubes with a pencil.

When using computer-generated labels, write your initials and the time collected on the computer label.

Observe Any Special Handling Instructions

Follow recommended special handling procedures for each specimen, such as putting it in crushed ice to cool (*eg*, protime); keeping it warm (*eg*, cold agglutinin); and protecting it from light (*eg*, bilirubin).

Check the Patient's Arm and Apply Bandage

Examine the patient's arm to see if bleeding has stopped. If the bleeding has stopped, apply an adhesive bandage (or tape over several folded gauze squares) over the site. Instruct the patient to remove the bandage after a minimum of 15 minutes to avoid irritation by the bandage. If the patient is allergic to adhesive bandages, apply paper tape over a clean folded gauze square or cotton ball.

If the patient has sensitive skin or is allergic to the paper tape, wrap gauze around the arm and place the tape over the gauze.

Some hospitals prefer not to bandage the site because bandages tend to irritate the skin and leave a sticky residue, which interferes with subsequent venipuncture. Follow hospital protocol.

Instruct an outpatient not to carry a purse or other heavy object, or lift heavy objects with that arm for approximately 1 hour.

Dispose of Contaminated Materials

Dispose of contaminated materials in proper biohazard containers. Do not leave other materials such as needle caps and wrappers in the patient's room. Check to see that you have your tourniquet and other equipment before exiting the patient's room.

Thank the Patient

Thanking patients for their cooperation is courteous and helps to leave the patient with a positive feeling about the laboratory.

Remove Gloves and Wash Hands

Remove gloves aseptically (Fig. 10-5) by grasping one glove at the wrist and pulling it inside out and off of the hand, ending up with it in the palm of the still gloved hand. Slip your nongloved fingers under the second glove at the wrist and pull it off of the hand, ending with one glove inside the other with the contaminated surfaces inside. Dispose of the gloves in a biohazard waste container. *Wash your hands before proceeding to the next patient.*

Check Specimen Collection Logs

Check the patient's name off of the specimen collection and diet restriction logs at the nursing station if applicable. In an outpatient setting, inform the patient that it is all right to go ahead and eat if no other tests are scheduled that require fasting.

Transport the Specimen to the Lab

Specimens should be transported to the laboratory in a timely fashion. Enter specimens into the computer system or log book. Collection of laboratory specimens must be documented and verified. The specimen collection process is not complete until the appropriate patient and specimen collection information is entered into a computer or manually recorded in a log book.

FAILURE TO OBTAIN BLOOD

Failure to obtain blood can be caused by any of a number of factors. Being aware of these factors and how to correct for them may determine whether you obtain blood on the first try or have to repeat the procedure. If you fail to obtain blood, it is

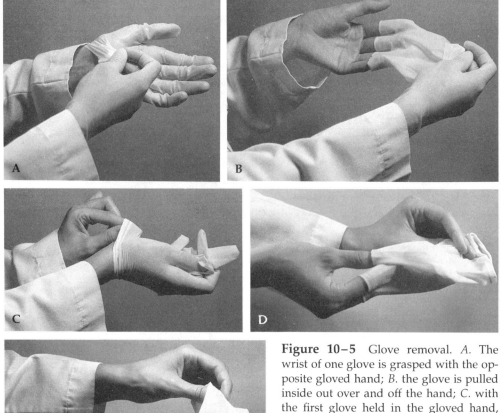

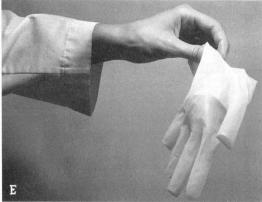

Figure 10–5 Glove removal. *A.* The wrist of one glove is grasped with the opposite gloved hand; *B.* the glove is pulled inside out over and off the hand; *C.* with the first glove held in the gloved hand, the fingers of the non-gloved hand are slipped under the wrist of the remaining glove without touching the exterior surfaces; *D.* the glove is then pulled inside out over the hand so that the first glove ends up inside of the second glove, no exterior glove surfaces are exposed; and *E.* the contaminated gloves can then be dropped into the proper waste receptacle.

important to remain calm so that you can clearly analyze the situation. Proceed to check the following.

Tube Position and Vacuum

Check the tube to see that it is properly seated and the needle has penetrated the stopper. Reseat the tube to make certain the needle sleeve is not pushing the tube off of the needle. If you suspect that the tube may have lost its vacuum, try another tube.

Needle Position

A seasoned phlebotomist uses visual cues to help determine proper needle position (Fig. 10-6). Try to determine visually if the following has occurred.

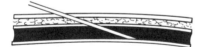

A. Correct insertion technique; blood flows freely into needle.

C. Bevel on vein lower wall does not allow blood to flow.

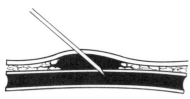

E. Needle partially inserted and causes blood leakage into tissue.

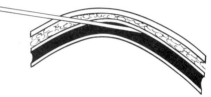

B. Bevel on vein upper wall does not allow blood to flow.

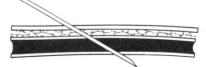

D. Needle inserted too far.

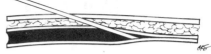

F. Collapsed.

Figure 10–6   Proper and improper needle positioning.
A. Proper needle position. *B.* Needle bevel against the upper wall of a vein. *C.* Needle bevel against or embedded in opposite wall of vein. *D.* Needle inserted all the way through a vein. *E.* Needle partially inserted into vein. *F.* Needle in collapsed vein.

NEEDLE TOO DEEP

The needle may have gone too deep and penetrated all the way through the vein. This can happen on needle insertion or as the tube is pushed onto the needle if the tube holder is not held steady. If this is the case, withdrawing the needle slightly should establish blood flow. If the needle position is not corrected quickly, blood will leak into the tissues and form a hematoma.

NEEDLE NOT DEEP ENOUGH

If the needle is not completely inserted into the vein, blood may fill the tube very slowly. Push the needle gently into the vein and correct blood flow should be established. Partial needle insertion can also cause blood to leak into the tissue and start to form a hematoma. If this occurs, immediately remove the tourniquet and withdraw the needle.

NEEDLE BEVEL AGAINST THE VEIN WALL

Blood flow can also be impaired if the needle bevel is up against either the upper or lower wall of the vein. This is very hard to tell. Try rotating the bevel slightly. If blood flow is established, this was probably the case.

NEEDLE HAS SLIPPED BESIDE THE VEIN

Veins are fairly tough and if not anchored well, the vein may move slightly and the needle may slip to the side of the vein instead of penetrating it. Sometimes the needle ends up to the side and slightly under the vein. In this situation, slip the tube off of the needle so that you do not risk losing the vacuum, and withdraw the needle until just the bevel is under the skin. Anchor the vein securely and redirect the needle into the vein.

NEEDLE POSITION CANNOT BE DETERMINED

If you can't determine the position of the needle and the above solutions do not help, you may have to use your fingers to relocate the vein. Remove the tube from the needle and withdraw the needle until the bevel is just under the skin.

If your gloved finger has been cleaned with alcohol, you may feel the arm above the point of needle insertion and try to determine needle position. *Do not* feel too close to the needle as this is painful to the patient.

Once you have relocated the vein, redirect the needle into the vein and proceed with the venipuncture. If you cannot relocate the vein, withdraw the needle in the proper manner and hold pressure over the site.

Do not blindly probe the arm in an attempt to locate a vein. Probing is painful to the patient and may cause damage to nerves and other tissues. It can also lead to inadvertent puncture of an artery.

Collapsed Vein

Sometimes the vacuum draw of a tube or the pressure created by pulling on a plunger of a syringe can be too much for a vein and cause it to collapse. You can often tell that a vein has collapsed because it will disappear as soon as the needle penetrates it. Tighten the tourniquet if possible by grasping the ends with one hand and twisting them together. That may be enough to reestablish blood flow. Remove the tube from the needle and wait a few seconds for the blood flow to reestablish. Try using a smaller volume tube or pull more slowly on the syringe plunger. If the blood flow does not reestablish, you will have to withdraw the needle and attempt a second venipuncture at another site.

PROCEDURE FOR USING A BUTTERFLY NEEDLE SET

The phlebotomist may elect to use a butterfly needle set (winged infusion set) when attempting to draw blood from antecubital veins of infants and small children or when drawing blood from difficult adult veins, such as small antecubital veins, wrist veins, or hand veins (Fig. 10-7).

Equipment Selection

A butterfly needle device with a threaded multiple sample **luer adapter** that can be attached directly to an evacuated tube holder is preferred. A 23-gauge needle will easily penetrate small veins and not rupture or "blow" them. Choose small volume **pediatric tubes** to collect the specimen. Large volume tubes may create too much vacuum draw on the vein and cause it to collapse. Large volume tubes used with a 23-gauge needle may also cause hemolysis of the specimen.

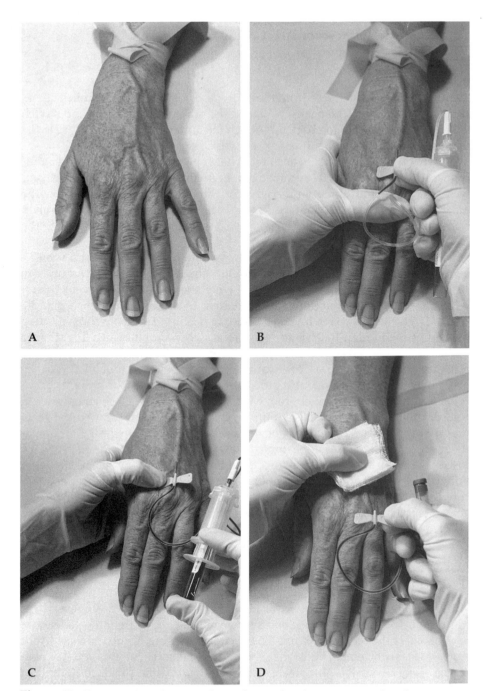

Figure 10-7 Procedure for using butterfly in a hand vein. *A.* Hand with tourniquet in place reveals prominent vein. *B.* With the skin pulled taut over the knuckles, the needle is inserted into the vein until there is a "flash" of blood in the tubing. *C.* Using the nondominant hand, a wing of the butterfly is held against the patient's hand to steady the needle while the blood collecting tube is pushed onto the blood collecting needle. *D.* Once the proper tubes have been drawn, gauze is placed over the vein and the needle is removed.

T method
15 —30
butterfly
10 - 15

Procedure

Remove the butterfly device from the package. The tubing will be coiled some-what because it was coiled in the package. Extend the tubing its full length and stretch slightly to help keep it from coiling back up. Attach the butterfly collection device to the evacuated tube holder. Seat the first tube in the holder.

When drawing the specimen from an antecubital vein, proceed as you would a routine venipuncture, being certain to anchor the vein securely. If drawing from a hand or wrist vein, apply the tourniquet to the wrist proximal to the wrist bone. Have the patient make a loose fist. Make certain the hand is well-supported on the bed, a rolled towel, or armrest. Choose a vein and cleanse the site. Anchor the vein by pulling the skin taut over the knuckles with the thumb.

With the needle bevel up and lined up with the vein, enter the vein at a shallow angle between 10 and 15 degrees. Be careful not to penetrate all the way through the vein. A "flash" of blood will appear in the tubing when the needle is in the vein. "Seat" the needle by threading it up the lumen (central area) of the vein slightly so that the needle will not twist out of the vein if you let go of the needle. Push the blood collecting tube to the end of the holder. Release the tourniquet when blood begins to flow into the tube.

Keep the tube and holder in a downward position so that the tube fills from the bottom up as in a regular venipuncture procedure. Follow the proper order of draw.

When the last tube has been filled, remove it from the needle. Place gauze and re-move the needle in the same manner as a routine venipuncture. If the draw was difficult and the tube is not completely full, it may be replaced on the needle to draw the remaining blood out of the tubing, if it is done immediately.

Dispose of the needle and tubing by dropping the needle into the sharps container while holding onto the still attached tube holder. Release the tubing from the luer adapter with a twisting motion and let it fall into the sharps container. The multiple sample adapter may then be released from the tube holder in the same manner as removing a regular needle.

SYRINGE VENIPUNCTURE PROCEDURE

Although the preferred method of obtaining venipuncture specimens is the evacuated tube method, use of a needle and syringe may be necessary if the patient has fragile or weak veins that collapse easily. The vacuum pressure of the evacuated tube may be too great for such veins. This is often the case with elderly patients and newborn infants. When using a syringe, the phlebotomist can control the pressure by pulling slowly on the syringe plunger.

When performing a venipuncture with needle and syringe, follow the same arm preparation procedures as for a routine venipuncture.

Prepare the needle and syringe by removing them from their sterile wrappers. Securely attach the needle to the syringe. *Do not* remove the needle cover. Pull on the syringe plunger to see that it moves freely. However, make certain the plunger is seated (pushed all the way into the barrel of the syringe) before attempting to draw the specimen. Remove the cap and visually inspect the needle for defects.

Enter the vein, bevel up in the same manner as routine venipuncture. When the vein has been entered you will see blood appear in the hub of the needle. Release the tourniquet.

Hold the syringe as you would the evacuated tube holder. Slowly pull back on the plunger of the syringe and allow the barrel of the syringe to fill with blood.

Filling More Than One Syringe

If more than one syringe is needed, place several thicknesses of gauze under the syringe at the point of needle attachment. While holding the needle very steady, twist the syringe off of the needle and quickly attach the second syringe. It is best to have someone assist with the procedure by filling the tubes from the first syringe while you are collecting blood in the second. When an adequate amount of blood has been collected, remove the needle in the same manner described for routine venipuncture.

Transferring the Blood to Tubes

Remove the needle from the syringe, being careful not to expel the contents of the syringe. Replace the needle with an 18-gauge needle. Place the tubes needed for the required tests in a rack or slot in the blood collecting tray. Penetrate the stopper of the tube to be filled with the syringe needle. Let the tube fill, using the vacuum draw of the tube.

- *Do not* hold the tubes in hand while filling from a syringe.
- *Do not* force the blood into the tube by pushing on the syringe plunger.

If the tube is not to be filled completely, pull back on the plunger to stop the flow. Fill the tubes following the proper order of draw for the syringe method as outlined in Chapter 7. Dispose of the syringe and needle as one unit by dropping it into a sharps container.

PROCEDURE FOR INABILITY TO OBTAIN A SPECIMEN

A phlebotomist who is unable to obtain a specimen on the first try should try again. If the second attempt is unsuccessful, the phlebotomist should *NOT* try a third time. Another phlebotomist should take over. Unsuccessful venipuncture attempts are frustrating to the patient as well as the phlebotomist. Unless it is for a stat, if the second phlebotomist is also unsuccessful, it is a good idea to give the patient a rest and come back at a later time.

ACCEPTABLE REASONS FOR INABILITY TO COLLECT A SPECIMEN

There are times when the phlebotomist will not be able to obtain a specimen from a patient. The following are acceptable reasons for the inability to obtain a specimen:

1. Patient refusal
2. Patient unavailability
3. Phlebotomist attempted, but was unable to draw blood.

Study & Review Questions

1. A tourniquet should be applied:
   a. away from open sores
   b. 8' to 10' above intended puncture
   c. for at least 2 minutes before releasing
   d. tight enough to stop all blood flow

2. Vigorous opening and closing (pumping) of the fist before and during specimen collection may cause:
   a. edema
   b. hemoconcentration
   c. hypertension
   d. petechiae

3. After cleansing the venipuncture site with alcohol, the phlebotomist should:
   a. blow on the site to help evaporate the alcohol
   b. dry the site with a regular gauze pad or cotton ball
   c. allow the alcohol to dry
   d. insert the needle before the alcohol has a chance to evaporate

4. Which of the following actions is NOT proper venipuncture technique?
   a. remove the tourniquet as soon as blood flows freely into tube
   b. maintain the tube in a downward position
   c. fill the tube from the stopper end first
   d. fill the tube until the vacuum is exhausted

5. Vigorous mixing of a tube filled with blood may cause:
   a. hemoglobin
   b. hemolysis
   c. hemoconcentration
   d. hemostasis

6. Collection tubes are labeled:
   a. before collecting the sample
   b. at the patient's bedside after collection
   c. in route to the patient
   d. at the nurse's station after collection

7. Failure to obtain blood may be caused by all of the following EXCEPT:
   a. needle bevel against the wall of the vein
   b. the needle penetrating through the opposite wall of the vein
   c. needle has not penetrated far enough into vein
   d. the needle is centered in the lumen of the vein

8. After penetrating a hand vein with a butterfly, the phlebotomist needs to "seat" the needle, meaning:
   a. have the patient make a tight fist to keep the needle in place
   b. keep the skin taut during the entire process
   c. slightly thread the needle up the central area of the vein
   d. push the needle up against the back wall of the vein

Suggested Laboratory Activities

1. Practice assembling equipment for collecting various tests.
2. Demonstrate proper venipuncture site selection on a fellow student.
3. Practice the performance of a routine venipuncture using an artificial arm.
4. Demonstrate proper venipuncture technique on a fellow student.
5. Practice the use of a butterfly device to obtain a specimen from the hand vein of an artificial arm.
6. Practice proper syringe usage on an artificial arm.

BIBLIOGRAPHY AND SUGGESTED READINGS

Bishop ML, Duben-Engelkirk JL, Fody EP: *Clinical Chemistry: Principles, Procedures, Correlations* (2nd ed.). Philadelphia: JB Lippincott Company, 1992.

Lotspeich-Steininger CA, Stiene-Martin EA, Koepke JA: *Clinical Hematology: Principles, Procedures, Correlations.* Philadelphia: JB Lippincott Company, 1992.

National Committee for Clinical Laboratory Standards, H3-A3: *Procedures for the Collection of Diagnostic Blood Specimens by Venipuncture* (3rd ed.). Villanova, PA: NCCLS, July 1991.

Skin Puncture Procedures and Blood Smear Preparation

11

OBJECTIVES

On successful completion of this chapter, the reader should be able to:

1   State the composition of skin puncture blood and list tests that cannot be performed on skin puncture specimens.
2   State indications for performing skin puncture.
3   Describe the proper procedure for skin puncture collection methods on infants and adults.
4   State precautions involved in skin puncture.
5   Describe the procedure for making a blood smear and the reason for making it at the collection site.

McCall: PHLEBOTOMY ESSENTIALS. © 1993
J. B. Lippincott Company.

COMPOSITION OF SKIN PUNCTURE BLOOD

Blood obtained through skin puncture is a mixture of arterial blood (from arterioles), venous blood (from venules), and capillary blood, along with **interstitial** and **intracellular fluids** from the surrounding tissues. It contains a higher proportion of arterial blood than venous blood because of the pressure with which the arterial blood enters the capillaries. Composition of skin puncture blood, therefore, more closely resembles arterial blood than venous blood obtained by venipuncture. This is especially true if the area has been warmed, as warming increases arterial flow into the area.

REFERENCE VALUES FOR SKIN PUNCTURE BLOOD

Because skin puncture blood differs in composition from regular venous blood, **reference** (normal) **values** for certain tests will be different for skin puncture blood. The most notable differences are for glucose, which is higher in skin puncture blood; and total protein (TP), calcium (Ca^{++}), and potassium (K^+), which are lower in skin puncture blood.

TESTS THAT CANNOT BE PERFORMED BY SKIN PUNCTURE

Although today's technology allows many tests to be performed on very small quantities of blood, and a wide selection of devices are available to make collection of skin puncture specimens relatively safe and easy, some tests cannot be performed on skin puncture specimens. These include erythrocyte sedimentation rate (ESR), most coagulation studies, blood cultures, and tests that still require large volumes of serum or plasma.

INDICATIONS FOR PERFORMING SKIN PUNCTURE

Adults

Skin puncture is performed on adults when there are no accessible veins, to save veins for other procedures such as chemotherapy, when the patient has thrombotic tendencies, and for certain bedside and home testing procedures such as glucose monitoring.

Infants and Children

Skin puncture is the preferred method of obtaining blood from infants and children. Obtaining blood from infants and children by venipuncture is difficult and may damage veins and surrounding tissues. Because infants and young children have such a small blood volume, removing large quantities of blood can also lead to anemia. Large quantities removed rapidly can cause cardiac arrest. In addition, some tests such as screening tests for **phenylketonuria (PKU)** and other inherited diseases are designed to be performed on skin puncture blood only.

SITE SELECTION FOR SKIN PUNCTURE

General Criteria

Skin puncture sites should be warm, pink, and free of scars, cuts, bruises, or rashes. *Do not* choose a site that is cold, **cyanotic**, or edematous (swollen).

INFANTS

The heel is the recommended site for collection of skin puncture specimens on infants less than 1 year old. However, it is important that the puncture be performed in an area of the heel where there is little risk of puncturing the bone.

Puncture of the bone can cause painful **osteomyelitis** (os'te-o-mi'el-i'tis) or bone infection, as well as **osteochondritis** (os'te-o-kon-dri'tis), inflammation of the bone and cartilage. Additional puncture through previous puncture sites may spread the infection.

Studies have shown that the **calcaneus** (heel bone) of premature infants may be as little as 2.4 mm below the skin surface on the bottom (**plantar surface**) of the heel and half that distance at the back (**posterior curvature**) of the heel.

For this reason, guidelines were developed to determine the safest areas, as well as the optimal depth for performing heel puncture. According to the guidelines recommended by NCCLS Document H4-A3 (National Committee for Clinical Laboratory Standards, 771 E. Lancaster Ave., Villanova, PA 19085), to avoid puncturing bone, heel puncture should only be performed on the plantar surface of the heel, medial to an imaginary line extending from the middle of the great (big) toe to the heel, or lateral to an imaginary line drawn from between the fourth and fifth toes to the heel (Fig. 11-1). In addition, the puncture should not exceed 2.4 mm in depth.

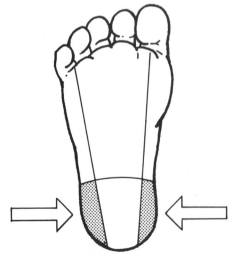

Figure 11-1   Infant heel. Shaded areas indicated by arrows represent recommended areas for infant heel puncture.

- *Do not* puncture deeper than 2.4 mm.
- *Do not* puncture through previous puncture sites.
- *Do not* puncture the area between the imaginary boundaries.
- *Do not* puncture the posterior curvature of the heel.
- *Do not* puncture in the area of the arch.
- *Do not* puncture areas of the foot other than the heel.

OLDER CHILDREN AND ADULTS

The recommended site for skin puncture on adults and older children is the palmar surface of the distal phalanx (end segment of the finger) of the middle or ring finger of the nondominant hand. The puncture should be made in the central, fleshy portion of the finger, slightly to the side of center and perpendicular to the whorls (grooves) of the fingerprint (Fig. 11-2).

- *Do not* puncture the side or very tip of the finger. The distance between the skin surface and the bone is half as much at the side and tip as it is in the central portion of the end of the finger.
- *Do not* puncture parallel to the grooves of the fingerprint. A puncture parallel to or along the lines of the fingerprint will cause blood to run down the finger and make collection difficult.
- *Do not* puncture the index finger. The index finger is more calloused and, therefore, harder to poke than the other fingers. Also, the patient will use that finger more and will notice the pain longer.
- *Do not* puncture the fifth or little finger. The amount of tissue between skin surface and bone is the thinnest in this finger.
- *Do not* puncture fingers of infants and very young children. The amount of tissue between skin surface and bone is so small that bone injury is very likely.

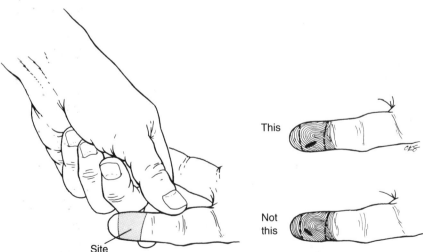

Figure 11–2   Recommended site and direction of finger puncture.

SKIN PUNCTURE EQUIPMENT

1. 70% isopropyl alcohol prep pads
2. Sterile gauze pads
3. Sterile lancet or automated skin puncture device
4. Heel warming device, if applicable
5. Collection devices (capillary tubes, microtainers, slides, etc.)

SITE WARMING PROCEDURES

Blood flow can be increased up to seven times by warming the site prior to skin puncture. Because warming primarily increases arterial flow into the area, the specimen obtained will be referred to as an "arterialized" specimen. When collecting *p*H or blood gas specimens by skin puncture, warming is an essential part of the procedure.

Warming can be accomplished by wrapping the site for a minimum of 3 minutes with a towel or diaper that has been moistened with comfortably warm water (no warmer than 42°C or 108°F). Commercial heel warmers are also available.

SITE CLEANING PROCEDURES

Skin puncture sites should be cleaned with 70% isopropanol. *Do not* use povidone iodine to clean skin puncture sites. Povidone iodine should not be used because it greatly interferes with a number of tests, most notably bilirubin, potassium, phosphorus, and uric acid.

Once cleaned, the site must be wiped dry with sterile gauze to eliminate alcohol residue. Alcohol residue, in addition to causing a stinging sensation, causes rapid hemolysis of red blood cells. Alcohol residue has also been shown to interfere with glucose testing.

PERFORMING A SKIN PUNCTURE

Finger Puncture (Fingerstick)

When performing a finger puncture (Fig. 11-3), the arm should be firmly supported and extended with the palmar surface of the hand facing up. Select, clean, and dry the site.

Grasp the finger firmly between your thumb and index finger and perform the puncture perpendicular to the whorls (lines) of the fingerprint. This will allow the blood to form a bead or drop that is easily collected.

Heel Puncture (Heelstick)

Grasp the heel firmly but gently with the index finger wrapped around the foot supporting the arch, and the thumb wrapped around the ankle and below the puncture

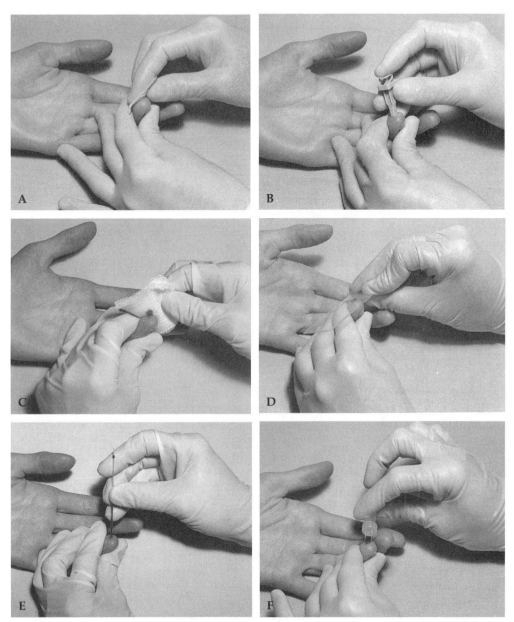

Figure 11–3   Finger puncture procedures. *A.* Cleaning the site. *B.* Puncturing the skin with an automatic safety lancet. *C.* Wiping the first drop. *D.* Making a slide from skin puncture by touching the slide to the drop of blood. *E.* Collecting skin puncture blood in a capillary tube. *F.* Collecting skin puncture blood in a microtainer.

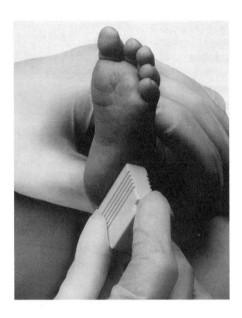

Figure 11–4   Infant heel puncture using Tender-foot® automatic incision device. (Courtesy of International Technidyne, Edison, NJ)

site (Fig. 11-4). Perform the puncture perpendicular to the lines of the footprint, using a recommended heel puncture device. Continue both heelsticks and fingersticks in the following manner.

Dispose of the puncture device promptly in a sharps container. Apply firm pressure toward the site. Wipe away the first drop of blood with a dry gauze. (The first drop is usually contaminated with tissue fluid.) This also gets rid of any remaining alcohol residue, which could hemolyze the specimen, as well as keep the blood from forming a well-rounded drop.

Position the site downward and continue to apply moderate pressure proximal to the puncture site. *Do not* squeeze or massage the site vigorously. Such activities introduce excess tissue fluid into the specimen and may also cause hemolysis of the specimen.

Proceed to collect the blood using devices appropriate for the type of test to be performed. Touch the collection device to the drop of blood formed on the surface of the skin. Capillary pipettes will fill by capillary action. When full, seal the ends of capillary pipettes with clay.

Touch the "scoop" of microcollection tubes to the drop of blood and let the drop of blood run down the walls of the tube. Tap the tube gently now and then to encourage the blood to settle to the bottom of the tube. *Do not* use a "scooping" motion against the surface of the skin. Scraping the scoop against the skin activates platelets and may also cause hemolysis. Cap microcollection tubes with the caps provided and mix additive tubes eight to ten times.

Some tests require blood smears made from a fresh drop of blood from a fingertip. An example is a leukocyte alkaline phosphatase (LAP) stain or score, which usually requires four fresh peripheral (a term used to indicate skin puncture blood as opposed to venous blood) blood smears. In addition, some hematologists prefer blood smears from blood that has not been in contact with anticoagulant. If such a blood smear is requested, it should be made first to avoid platelet clumping. EDTA tubes for hematology specimens should be collected next for the same reason.

When finished, apply pressure to the site with a clean gauze until bleeding stops. Keep the site elevated. Label the containers with the appropriate information.

Do not apply bandages to skin puncture sites of infants under 2 years of age. Adhesive bandages may irritate the skin of young children and may even tear the skin of newborns, especially premature infants, when removed. In addition, an infant or young child could aspirate the bandage and choke.

BLOOD SMEAR PREPARATION

A blood smear (Fig. 11-5) is needed when a manual **differential** is part of a complete blood count. Blood smears are rarely made at the patient's bedside. They are

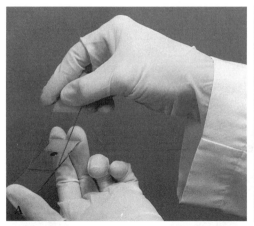
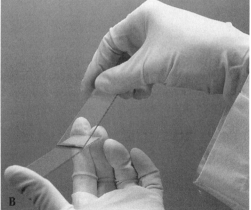
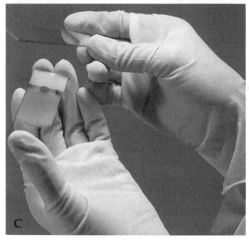

Figure 11–5 Blood smear preparation. *A.* Drop of blood on slide with pusher slide placed in front. *B.* Pusher slide with drop of blood spreading to its edges. *C.* Completed blood smear.

generally made in the hematology department from the EDTA specimen tube. They are often made using an automated machine that makes a uniform smear from a single drop of blood. Blood smears made from EDTA-anticoagulated blood should be made within 1 hour of collection to eliminate cell distortion caused by the anticoagulant.

A blood smear may be made at the patient's bedside when a CBC is collected by skin puncture. When making a blood smear from a skin puncture, the first drop is wiped away as usual. The slide is then touched to the next drop in such a manner that the drop ends up ½ to 1 inch from the end of the slide, or right after the end of the frosted area. The drop should be about 1 to 2 mm in diameter and centered on the slide. If the smear is made manually from anticoagulated blood, a capillary tube or pipette is used to dispense a drop of blood onto the slide in the same position.

Next a second (or spreader) slide is placed in front of the drop at approximately a 30-degree angle. The spreader slide is then pulled back into the drop. It should be stopped as soon as it touches the drop and the blood should be allowed to run along its entire width. As soon as the blood spreads to the edges, the spreader slide should be pushed forward in one smooth motion.

Do not push down on the spreader slide. Let the weight of the spreader slide carry the blood and make the smear. The smear should be allowed to dry naturally. *Never* blow on a slide to dry it because this results in red blood cell distortion.

Making a good blood smear is a skill that takes practice to perfect. An acceptable smear will cover about one-half the surface of the slide and have no holes, jagged edges, or lines. It will have the appearance of a **feather** in that there will be a smooth gradient from thick to thin when held up to the light. The thinnest area, often referred to as the "feather," is the most important because that is where a differential is performed.

Smears that are too long (cover the entire length of the slide) or too short are not acceptable. The length of the smear can be controlled by the size of the drop and the angle of the spreader slide.

Holes in the smear can be caused by fingerprints or dirt on the slide. Ragged edges can be caused by a chipped pusher slide, a blood drop that has started to dry, or uneven pressure as the smear is made.

Study & Review Questions

1. Skin puncture blood is:
   a. venous
   b. arterial
   c. interstitial fluid
   d. all of the above

2. Which of the following has a higher concentration in capillary blood than in venous?
   a. blood urea nitrogen
   b. carotene
   c. glucose
   d. total protein

3. A blood test that cannot normally be performed by skin puncture is:
   a. CBC
   b. erythrocyte sedimentation rate
   c. potassium
   d. thyroid panel

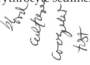

4. The least hazardous area of an infant's foot on which to perform skin puncture is the:
   a. arch
   b. central area of the heel
   c. posterior curvature of the heel
   d. medial or lateral area of the plantar surface of the heel

5. It is necessary to control the depth of lancet insertion during heel puncture to avoid:
   a. puncturing a vein
   b. excessive bleeding
   c. bone injury
   d. bacterial contamination

6. Povidone iodine used to clean a skin puncture site is known to cause erroneous results for which of the following tests?
   a. albumin
   b. bilirubin
   c. CBC
   d. triglycerides

7. When collecting skin puncture tests, which of the following should be collected first?
   a. CBC
   b. electrolytes
   c. glucose
   d. phosphorus

8. A blood smear "pusher slide" should be at a:
   a. 15-degree angle
   b. 30-degree angle
   c. 45-degree angle
   d. 60-degree angle

Suggested Laboratory Activities

1. Identify the proper sites for adult skin puncture on a fellow student.

2. Identify the proper sites for skin puncture on an infant, using an infant anatomic model.

3. Perform a finger puncture on another student and collect the blood using the various types of microcollection equipment.

4. Practice proper collection of blood for newborn screening, substituting blood obtained by finger puncture to fill the circles.

5. Practice making and labeling blood smears.

BIBLIOGRAPHY AND SUGGESTED READINGS

Bishop ML, Duben-Engelkirk JL, Fody EP: *Clinical Chemistry: Principles, Procedures, Correlations* (2nd ed.). Philadelphia: JB Lippincott Company, 1992.

Lotspeich-Steininger CA, Stiene-Martin EA, Koepke JA: *Clinical Hematology: Principles, Procedure, Correlations*. Philadelphia: JB Lippincott Company, 1992.

National Committee for Clinical Laboratory Standards, H4-A3: *Procedures for the Collection of Diagnostic Blood Specimens by Skin Puncture* (3rd ed.). Villanova, PA: NCCLS, July 1991.

National Committee for Clinical Laboratory Standards, H14-A2: *Devices for Collection of Skin Puncture Blood Specimens* (2nd ed.). Villanova, PA: NCCLS, July 1990.

Special Blood Tests and Procedures

12

OBJECTIVES

On successful completion of this chapter, the reader should be able to:

1 State the theory behind and describe the importance of each of the special tests.
2 Identify equipment and describe the procedure for each of the special tests.
3 Identify potential sources of error associated with each of the special tests.
4 List identification information required when collecting and labeling blood bank specimens and explain why this is so important.
5 State criteria for routine and autologous donor selection.
6 State the importance of timing for blood cultures, tolerance tests, and therapeutic drug monitoring.

KEY TERMS

activated coagulation time (ACT)
aerobic
anaerobic
ancillary blood glucose testing (ABGT)
antimicrobial removal device (ARD)
antimicrobial therapy
bacteremia
bleeding time (BT)
chain of custody
compatibility
fever of unknown origin (FUO)
glucose tolerance test
peak levels
postprandial (PP)
septicemia
skin antisepsis
therapeutic drug monitoring (TDM)
trough levels

McCall: PHLEBOTOMY ESSENTIALS. © 1993
J. B. Lippincott Company.

SPECIAL VENIPUNCTURE PROCEDURES

Blood specimens for most laboratory tests can be collected using routine venipuncture or skin puncture procedures. Some tests, however, require special collection procedures. Collecting specimens for these tests may require special preparation, equipment, handling, or timing. Several tests are actually performed by the phlebotomist at bedside (or in the outpatient setting) with results immediately available and reported by the phlebotomist. Some of the most commonly encountered special blood test procedures are listed below.

Activated Coagulation Time

Activated coagulation time (ACT), also called activated clotting time, tests the activity of the intrinsic coagulation factors and is used to monitor heparin therapy. Heparin is given intravenously to patients who have blood clots, to patients whose blood is apt to clot too easily, or as a precaution following certain surgeries. When given intravenously, heparin therapy results are immediate but difficult to control. Too much heparin can cause the patient to bleed, therefore, heparin therapy is closely monitored. Once a patient's condition is stabilized, the patient is placed on oral anticoagulant therapy, such as coumadin, which can be monitored by the **prothrombin test (PT)**.

The ACT test is performed at the bedside with results available within minutes. The phlebotomist who performs the test is responsible for reporting the results to the patient's nurse, as well as to the coagulation department of the lab.

Test procedure involves expediting coagulation time by use of a clot enhancing substance (activator), such as siliceous earth, silica, or celite contained in a special gray top tube. Other equipment needed to perform the test includes regular venipuncture equipment, a heat block or incubator, and a stopwatch or timer.

TEST PROCEDURE
1. A routine venipuncture is performed and a 4-ml discard tube is drawn.
2. Blood is then drawn into a prewarmed tube containing the clot activator. A timer is started as soon as blood flows into the tube.
3. As soon as the tube vacuum is exhausted, the tube is mixed well and placed in the heat block for 60 seconds. *Note*: although the tube may look like one that draws a larger volume, ACT tubes draw only a small volume of blood (approximately 2 ml).
4. At the end of 60 seconds, the tube is rocked gently back and forth and visually inspected for the first visible sign of a clot.
5. If no clot formation is seen, it is placed back in the heat block for 5 seconds after which it is removed and inspected again.
6. The procedure is repeated every 5 seconds until the first visible clot is observed, at which point the timer is stopped and the time recorded.
7. Results are recorded at the nurses station and also reported to the coagulation department.

   Sources of error include:

1. Failure to start the timer as soon as the blood flow starts will decrease values.
2. Failure to adequately mix the tube properly will result in increased values.

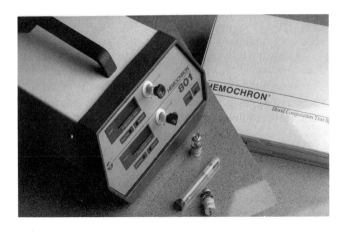

Figure 12–1 The Hemachron® machine for ACT determinations. (Courtesy of International Technidyne, Edison, NJ.)

3. A sample obtained by a traumatic draw, as well as an inadequate sample, will cause decreased values.
4. Anticoagulant drugs, antibiotics, steroids, and barbiturates can lead to erroneous results.

An automated variation of the ACT procedure, the Hemochron system (Fig. 12–1) is available from International Technidyne Corporation, Edison, NJ. With this system, a machine does the mixing and timing automatically. In addition, this system requires the use of a special tube with a black plastic cap, which is supplied by the manufacturer.

Blood Alcohol (Ethanol) Specimens

The 70% isopropyl alcohol used in skin preparation for routine venipuncture may interfere with test results of specimens drawn for blood alcohol determinations. A nonalcohol-containing alternative antiseptic or regular soap and water should be used to clean the site instead. A gray top, sodium fluoride tube is generally required for the test.

Forensic Specimens

Occasionally a blood specimen is requested by law enforcement officials for forensic or legal reasons. Examples are specimens for blood alcohol levels and specimens for drug testing. In such an event, special protocol referred to as "**chain of custody**" must be strictly followed. Chain of custody requires documentation that the specimen is accounted for at all times. A special form is used to identify the specimen and the person or persons who obtained and processed the specimen. Information on the form also includes the time, date, and place the specimen was obtained, along with the signature of the person from whom the specimen was obtained. If documentation is incomplete, any legal action may be impaired. A phlebotomist involved in drawing a blood alcohol for legal reasons can be summoned to appear in court.

Blood Bank Specimens for Type and Crossmatch

A blood type and crossmatch is performed to determine the **compatibility** of blood to be used in a transfusion. A transfusion of incompatible blood can be fatal due

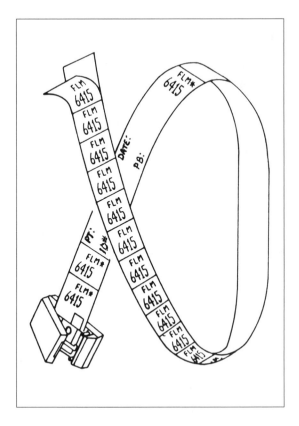

Figure 12–2 Typenex bloodbank identification bracelet. (Courtesy of Fenwal Laboratories, a division of Travenol Laboratories, Chicago, IL.)

to agglutination (clumping) and lysis (rupturing) of the red blood cells within the patient's circulatory system (see Chapter 5). For this reason, hospitals require *strict* identification and labeling procedures when obtaining specimens for crossmatch. One such procedure requires attachment to the patient's wrist of a special identification (ID) bracelet such as the Typenex Blood Recipient Identification Band (Fenwal Biotech Division, a division of Travenol Laboratories, Chicago, IL) (Fig. 12–2).

In this procedure, the patient's identity is confirmed and the information placed on the special bracelet, which contains an ID number. An adhesive label from the bracelet, which also contains the ID number and the patient's ID, is placed on the specimen drawn from the patient. Additional ID number labels from the bracelet are sent to the lab with the specimen to be used in the crossmatch process and eventually attached to the unit of blood used for transfusion. Before the transfusion is given, the nurse *must* match the number on the patient's ID bracelet with the number on the unit of blood.

One of the latest identification systems for blood bank patients, the Bloodloc Safety System (Fig. 12–3) from Novatek Medical Inc. (Greenwich, CT), consists of four elements: a unique three-letter code printed on a colored adhesive sticker; a single-use plastic combination lock designed to seal the opening of a plastic bag; a back-plate that works in conjunction with the lock; and a 5 × 13-inch clear plastic bag. On admission to the hospital, a coded sticker is applied to the patient's ID wristband. When a specimen

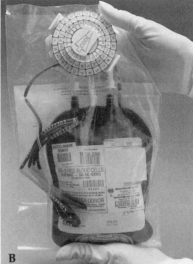
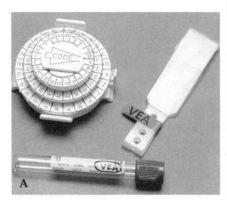

Figure 12–3 Components of the Blood-Loc® safety system showing: *A.* the blood bag combination lock, a wrist band with unique code, and a tube with the code circled; *B.* a Blood-Loc® safety bag with lock in place containing a unit of blood.

is drawn for a crossmatch, the phlebotomist must copy this unique code onto the specimen label. The code is circled so it is not confused with the phlebotomist's initials on the label, and then sent to the lab and the crossmatch performed. When the unit of blood is needed for transfusion, it is put into a bag and sealed with the disposable lock, which is then permanently set with the patient's unique code. Before the unit is given to the patient, the nurse must use the code from the patient's wristband to be able to open the lock and remove the unit from the plastic bag.

Identification information for blood bank specimens includes:

1. Patient's full name (including middle initial).
2. Patient's hospital identification number (or social security number for outpatients)
3. Patient's date of birth
4. Date and time of collection
5. Phlebotomist's initials
6. Room number and bed number (optional)
7. Patient's Blood-Loc code, if applicable

A crossmatch normally requires a large, plain (no serum separator gel) red stopper tube. Tubes with incomplete or inaccurate information are not accepted by blood bank personnel for processing.

Blood Donor Collection

Blood donor collection involves collecting blood in amounts referred to as *units* to be used for transfusion purposes rather than for diagnostic testing. Donor collection requires special training and exceptional venipuncture skills. Facilities (blood banks) that provide blood donor services follow guidelines of the American Association of Blood Banks (AABB).

DONOR ELIGIBILITY

Anyone wishing to donate blood must be interviewed to determine eligibility to donate blood, as well as to obtain information for the record that must be kept for all blood donors. To donate blood, a person must be within the ages of 17 and 66 years and weigh at least 110 pounds. Minors must have written permission from their parents. Adults over the age of 66 years may be allowed to donate at the discretion of the blood bank physician. A brief physical examination, as well as a complete medical history, is needed to determine a patient's state of health. This information is needed each time a person donates, no matter how many times a person has donated before. All donor information is strictly confidential. In addition, the donor must give written permission for the blood bank to use his or her blood.

PROCEDURE

Donor units are normally collected from a large antecubital vein. The vein is selected in a similar manner as for routine venipuncture. Skin preparation involves a two-step cleaning process with a povidone iodine preparation in a similar manner to blood culture collection. The collection unit is a sterile, closed system consisting of a bag to contain the blood connected by a length of tubing to a sterile needle. A 16-gauge needle is most commonly used. The bag fills by gravity and must be placed lower than the patient's arm. The collection bag contains an anticoagulant, generally a citrate phosphate dextrose solution, and is commonly placed on a mixing unit as the blood is being drawn. The unit is often filled by weight but generally contains about 450 ml when full. Only one needle puncture can be used to fill a unit. If the unit only partially fills and the procedure must be repeated, an entire new unit must be used. Average time to collect a unit is around 7 minutes.

A unit of blood can be separated into several components: red blood cells, plasma, and platelets. All components of the unit must be easily traceable to the donor.

Autologous Blood Donation

Autologous donation is the process by which a person donates blood for his or her own use. This is done for elective surgeries where possibility of transfusion is likely or anticipated. Using one's own blood eliminates many associated risks such as disease transmission and blood or plasma incompatibilities. Blood is generally collected several weeks prior to the scheduled surgery, however, minimum time between donation and surgery can be as little as 72 hours. To be eligible to make an autologous donation, a person must have a written order from a physician, be in reasonably good health, be able to regenerate red blood cells, and have a hemoglobin of at least 11 g. If the patient meets regular donor requirements and the blood is not used, the blood may be used for the general population with the donor's permission.

Blood Cultures

Blood cultures are ordered by the physician when there is **"fever of unknown origin" (FUO)** or reason to suspect **bacteremia** or **septicemia** (pathogenic bacteria in the blood). Blood cultures help determine the presence and extent of infection, as well as indicate the type of organism responsible and the antibiotic to which it is most susceptible.

Collecting blood cultures in a timely fashion is important as cultures are commonly ordered immediately before anticipated fever spikes, as well as immediately after. Bacteria are most likely to be present in the bloodstream at these times.

Blood cultures are generally collected in sets of two: one **anaerobic** (without air) and one **aerobic** (Fig. 12–4). Anaerobic culture bottles are filled first. When more than one set is ordered for the same time, the second set should be obtained from a separately prepared site on the opposite arm. However, in some cases, "second sight" blood cultures are more useful when drawn 30 minutes apart. If timing is not specified on the laboratory slip, follow laboratory protocol.

Skin antisepsis is a very important part of the blood culture collection procedure. Failure to follow sterile technique can introduce skin surface bacteria into the blood culture bottle and interfere with interpretation of results. Because all microorganisms isolated from blood cultures must be reported by the laboratory, it is up to the patient's physician to determine if the organism is clinically significant or merely a contaminant. If an organism is misinterpreted as pathogenic, it could result in inappropriate treatment and additional expense. Sterile technique methods vary slightly from one laboratory to another. The procedure for one commonly accepted method follows.

TEST PROCEDURE

1. After selecting the venipuncture site, the tourniquet is released (if applicable) and the site is cleansed using a povidone- iodine swabstick for a minimum of 2 minutes and covering an area 3 to 4 square inches in diameter. (Some clinicians recommend cleaning the site with an alcohol prep pad prior to Step 1 to initially rid the site of excess dirt and surface debris.)

2. The venipuncture site is cleansed again with a second povidone-iodine swabstick, beginning in the center and moving outward in concentric circles. The area is then allowed to air dry. Touching or palpating the site once it has been prepared is not recommended. However, if the necessity to repalpate is anticipated, the phlebotomist's gloved finger should be cleaned in the same manner as the venipuncture site. Note that antisepsis does not occur instantly. The scrubbing process in Step 1, as well as the drying process in Step 2, allows time for the antiseptic agent to be effective against skin surface bacteria.

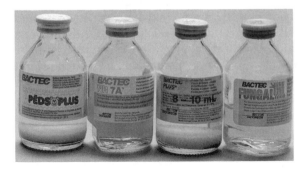

Figure 12–4   Blood culture bottles.

3. While the area is drying, the tops of blood culture containers are cleaned with a third swabstick and venipuncture equipment is prepared. (Blood culture containers equipped with plastic caps can be cleaned with 70% isopropyl alcohol after removing the cap.) When preparing venipuncture equipment, needles and so on should be handled carefully so as not to destroy sterility. If a syringe is used, an 18-gauge needle should be available for specimen transfer.

4. Prior to inoculation with blood, the tops of the blood culture bottles are wiped with 70% alcohol to prevent introduction of iodine residue into the blood culture media. Contamination of the media with iodine can inhibit growth of microorganisms and lead to false-negative culture results.

5. The tourniquet is reapplied, taking care that nothing touches the prepped area in the process.

6. Venipuncture is performed. Blood may be collected directly into blood culture media when using specially designed tubes or a blood transfer system. Care must be taken to avoid backflow.

7. When the syringe method is used, a new needle must be used to transfer blood into the collection bottles to prevent contamination of the blood culture media with bacteria picked up from skin pores and recesses during needle withdrawal. An 18-gauge needle is commonly used for the transfer process to minimize further trauma to the red blood cells and to prevent possible hemolysis. To prevent accidental needle sticks when using a transfer set or needle and syringe, the culture bottle should *not* be held in the phlebotomist's hand during the inoculation process.

Antimicrobial Removal Device

It is not unusual for patients to be on **antimicrobial** (antibiotic) **therapy** at the time blood culture specimens are collected. Antimicrobial agents in the patient's blood can inhibit the growth of the microorganisms in the blood culture bottle. In such cases, the physician may order blood cultures to be collected in an **antimicrobial removal device (ARD)**. The ARD contains a resin that removes antimicrobials from the blood. The blood can then be processed by conventional technique without inhibiting the growth of microorganisms. The ARD should be delivered to the lab for processing as soon as possible because blood should not be exposed to the device for more than 2 hours. Some new blood culture media eliminate the need for special ARD media.

Postprandial Glucose Testing

Postprandial (PP) means "after a meal." Glucose levels in blood specimens obtained 2 hours after a meal are rarely elevated in normal persons but may be significantly increased in diabetic patients. Therefore, a glucose test collected 2 hours after a meal, a 2-hour PP, is an excellent screening test for diabetes. The test is also used to monitor insulin therapy. Correct timing of specimen collection is important. Glucose levels, if collected too early, may still be elevated and lead to misinterpretation of results.

TEST PROCEDURE

1. Preparation for the test involves placing the patient on a high carbohydrate diet for 2 to 3 days prior to the test.

2. It is important for the patient to be fasting prior to the test. This means no eating, smoking, or drinking other than water at least 10 hours before the test.

3. The day of the test, the patient is instructed to eat a special breakfast containing the equivalent of 100 g of glucose.
4. A blood specimen for glucose determination is collected 2 hours after the patient finishes eating.

Glucose Tolerance Test

A **glucose tolerance test (GTT)** is performed to check for carbohydrate metabolism problems. The major carbohydrate in the blood is glucose. The major types of disorders involving glucose metabolism are those in which the blood glucose level is increased (hyperglycemia) as in diabetes mellitus, and those in which the blood glucose levels are decreased (hypoglycemia). The enzyme insulin produced by the pancreas is primarily responsible for regulating blood glucose levels. The GTT evaluates insulin response to a measured dose of glucose by recording glucose levels at specific time intervals (Fig. 12–5).

Patient preparation for a GTT is very important. A patient should receive verbal as well as written instructions.

TEST PROCEDURE

1. The patient is instructed to eat balanced meals containing approximately 150 g of carbohydrates for 3 days prior to the test.
2. The patient must then fast at least 12 hours preceding the test but not for more than 16 hours. The patient is allowed and encouraged to drink water during the fast because urine specimens are usually collected as part of the procedure. No other food or beverages are allowed. The patient is also not allowed to smoke or chew gum because these activities stimulate the digestive process and may cause erroneous test results.

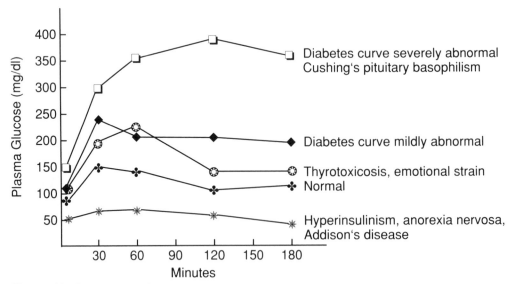

Figure 12–5   Glucose tolerance test curves.

3. A fasting blood specimen is drawn and checked for glucose. (If the fasting blood glucose is over 200 mg/dl, the test is usually not performed.) A fasting urine specimen may also be collected.
4. An adult patient is given a commercial glucose beverage containing approximately 100 g of glucose. Children and small adults are given approximately 1 g/kg of weight. The patient must consume the drink within 5 minutes.
5. Timing for the test is started as soon as the patient finishes the glucose beverage. Both blood and urine specimens are normally collected at 30 minutes, 1 hour, 2 hours, 3 hours, and so on, for however long the physician has specified the test. Specimens should be labeled with both the exact time collected and the time interval of the test, such as 1 hour, and so on.
6. No food, alcohol, smoking, or chewing gum is allowed throughout the test period. Water intake is allowed and encouraged.

In normal patients, blood glucose levels peak within 30 minutes to 1 hour following glucose ingestion. The peak in glucose levels triggers the release of insulin, which brings glucose levels back down to fasting levels within about 2 hours and no glucose spills over into the urine. Because diabetics have inadequate or absent insulin response, glucose levels peak at higher levels and are slower to return to fasting levels. If blood is not drawn on time, it is important for the phlebotomist to note the discrepancy so that the physician will take this into consideration.

The method used to collect specimens should be consistent for all specimens. That is, if the first specimen is collected by venipuncture, all succeeding specimens should be venipuncture specimens. If skin puncture is used to collect the first specimen, all succeeding specimens should also be skin puncture specimens.

Other Tolerance Tests

LACTOSE TOLERANCE TEST

A lactose tolerance test is used to determine if a patient lacks the enzyme (mucosal lactase) that is necessary to convert the milk sugar lactose into glucose and galactose. A person lacking the enzyme suffers from gastrointestinal distress and diarrhea following ingestion of milk and other lactose-containing foods.

Symptoms are relieved by eliminating milk from the diet.

TEST PROCEDURE

1. A 3-hour GTT is performed the day before the lactose tolerance test.
2. The 3-hour lactose tolerance test is performed in the same manner as the GTT, however, an equal amount of lactose is substituted for the glucose.
3. Blood samples for glucose testing are drawn at the same times used in the GTT test the day before. If the patient has mucosal lactase, the resulting glucose curve will be similar to the GTT curve from the day before. If the patient lacks the enzyme (lactose intolerant) glucose levels will rise no more than 20 mg/dl from the fasting level resulting in a "flat" curve. False-positive results have been demonstrated in patients with slow gastric emptying.

EPINEPHRINE TOLERANCE TEST

The epinephrine tolerance test is used to evaluate the presence and availability of glycogen stores in the liver. Glycogen is stored in the liver and converted to glucose when needed. Epinephrine accelerates the conversion of glycogen to glucose (glycogenolysis).

TEST PROCEDURE

1. A fasting glucose specimen is collected.
2. A solution of epinephrine hydrochloride is injected intravenously by a physician or other qualified person.
3. A blood glucose specimen is collected 30 minutes later.

In a patient with normal glycogen stores, blood glucose levels at 30 minutes will increase at least 30 mg/dL above fasting levels. Little or no increase in blood sugar levels indicates depletion of glycogen stores or an interference in the conversion of available glycogen stores, such as caused by Von Gierke's disease.

GLUCAGON TOLERANCE TEST

A glucagon tolerance test also tests the presence and availability of liver glycogen stores. The test is conducted in the same way as the epinephrine tolerance test above, substituting glucagon for epinephrine. Results are also interpreted in the same manner.

D-XYLOSE TOLERANCE TEST

The D-xylose tolerance test is used to diagnose problems with intestinal absorption. This condition is frequently seen in elderly patients. D-xylose is a simple sugar called a pentose that is present in certain fruits. It is not metabolized by the body and is not normally present in blood or urine.

TEST PROCEDURE

1. The patient is instructed not to eat fruits containing D-xylose for 3 days prior to the test.
2. The patient must fast after midnight the day of the test.
3. The patient is instructed to void and discard urine prior to the test.
4. The patient is given an oral dose of 25 g of D-xylose dissolved in 500 ml (approximately 16 ounces) of water. Timing is started as soon as the patient finishes the D-xylose solution. The patient remains fasting until the test is completed 5 hours later.
5. A blood specimen for D-xylose determination is collected 2 hours following the ingestion of the D-xylose solution.
6. All urine voided by the patient is collected, pooled, and refrigerated for the duration of the test. A final urine specimen is collected at the end of 5 hours and added to the pool. A D-xylose determination is performed on the pooled specimen.

If absorption is normal, D-xylose will be absorbed into the bloodstream from the small intestine, pass through the liver and be excreted by the kidneys, thus appearing in the blood and urine. If absorption is abnormal (malabsorption), low blood and urine values will be obtained. Falsely low blood and urine values may result from bacterial overgrowth of the small intestine. Normal blood levels and low urine levels may result from impaired renal function.

Therapeutic Drug Monitoring

Because the dosage of drug necessary to produce the desired effect varies widely among patients, **therapeutic drug monitoring (TDM)** is used by the physician to manage individual patient drug treatment. It is used to help establish drug dosages and to maintain dosages at beneficial levels and avoid drug toxicity. Timing of specimen collection in regard to dosage administration is critical for safe and beneficial treatment and, therefore, must be consistent. A team effort is essential and requires coordination with pharmacy, nursing, and the lab. The phlebotomist is a key player in this team effort.

Some therapeutic drugs require the monitoring and evaluation of "peak" and "trough"—drug levels for the physician to determine a safe and effective dosage for the patient.

Peak (or maximum) **levels** are collected when the highest serum concentration of the drug is anticipated, about 15 to 30 minutes after administration of the drug. Peak levels screen for drug intoxication.

Trough (or minimum) **levels** are collected when the lowest serum concentration of the drug is expected, usually immediately prior to administration of the next scheduled dose. Trough levels are monitored to assure that levels of the drug stay within the therapeutic (or effective) range.

Therapeutic Phlebotomy

Therapeutic phlebotomy involves the withdrawal of a large volume of blood usually measured by the unit as in blood donation. It is performed as a treatment for certain medical conditions such as polycythemia. (Polycythemia is an overproduction of red blood cells, which is detrimental to the patient's health). Therapeutic phlebotomy is performed in a manner similar to donor collection; however, the blood is usually discarded. Therapeutic phlebotomy is only performed by phlebotomists who have been specially trained in the procedure, such as those trained in donor phlebotomy.

SPECIAL SKIN PUNCTURE PROCEDURES

Ancillary Blood Glucose Testing or Bedside Glucose Testing

Reliable, instant glucose testing became available with the advent of small, portable, and relatively inexpensive glucose analyzers such as the Glucometer II (Ames division, Miles Laboratories, Elkhart, IN), Accu-check II (Boehringer Mannheim Diagnostics, Indianapolis, IN) and ONE TOUCH II (LifeScan, Inc., Milpitas, CA) (Fig. 12–6).

Ancillary blood glucose testing (ABGT) analyzers use whole blood specimens most commonly obtained by routine skin puncture. A drop of blood is applied to a reagent strip, which is then inserted into the analyzer. The level of glucose in the blood is determined by the machine and the result appears on a screen.

Phlebotomists are often required to perform bedside testing. However, before being eligible to perform ABGT, NCCLS guidelines recommend that a phlebotomist receive institution authorization to do so only after completing formal training in ABGT procedures under the supervision of or sponsored by the particular health care institution.

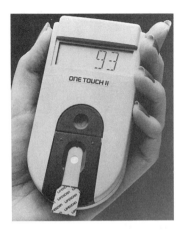

Figure 12–6 ONE TOUCH II® Blood Glucose Meter. (Courtesy of LifeScan Inc., Milpitas, CA.)

Daily maintenance and quality control procedures must be performed and recorded before an ABGT analyzer is used. These procedures should be repeated if the unit is dropped, the battery is replaced, patient results are questioned, or any time functioning of the unit is questioned.

Bleeding Time Test

The **bleeding time (BT)** test (Fig. 12–7) detects platelet function disorders by testing platelet plug formation in the capillaries. It is used in diagnosing problems with hemostasis and as a presurgical screening test.

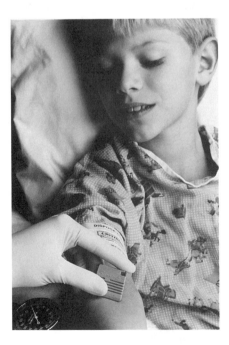

Figure 12–7 Bleeding time being performed. (Courtesy of International Technidyne, Edison, NJ.)

Bleeding time is the time required for bleeding to stop flowing from a standardized puncture in either the earlobe, finger, or the inner surface of the forearm. Prolonged bleeding can be caused by abnormal platelet function or the ingestion of aspirin or other salicylate-containing drugs within 2 weeks prior to the test. A number of other drugs such as ethanol, dextran, and streptokinase may also prolong bleeding time.

Bleeding time on the earlobe, originally described by Duke in 1910, is rarely ordered today. However, the test is still ordered by some facial surgeons who feel that the circulation of the ear more closely resembles that of the face.

The Duke bleeding time was modified by Ivy in 1941. The Ivy bleeding time is performed on the volar (inner) surface of the forearm using a blood pressure cuff to maintain constant pressure. The incision is made with a sterile lancet.

Most laboratories today use a modification of the Ivy procedure, controlling the width and depth of the incision by use of an automated incision device such as the Surgicutt (International Technidyne, Edison, NJ), Hemalet (Medprobe Laboratories, New York, NY), or Simplate II (Organon Teknika Corp., Durham, NC) (Fig. 12–8).

Materials needed for the the modified Ivy are:

1. Automated bleeding time device
2. Sphygmomanometer (blood pressure cuff)
3. Stopwatch, timer, or watch with sweep second hand
4. Filter paper (#1 watman or equivalent)
5. Alcohol prep pad
6. Butterfly bandage or steri-strip

TEST PROCEDURE
1. The patient is asked if he or she has taken aspirin or any other salicylate-containing drug within the last 2 weeks. The patient is advised of potential for scarring.
2. The patient's arm is supported on a steady surface.

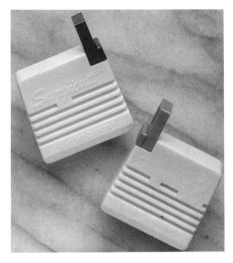

Figure 12–8 Surgicutt automated bleeding time device. (Courtesy of International Technidyne, Edison, NJ.)

3. An area of the inner (volar) surface of the forearm, distal to the antecubital area and devoid of surface veins scars or bruises, is selected for the procedure.
4. The area selected is cleaned with alcohol and allowed to dry.
5. The blood pressure cuff is placed around the arm.
6. The puncture device is removed from its package, being careful not to touch or rest the blade slot on any unsterile surface.
7. The blood pressure cuff is inflated to 40 mm Hg. (Time between inflation of the blood pressure cuff and making the incision should be between 30 and 60 seconds.) A pressure of 40 mm Hg *must* be maintained throughout the entire procedure.
8. The safety clip is removed and the puncture device is placed firmly on the forearm without pressing. A horizontal incision parallel to the antecubital crease is recommended.
9. The trigger is depressed while simultaneously starting the timer. The device is removed from the arm as soon as the blade has retracted.
10. The blood flow is blotted after 30 seconds by bringing the filter paper close to the incision and absorbing or "wicking" the blood onto the filter paper without touching the wound. (Touching the wound will disturb platelet plug formation.)
11. The blood flow is blotted every 30 seconds until the blood no longer stains the filter paper. At this point, the timer is stopped and the time recorded to the nearest 30 seconds. (Normal ranges are usually about 2 to 8 minutes, depending on the method used.
12. If bleeding persists after 30 minutes, the test is stopped and the time is recorded as 30 minutes or greater.
13. The blood pressure cuff is removed, the arm is cleaned, and a butterfly bandage is applied covered with an adhesive bandage. The patient is instructed not to remove either bandage for 24 hours.

The following are sources of error:

1. Disturbing platelet plug formation will increase the bleeding time.
2. Failure to maintain a pressure of 40 mm Hg will decrease the bleeding time.
3. Failure to start the timing as soon as the incision is made will decrease the bleeding time.

Capillary Blood Gases

Arterial punctures can be hazardous to infants and young children. For this reason, blood gas determinations on infants and young children are usually performed on arterialized skin puncture specimens. Arterialized skin puncture specimens for blood gas determinations are commonly called **capillary blood gases (CBGs)**.

Skin puncture blood is less desirable for blood gases not only because of its partial arterial composition, but also because it is temporarily exposed to air during collection, possibly altering blood gas results. Proper collection techniques are essential to minimize this exposure.

Skin puncture specimens for blood gas determinations are collected from the same sites as routine skin puncture specimens. Warming the site for 5 to 10 minutes prior to skin puncture helps arterialize the specimen.

TEST PROCEDURE

1. The site is selected, warmed, and skin puncture performed following routine skin puncture procedure.
2. After wiping away the first drop, blood is collected in special heparinized glass capillary tubes. Blood must be collected carefully so as to not introduce air bubbles into the capillary tube while obtaining the specimen. (Exposure of blood to air for as little as 10 seconds can cause erroneous results.)
3. After collecting the specimen, one end of the tube should be immediately sealed with clay or a special cap.
4. A small magnetic mixing bar or several magnetic "fleas" are then placed into the capillary tube.
5. The other end is quickly sealed and the blood mixed by running a magnet from one end of the tube to the other several times. (This procedure mixes the heparin with the specimen to prevent clotting.)
6. The specimen is labeled and immediately placed horizontally in a mixture of ice and water to prevent changes in pH and blood gas values.
7. The specimen should then be immediately transported to the lab.

Newborn Screening

Newborn screening is performed to test for the presence of genetic, or inherited, diseases, the most common of which is PKU or phenylketonuria (fen'il-kee'to-nu'ree-ah). Incidence of PKU in the United States is approximately 1 in 40,000 births. PKU results from a defect in the enzyme that converts the amino acid phenylalanine to tyrosine. PKU cannot be cured but it can be treated with a diet low in phenylalanine. If left untreated or not treated early, PKU can lead to brain damage and mental retardation. PKU testing requires the collection of two specimens, one shortly after the infant is born and the other when the infant is 10 to 15 days old. In many states PKU testing of newborns is required by law.

Blood samples for newborn screening are commonly collected by absorption onto a special filter paper which is part of the test requisition. The filter paper contains printed circles which must be filled with blood. The circles are filled by touching the paper to drops of blood obtained by heel puncture. A large drop of blood must be applied from only one side of the filter paper and blood must soak completely through to the other side. Blood should *not* be applied more than once or layered with successive drops in the same collection circle. The drops should not be smeared or touched. The phlebotomist must also be careful not to touch the filter paper with gloves or any other object or substance. The specimen should be allowed to air dry in an elevated horizontal position away from heat or sunlight and should not be stacked with other specimens.

Study & Review Questions

1. The ACT test is for:
   a. glucose measurements
   b. hemoglobin determinations
   c. monitoring heparin therapy
   d. screening for drugs

2. When drawing a blood alcohol, the arm cannot be prepped with:
   a. chlorhexidine
   b. isopropyl alcohol
   c. povidone iodine
   d. soap and water

3. Patient information that must be used for blood bank identification includes all of the following EXCEPT:
   a. full name
   b. hospital number
   c. phlebotomist's initials
   d. physician's name

4. The most important part of blood culture collection is:
   a. adequately filling two media vials
   b. cleansing the arm after the test is complete
   c. preparation of the site
   d. timing of the second set of cultures

5. Peak concentration may be defined as:
   a. the highest concentration during a dosing interval
   b. time when the amount of drug entering the body is equal to amount leaving
   c. the lowest concentration during a dosing interval
   d. the effectiveness of the drug

6. When performing a glucose tolerance test:
   a. all specimens are timed from the fasting draw
   b. a standard amount of glucose drink must be given to patients
   c. fasting blood sample is not part of the test
   d. blood and urine should be collected every half hour

7. The purpose of a bleeding time is to:
   a. check for diabetes mellitus
   b. screen for platelet and vascular function
   c. test a patient's vascular pressure
   d. look for abnormalities in drug metabolism

8. Which of the following tests uses an automated incision device to obtain blood for testing platelet integrity?
   a. bleeding time
   b. blood culture
   c. complete blood count
   d. therapeutic drug monitoring

Suggested Laboratory Activities

1. Practice performing an ACT on a fellow student using a manual or automated method.

2. Perform ABO typing.

3. Practice proper cleansing for blood culture collection on a fellow student.

4. Practice performing an ABGT on a fellow student.

5. Practice proper blood pressure cuff inflation for a bleeding time test. Practice performing the test, simulating the incision, and blotting steps.

BIBLIOGRAPHY AND SUGGESTED READINGS

Bishop ML, Duben-Engelkirk JL, Fody EP: *Clinical Chemistry: Principles, Procedures, Correlations* (2nd ed.). Philadelphia: JB Lippincott Company, 1992.

Davis B, Bishop ML, Mass D: *Clinical Laboratory Science: Strategies for Practice*. Philadelphia: JB Lippincott Company, 1989.

Fischbach F: *Laboratory Diagnostic Tests* (4th ed.). Philadelphia: JB Lippincott Company, 1992.

National Committee for Clinical Laboratory Standards, C30-T: *Ancillary Blood Testing in Acute and Chronic Care Facilities*. Villanova, PA: NCCLS Tentative Guideline, 1991.

Arterial Blood Gases

13

OBJECTIVES

On successful completion of this chapter, the reader should be able to:

1 State the primary reason for performing an arterial puncture procedure.
2 Identify the sites that can be used for arterial puncture, the criteria used for selection of the site, and the advantages and disadvantages of using each site.
3 Describe the need for collateral circulation and the tests used to determine the presence of collateral blood flow.
4 List equipment and supplies needed for arterial puncture.
5 Describe patient assessment and preparation procedures, including the administration of local anesthetic, prior to performing arterial puncture for arterial blood gases (ABGs).
6 Describe the proper performance of radial arterial blood gases.
7 List complications associated with arterial puncture.
8 List factors that may affect the integrity of the blood gas sample and the criteria for sample rejection.

KEY TERMS

Allen test
arterial blood gases
   (ABGs)
arteriospasm
brachial artery
collateral circulation
femoral artery
radial artery
steady state
thrombus formation

McCall: PHLEBOTOMY ESSENTIALS. © 1993
J. B. Lippincott Company.

INTRODUCTION

The composition of arterial blood is consistent throughout the body, while the composition of venous blood varies relative to the metabolic needs of the areas of the body it services. However, because arterial puncture is technically more difficult to perform and potentially more painful and hazardous to the patient than venipuncture, arterial specimens are not used for routine blood tests. The primary reason for performing arterial puncture is to obtain blood for evaluation of **arterial blood gases (ABGs)**. Arterial blood gas evaluation is used in the diagnosis and management of respiratory disease, and provides valuable information about a patient's oxygenation, ventilation, and acid–base balance.

Unlike venipuncture procedures, which have been performed for centuries, arterial puncture has a relatively recent history. The first recorded human arterial puncture was performed in 1912. Although the first arterial sample used for blood gas analysis was obtained in 1919, routine blood gas analysis did not occur until after 1953 with the introduction of the Clark platinum electrode used to measure oxygen pressure.

PERSONNEL WHO PERFORM ARTERIAL PUNCTURES

Paramedical personnel (health care workers other than physicians) who may be required to perform ABGs include nurses, medical technologists and technicians, respiratory therapists, emergency medical technicians, and level II phlebotomists. According to NCCLS, all personnel who perform ABG procedures should be certified by the health care institution after successfully completing training involving theory, demonstration of technique, observation of the actual procedure, and performance of arterial puncture under the supervision of qualified personnel.

SITE SELECTION

Several different sites can be used for arterial puncture. The criteria for site selection include the presence of collateral circulation, how large and accessible the artery is, and the type of tissue surrounding the puncture site. The site chosen should not be inflamed, irritated, edematous, or in close proximity to a wound. In addition, *never* select a site in a limb with an A-V shunt or fistula. The following are sites commonly chosen for arterial puncture.

The Radial Artery

The first choice and most common site used for arterial puncture is the **radial artery**, located in the thumb side of the wrist (Fig. 13–1). Although smaller than arteries in other sites, the radial artery is readily accessible in most patients.

ADVANTAGES OF RADIAL ARTERY PUNCTURE

The biggest advantage of using the radial artery is the presence of **collateral circulation**. Having collateral circulation means that the area is supplied with blood

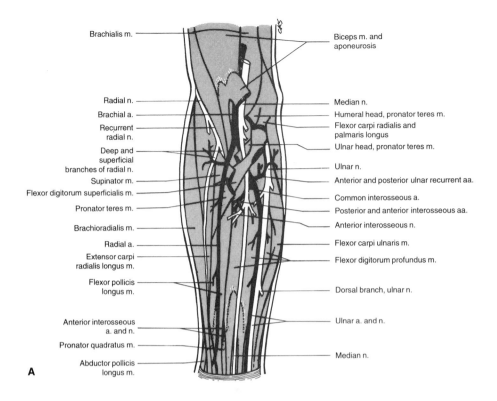

Brachialis m.

Biceps m. and
aponeurosis

Radial n.

Median n.

Brachial a.

Humeral head, pronator teres m.

Recurrent
radial n.

Flexor carpi radialis and
palmaris longus

Deep and
superficial
branches of radial n.

Ulnar head, pronator teres m.

Ulnar n.

Supinator m.

Anterior and posterior ulnar recurrent aa.

Flexor digitorum superficialis m.

Common interosseous a.

Pronator teres m.

Posterior and anterior interosseous aa.

Brachioradialis m.

Anterior interosseous n.

Radial a.

Flexor carpi ulnaris m.

Extensor carpi
radialis longus m.

Flexor digitorum profundus m.

Flexor pollicis
longus m.

Dorsal branch, ulnar n.

Anterior interosseous
a. and n.

Ulnar a. and n.

Pronator quadratus m.

Abductor pollicis
longus m.

Median n.

A

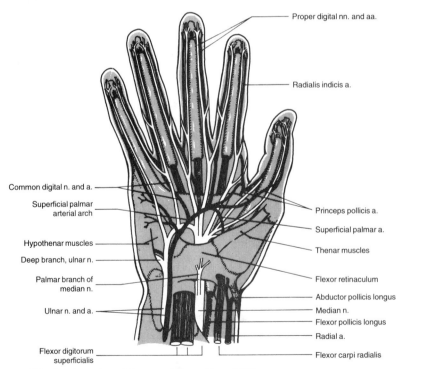

Proper digital nn. and aa.

Radialis indicis a.

Common digital n. and a.

Superficial palmar
arterial arch

Princeps pollicis a.

Superficial palmar a.

Hypothenar muscles

Thenar muscles

Deep branch, ulnar n.

Palmar branch of
median n.

Flexor retinaculum

Abductor pollicis longus

Ulnar n. and a.

Median n.

Flexor pollicis longus

Radial a.

Flexor digitorum
superficialis

Flexor carpi radialis

B

Figure 13–1   Arteries of the arm (*A*) and hand (*B*).

from more than one artery. Under normal circumstances, both the radial and the ulnar artery supply the hand with blood. If the radial artery were to be inadvertently damaged as a consequence of arterial puncture, the ulnar artery could supply blood to the hand. For this reason, the ulnar artery is *never* used for arterial puncture. If collateral circulation (which can be determined by an instrument called the Doppler ultrasonic flow indicator or by performing the Allen test described below) is absent, the radial artery should not be punctured.

Another advantage of using the radial artery is that there is less chance of hematoma formation following the procedure because the radial artery can be easily compressed over the ligaments and bones of the wrist.

DISADVANTAGES OF RADIAL ARTERY PUNCTURE

Disadvantages of using the radial artery include its small size, which requires considerable skill to puncture successfully, and the fact that it may be difficult or impossible to locate on patients with low cardiac output.

The Brachial Artery

The **brachial artery** (see Figure 13–1) is the second choice for arterial puncture. It is located in the medial anterior aspect of the antecubital fossa near the insertion of the biceps muscle.

ADVANTAGES OF BRACHIAL ARTERY PUNCTURE

Advantages of the brachial artery are that it is large and easy to palpate and puncture. The brachial artery has adequate collateral circulation, though not as much as the radial artery.

DISADVANTAGES OF BRACHIAL ARTERY PUNCTURE

There are several disadvantages to puncturing the brachial artery: 1) it is deeper than the radial artery; and 2) it lies close to a large vein (the basilic) and the median nerve, both of which may be inadvertently punctured.

Unlike the radial artery, there are no underlying ligaments or bone to support compression of the brachial artery, resulting in an increased risk of hematoma formation following the procedure.

The Femoral Artery

The **femoral artery** (Fig. 13–2) is the largest artery used for arterial puncture. It is located superficially in the groin, lateral to the pubis bone. Femoral puncture is performed primarily by physicians or specially trained emergency room personnel.

ADVANTAGES OF FEMORAL PUNCTURE

The femoral artery is large and easily palpated and punctured. It is sometimes the only site where arterial sampling is possible, especially on patients with low cardiac output.

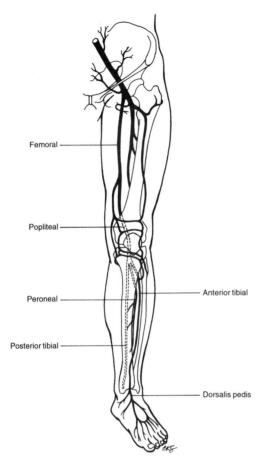

Figure 13–2   Arteries of the leg.

DISADVANTAGES OF FEMORAL PUNCTURE

Disadvantages of femoral arterial puncture include poor collateral circulation, increased risk of infection due to the location of the site, difficulty in achieving aseptic technique due to the presence of pubic hair, and the possibility of dislodging plaque build-up from the inner artery walls of older patients. In addition, the femoral artery lies close to the femoral vein, which may be inadvertently punctured.

Because of the numerous disadvantages associated with femoral puncture, it is used for obtaining ABGs only in emergency situations or when other sites are not available.

Other Sites

Other sites where arterial specimens may be obtained include the scalp and umbilical arteries in infants and the dorsalis pedis arteries of the adult. The phlebotomist is not trained to perform arterial punctures at these locations or to obtain specimens from cannulae, catheters, or other indwelling devices at these or any other locations.

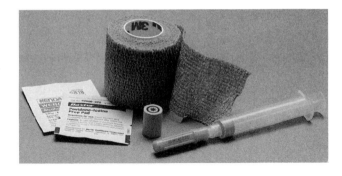

Figure 13–3 ABG equipment.

EQUIPMENT AND SUPPLIES

The following equipment and supplies are needed to collect arterial blood gas specimens (Fig. 13–3):

1. Antiseptic solution for cleaning the site: NCCLS recommended antiseptics are povidone iodine or chlorhexidine.
2. Anesthetic solution: local anesthetic solution such as 0.5% lidocaine may be used to numb the site.
3. Hypodermic needles: needle gauge and length depends on the site selected, the size of the artery selected, and the amount of blood needed. Needle sizes used include 20, 21, 22, 23, and 25 gauge, in lengths from $\frac{5}{8}$ to $1\frac{1}{2}$ inches. A 22-gauge, 1-inch needle is most commonly used for radial and brachial puncture; a $1\frac{1}{2}$-inch needle is used for femoral puncture.
4. Syringes: ABGs are collected in 1- to 5-ml syringes, depending on the amount of blood required. Special glass or plastic syringes are suitable. Heparin-containing syringes are available. Syringes most commonly contained in blood gas kits are prefilled with heparin and are designed to fill spontaneously on arterial penetration. A 1- or 2-ml plastic syringe with a 25- or 26-gauge needle, $\frac{1}{2}$ to $\frac{5}{8}$ inch long, is used for administration of anesthetic solution.
5. A small block of rubber or latex to insert the needle into following specimen collection.
6. Luer tip cap: a luer tip cap or other suitable device is used to cover the end of the syringe after needle removal to maintain anaerobic conditions within the specimen.
7. Lithium (or sodium) heparin: 1,000 units/ml heparin solution is used to prevent the specimen from clotting.
8. Coolant: a coolant capable of maintaining a temperature of 1°C to 5°C is necessary to slow the metabolism of white blood cells, which consume oxygen. A container of ice water is most commonly used. The container should be large enough to allow the complete immersion of the barrel of the collection syringe.
9. Gauze: 2 × 2 gauze squares are used to hold pressure over the site until bleeding has stopped.

10. Identification materials: labels and waterproof ink pens or markers are needed for specimen identification.
11. Oxygen analyzer: an oxygen measuring device is needed when patients are breathing oxygen-enriched gas mixtures instead of room air.

PREPARATION

General Instructions

As with any other test, a physician's order is needed before performing the test. The patient must then be properly identified and informed of the procedure. In addition, it should be determined if the patient is on anticoagulant therapy or is allergic to the anesthetic.

Steady State

A patient's temperature and breathing pattern, as well as the concentration of oxygen inhaled, affect the amount of oxygen and carbon dioxide in the blood. Ideally, a patient should have been in a stable or "**steady state**" (*ie,* no exercise, suctioning, or respirator changes) for at least 30 minutes prior to obtaining blood gases.

Administration of Local Anesthetics

Although administration of local anesthetics may be slightly painful, it minimizes discomfort associated with the arterial puncture and is reassuring to the patient, making him or her less fearful of the procedure. A fearful patient may respond by breath-holding, crying, or hyperventilation, all of which may affect blood gas results. Administration of anesthetic may be omitted for patients who have had the procedure before and are not apprehensive of it, and patients who are unconscious and do not respond to pain.

PROCEDURE FOR RADIAL ABGs

1. Receive physician's order and note the time ABGs are to be drawn.
2. Assemble and transport equipment to the patient's bedside.
3. Identify the patient and explain the procedure.
4. Record the patient's temperature, respiratory rate, and breathing mixture (*ie,* room air) on the laboratory slip.
5. Wash hands and put on gloves.
6. Prepare the ABG syringe with heparin, if applicable, in the following manner:
   a. Check the syringe for free movement and attach a 20-gauge needle.
   b. Clean the top of the heparin bottle with alcohol.
   c. Draw 0.5 to 1 ml heparin into the syringe. Pull back on the plunger, rotating it at the same time to wet the entire barrel of the syringe.
   d. With the syringe held vertically, expel the majority of the heparin.
   e. Replace the needle with another needle selected for arterial puncture.
7. Prepare the anesthetic syringe in the following manner: After cleaning the top of the

bottle, draw 0.5 ml of anesthetic (*ie*, lidocaine) into a 1-ml syringe using a 25-gauge needle. Carefully replace the cap and leave the syringe in a horizontal position.

8. Position the patient's arm with the palm facing up. A rolled towel may be placed under the wrist for support.

9. Assess collateral circulation using the **Allen test** (Fig. 13–4) or Doppler ultrasonic flow indicator.
   a. Allen Test
      1. Have the patient make a fist.
      2. Occlude both the radial and ulnar arteries of the patient at the same time with the middle and index fingers of both hands.
      3. While maintaining pressure, have the patient open and close the hand slowly several times. The hand should appear blanched or drained of color.
      4. Lower the patient's hand and release pressure on the ulnar artery.
      5. The patient's hand should flush pink within 15 seconds.
      6. Record the results on the request slip.
   b. *Positive Allen test:* The hand flushes pink within 15 seconds, indicating the presence of collateral circulation. If the Allen test is positive, proceed with step 10.
   c. *Negative Allen test:* The hand does not flush pink, indicating the inability of the ulnar artery to adequately supply blood to the hand and, therefore, the absence of collateral circulation. If the Allen test is negative, the radial artery should not be used and another site should be selected.

10. With the palm still facing up, have the patient flex the wrist at a 30 to 45 degree angle.

11. Locate the radial artery on the thumb side of the wrist, using the index and middle fingers of the left hand. Palpate the artery to determine its size, depth, and direction. *Never* use the thumb to palpate; it has a pulse, which can be misleading.

12. Prepare the site by cleaning first with alcohol and then with povidone iodine. Prep the fingers used to palpate in the same manner. Allow the site to dry, being careful not to touch it with any unsterile object.

13. If local anesthetic is to be administered, infiltrate the skin over the selected site, entering the skin with the needle at an approximately 10-degree angle with the skin. Pull back slightly on the plunger to be certain a vein was not inadvertently penetrated. If blood appears in the syringe, withdraw the syringe, prepare a fresh syringe and needle, and repeat the procedure in a slightly different spot. If no blood appears in the syringe, slowly expel the contents into the skin, forming a raised "wheal." Wait 1 to 2 minutes for the anesthetic to take effect before proceeding with arterial puncture. Note the lidocaine application on the request form.

14. Expel the remaining heparin from the ABG syringe. Be careful to not draw air into the syringe. Hold the syringe in the dominant hand as if holding a dart. Relocate the artery with the index finger of the opposite hand.

15. Warn the patient. Insert the needle bevel up, into the skin at a 45-degree angle (femoral ABGs require a 90-degree angle), approximately 5 to 10 mm distal to the finger locating the artery. Direct the needle away from the hand with the bevel facing the blood flow (Fig. 13–5).

16. Slowly advance the needle, directing it toward the artery just under the finger. When the artery is pierced, a "flash" of blood will appear in the hub of the needle.

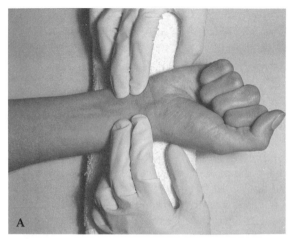

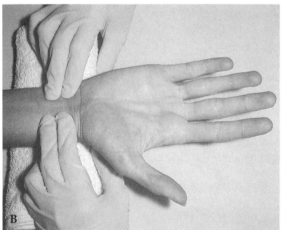

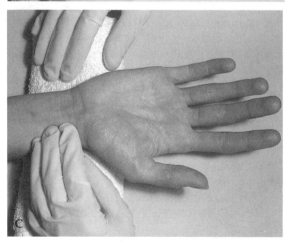

Figure 13-4 Allen test. *A.* Occluding the radial and ulnar arteries by pressing with fingertips while the patient makes a fist. *B.* Observing a blanched appearance to the hand when opened as both arteries are being pressed. *C.* Releasing the ulnar artery and checking for the patient's hand to flush with color.

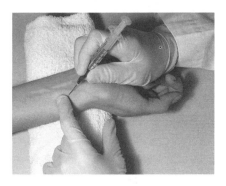

Figure 13–5   Performing an arterial puncture.

When the flash appears, stop advancing the needle. The blood will continue to "pump" into the syringe. Do not pull back on the plunger. Hold the syringe very steady until the desired amount of blood has been collected.

17. If the artery is missed, slowly withdraw the needle until just the bevel is under the skin. Redirect the needle into the artery as above. Do not probe; probing is painful and may lead to hematoma or thrombus formation and damage to the artery.

18. After the desired amount of blood has been obtained, quickly withdraw the needle, immediately placing a clean, dry gauze square over the site and applying firm pressure for a minimum of 5 minutes. Longer application of pressure is required for patients on anticoagulant therapy. *Never* allow the patient to apply the pressure; a patient may not apply pressure firmly enough.

19. With your free hand, immediately eject any air bubbles from the specimen and embed the needle into the small latex cube (Fig. 13–6).

20. Gently mix the specimen by inversion or rolling.

21. Remove the needle, being careful not to introduce bubbles into the syringe. Replace the needle with the luer cap.

22. Label the specimen and place in a bag or tray of crushed ice and water or other coolant.

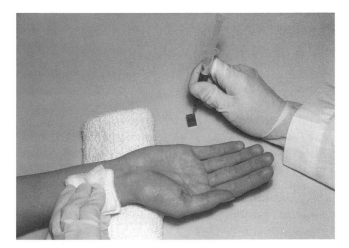

Figure 13–6   Embedding the point of the ABG needle in the latex cube while holding pressure over the patient's artery.

23. After pressure has been applied to the site for 5 minutes, check the site for swelling or bruising. If none is noted, clean the povidone iodine from the site with an alcohol prep pad, wait 2 minutes, and check the site again. Check the pulse distal to the site. If absent or faint, alert the patient's nurse to call the physician immediately. If the site appears normal, apply a pressure bandage.
24. Dispose of used equipment properly. Remove gloves and wash hands.
25. Thank the patient.
26. Deliver the specimen to the lab as soon as possible.

ABG COLLECTION FROM OTHER SITES

Collection of ABGs from other sites is similar to the procedure for radial ABGs. Because phlebotomists are not normally trained to collect specimens from these sites, specific procedures are not given in this text. Phlebotomists may, however, be asked to provide the equipment and assist in labeling and transporting specimens collected from these sites by others (*eg*, an emergency room physician).

COMPLICATIONS ASSOCIATED WITH ARTERIAL PUNCTURE

Discomfort: Some discomfort is generally associated with arterial puncture, even with use of a local anesthetic.

Infection: Proper antiseptic preparation of the site minimizes the chance of infection.

Hematoma: Because the blood is under considerable pressure in the arteries, blood is initially more apt to leak from an arterial puncture site than from a venipuncture site. However, arterial puncture sites tend to close more rapidly due to the elastic nature of the arterial wall. Because this elasticity tends to decrease with age, the probability of hematoma formation is greater in older patients or in patients receiving anticoagulant therapy.

Arteriospasm: Irritation caused by needle penetration of the artery muscle can cause a reflex constriction of the artery or arteriospasm. The condition is transitory but may make it difficult to obtain a specimen.

Thrombus formation: Injury to the intima of the artery can lead to clot (thrombus) formation. A large thrombus can obstruct the flow of blood and impair circulation.

SAMPLING ERRORS

A number of factors can affect the integrity of a blood gas sample and lead to erroneous results.

Air bubbles: If air bubbles are not immediately or completely expelled from the sample, oxygen from the air bubbles can diffuse into the sample and CO_2 can escape from the sample, changing the results.

Delay in cooling or analysis: Blood cells continue to consume oxygen and nutrients and produce acids and carbon dioxide at room temperature. If the specimen remains at room temperature for more than 5 to 10 minutes, the *pH*, blood gases, and glucose values will change. Cooling to between 1°C to 5°C slows this metabolism and helps stabilize the specimen. Processing the specimen as soon after obtaining as possible will ensure the most accurate results.

Obtaining a venous sample by mistake: Markedly inaccurate ABG values will result if a venous sample is obtained by mistake. Normal arterial blood is bright cherry red in color. However, it is sometimes difficult to distinguish between arterial and venous blood in poorly ventilated patients because their arterial blood may appear as dark as venous blood. The best way to be certain that a specimen is arterial is if the blood pulses into the syringe. In some instances, such as with low cardiac output, a specimen may need to be aspirated. In such cases, it is hard to be certain that the specimen is truly arterial.

Use of improper anticoagulant: Heparin is the acceptable anticoagulant for blood gases. Oxalates, EDTA, and citrates may alter results, especially *pH*.

Use of too much or too little anticoagulant: Too much heparin can cause erroneous results due to acidosis. Too little heparin can result in clotting of the specimen.

Improper mixing: Inadequate or delayed mixing of the sample can lead to clotting, making the sample unacceptable for testing. Undetected micro-clots can lead to erroneous results.

Improper syringe: Use of regular plastic syringes will lead to erroneous values. Use only plastic syringes especially designed for ABG procedures.

CRITERIA FOR SPECIMEN REJECTION

1. Inadequate volume of specimen for the test
2. Clotted specimen
3. Improper or absent labeling
4. Use of wrong syringe
5. Too long of a delay in delivering specimen to the lab
6. Specimen not on ice
7. Air bubbles in specimen

Study & Review Questions

1. Locations to obtain arterial blood gases are all of the following EXCEPT:
   a. brachial artery
   b. ulnar artery
   c. femoral artery
   d. radial artery

2. The equipment used for ABGs is all of the following EXCEPT:
   a. povidone iodine
   b. heparin
   c. syringe
   d. tourniquet

3. The purpose of the Allen test is to determine:
   a. blood pressure in the radial artery
   b. the presence of collateral circulation of
      the radial or ulnar arteries

   c. if the patient is absorbing oxygen
   d. the coagulation time of the arteries

4. The angle of needle insertion for radial ABGs is:
   a. 5 degrees
   b. 15 degrees

   c. 45 degrees
   d. 75 degrees

5. Which of the following complications are associated with ABGs?
   a. hematoma
   b. infection

   c. arteriospasm
   d. all of the above

6. Which of the following will NOT produce erroneous ABG values?
   a. cooling the specimen
   b. improper mixing

   c. air bubbles in the sample
   d. too much heparin

Suggested Laboratory Activities

1. Identify the common sites for ABG collection and locate the radial, ulnar, and brachial pulses.

2. Perform the Allen test on a fellow student.

3. Identify and assemble the proper equipment for ABG collection.

4. Practice ABG technique on an artificial arm with a simulated pulse.

5. Assemble equipment necessary to perform an ABG, practice filling a Natelson tube without bubbles and mixing it properly with fleas and magnet, using the procedure outlined in Chapter 12.

BIBLIOGRAPHY AND SUGGESTED READINGS

Burton GG, Hodgkin JE, Ward JJ: *Respiratory Care: A Guide to Clinical Practice* (3rd ed.). Philadelphia: JB Lippincott Company, 1991.

National Committee for Clinical Laboratory Standards, H11-A: *Percutaneous Collection of Arterial Blood for Laboratory Analysis.* Villanova, PA: NCCLS, April 1985.

Nonblood Specimens and Tests

14

OBJECTIVES

On successful completion of this chapter, the reader should be able to:

1 Describe nonblood specimen labeling and handling.
2 Name three types of urine collection procedures used by the laboratory and describe the differences.
3 List types of specimens other than blood received by the laboratory, and describe associated collection on testing procedures.
4 Describe the gastric analysis test and the role of the phlebotomist.
5 Name skin tests used to determine patient immune status and describe procedure.
6 Describe the purpose of the sweat chloride test.
7 Differentiate between the throat culture collection procedure and the nasopharyngeal culture procedure.

KEY TERMS

amniotic fluid
antibiotic susceptibility
body cavity fluids
cerebrospinal fluid (CSF)
clean catch
culture and sensitivity
erythema
induration
midstream collection
nasopharyngeal culture
occult blood
semen analysis
sweat chloride
urinary tract infection
 (UTI)

McCall: PHLEBOTOMY ESSENTIALS. © 1993
J. B. Lippincott Company.

NONBLOOD SPECIMEN LABELING AND HANDLING

Although blood is the type of specimen most frequently analyzed in the medical laboratory, other body fluids are also analyzed. The phlebotomist may be involved in obtaining the specimen (as in throat swab collection); test administration (as in sweat chloride collection); instruction (as in urine collection); or merely labeling and transporting specimens to the lab.

As a minimum, nonblood specimens should be labeled with the same identifying information as blood specimens. Most institutions also require information on the type and source of the specimen. Before accepting specimens collected by other hospital personnel, the phlebotomist must check to see that the specimen is properly labeled. Universal precautions should be observed when handling nonblood specimens as many body fluids are potentially infectious.

TYPES OF NONBLOOD SPECIMENS

Urine

Urine is perhaps the most commonly analyzed nonblood body fluid. Analysis of urine can aid in the diagnosis and treatment of urinary tract infections and the detection of metabolic disease. The type of specimen preferred for most urine studies is the first urine voided (passed naturally from the bladder or urinated) in the morning. This specimen is the most concentrated. Urine specimens collected at other times (random specimens) are acceptable, however. Collection of urine specimens on hospitalized patients is usually handled by nursing personnel. Outpatient urine specimen collection, however, is often handled by a phlebotomist who must be able to explain proper collection procedures to the patient. The phlebotomist must be able to explain procedures to the patient without causing the patient embarrassment. Oral instructions should be followed by written instructions, preferably with illustrations. The procedure for collecting a urine specimen depends on the type of test for which the specimen is intended. The most common types of urine tests and the procedure for collecting each test follow.

ROUTINE URINALYSIS

A routine urinalysis (UA) includes a physical, chemical, and microscopic analysis of the specimen. Physical characteristics noted include color, odor, transparency, and specific gravity or concentration. Chemical composition is most commonly determined by use of a plastic strip containing areas impregnated with reagents that test for the presence of bacteria, blood, white blood cells, protein, glucose, and other substances. The strip is dipped into the urine and compared to a color chart, usually found on the label of the reagent strip container. The manner in which the results are to be reported is indicated on the reagent label. Most results are reported using the terms *trace, 1+, 2+,* and so on, indicating the degree of a positive result, and *negative* (neg) when no reaction is noted. The strip is used once and discarded.

Urine components such as cells, crystals, and microorganisms can be seen by microscopic examination of a sample of urine sediment obtained through centrifugation. A measured portion of urine is centrifuged in a special plastic tube, after which the "supernatant"—or top portion of the specimen is discarded and a drop of the remaining sediment is placed on a glass slide, covered with a small square of glass called a coverslip, and examined under the microscope by either a laboratory technician or technologist.

Routine UA collection procedure.   Specimens for routine UA should be collected in clear, chemically clean containers with tight fitting lids. If a culture and sensitivity (C&S) is also ordered, the container should be sterile. Urine specimens should be transported to the lab promptly. Specimens for routine UA that cannot be transported or analyzed promptly can be held at room temperature and protected from light for up to 2 hours. Specimens held longer should be refrigerated. Specimens requiring a C&S and UA should be refrigerated if immediate processing is not possible.

A regular voided specimen is acceptable for routine UA. However, to avoid contamination of the specimen by genital secretions, pubic hair, and bacteria surrounding the urinary opening, the ideal procedure for collecting a specimen for routine UA is referred to as a **"midstream" collection**.

To collect a midstream specimen, the patient starts to void (urinate) into the toilet. The urine flow is interrupted and the specimen collected into the container (Fig. 14–1). The last of the urine flow is again voided into the toilet.

URINE CULTURE AND SENSITIVITY (C&S)

A urine **culture and sensitivity** may be requested on a patient with symptoms of **urinary tract infection (UTI)**. A urine culture is performed by transferring a measured portion of urine onto a special nutrient media. The media is incubated for 18 to 24 hours and then checked for bacterial growth. If an organism is identified, a sensitivity **(antibiotic susceptibility)** test is performed to determine which antibiotics will be effective against the organism.

Urine C&S collection procedures.   Urine for C&S should be collected in a sterile container following "**clean-catch**," midstream procedures.

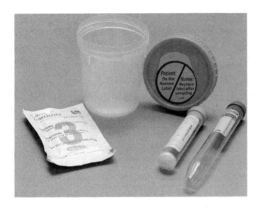

Figure   14–1   Becton-Dickinson   (Franklin Lakes, NJ) midstream urine collection sampling container and evacuated tubes for transporting and storing urine specimens.

Clean-catch procedures are necessary to ensure that the specimen is free of contaminating matter from the external genital areas. The phlebotomist must be able to explain the proper procedure to both male and female patients.

Clean-catch procedure for males:

1. Wash hands thoroughly.
2. Cleanse the end of the penis with sterile, soapy cotton balls (or special towelettes) beginning at the urethral opening and working away from it. (The foreskin of an uncircumcised male must first be retracted.)
3. Repeat the above procedure using two successive sterile, water-soaked cotton balls (or clean towelettes).
4. Void the first portion of urine into the toilet. Collect a portion of urine into the container, being careful not to touch the inside or lip of the container with the hands or any other portion of the body.
5. Void the remainder of urine into the toilet.
6. Cover the container with the sterile lid, touching only the *outside* surfaces of the lid and container.

Clean-catch procedure for females:

1. Stand in a squatting position over the toilet.
2. Separate the folds of skin around the urinary opening. Cleanse the area around the opening with special towelettes (or sterile, soapy cotton balls).
3. Cleanse area again with clean towelettes (or water-soaked sterile cotton balls), wiping from front to back.
4. Void the first portion of urine into the toilet. Collect a portion of urine into the container, being careful not to touch the inside or lip of the container with the hands or any other part of the body.
5. Void the remainder of urine into the toilet.
6. Cover the specimen with the lid provided, touching only *outside* surfaces of the lid and container.

Specimens for C&S and other microbiologic studies should be transported to the lab and processed immediately. If a delay in transportation or processing is unavoidable, the specimen should be refrigerated.

TIMED URINE TESTS

Some tests, such as tolerance tests, require the collection of urine at specific times. Tolerance test specimens are individual specimens collected at specific times. Other tests require urine to be collected and pooled over an extended period of time, most commonly 24 hours. The procedure for collecting a 24-hour urine specimen follows; it is similar for other extended time specimens.

TWENTY-FOUR HOUR URINE COLLECTION

A 24-hour urine specimen is collected in a large, clean, disposable, wide-mouth container capable of holding several liters. Some 24-hour specimens require the addition of a preservative prior to collection. Others should simply be kept refrigerated throughout collection. Whether or not a preservative is required can be determined by consulting the laboratory procedure manual. In addition to standard patient identification, the container label must state the length of time of the collection (*ie*, 12 hours, 24 hours, and so on), and what preservative has been added, including any precautions associated with the preservative.

PROCEDURE
1. The best time to begin a 24-hour collection is when the patient wakes in the morning. Have the patient void as usual into the toilet and note the time and date on the container label.
2. Collect all urine voided for the next 24-hour period. Refrigerate the specimen throughout the collection period, unless urate testing is ordered. This can be accomplished by placing the specimen container in an ice chest in the bathtub, for example.
3. To prevent contamination of the specimen by fecal material, it is best that the patient urinate *before* having a bowel movement, rather than after.
4. At the end of the 24-hour period, instruct the patient to void one last time and add this specimen to the collection container.
5. Put the container in a portable cooler and transport the specimen to the lab as soon as possible.

Amniotic Fluid

Amniotic fluid is the fluid that surrounds a fetus in the uterus. Normal amniotic fluid is a clear, almost colorless-to-pale yellow liquid. It is obtained by inserting a needle through the mother's abdominal wall into the uterus and extracting the fluid from within the membrane (amniotic sac) that contains the fetus. Amniotic fluid is normally sterile and must be delivered to the lab in a sterile container.

The specimen should *not* be opened and should be kept at room temperature (not refrigerated), so that the cells will grow more quickly when cultured.

Amniotic fluid is most commonly obtained at approximately 16 weeks' gestation and is used for fetal chromosome analysis to detect genetic defects and to assess fetal development. Cells from the fluid are removed and grown in culture for 3 to 7 days before the chromosomes are analyzed. The fluid portion of the specimen is analyzed for alpha-fetoprotein (AFP) after the cell culture is set up. Alpha-fetoprotein is an antigen normally present in the human fetus; it is also found in maternal serum. The test is performed to see if the fetus is developing normally. (Elevated serum levels of AFP in males and nonpregnant females is a sign of certain cancers.) Normal values for fetal AFP are different for each week of gestation. For this reason, the gestational age of the fetus must be included on the specimen label along with the identification information.

Amniotic fluid is also commonly obtained on or near the patient's due date to determine the lung maturity of the fetus. This type of test is often ordered "stat" when the fetus is in distress.

Stool

Examination of stool (feces) is helpful in the evaluation of gastrointestinal disorders. Stool specimens can be evaluated for the presence of fat and intestinal parasites (ova & parasite; O & P); cultured to detect the presence of pathogenic bacteria; and tested for the presence of **occult** (hidden) **blood** by means of the guaiac test.

Stool specimens are normally collected in clean, dry containers. They should be covered and sent to the laboratory immediately. Most specimens, especially those for detection of parasites should be kept at body temperature (37°C). Twenty-four, forty-eight or seventy-two hour stool collections for fat and urobilinogen are collected in large gallon containers similar to paint cans, and refrigerated throughout the collection period.

Stool specimens for occult blood collected by outpatients are most often collected on special test cards such as Hematest (Miles Inc., Elkhart, IN), and Hemacult (Smith-Kline Diagnostics, San Jose, CA). The patient is usually instructed to have a meat-free diet for 3 days prior to the test. Patients are then instructed to collect separate specimens for 3 successive days. Cards can be mailed or brought to the lab after collection.

Semen

Semen analysis is used to assess fertility and also to determine the effectiveness of sterilization following vasectomy. Semen specimens are collected in sterile containers, similar to sterile urine containers. A semen specimen should *never* be collected in a condom. Condoms often contain substances which kill sperm (spermicides) and invalidate test results. Semen specimens should be kept warm and delivered to the lab immediately.

Gastric Secretions

Gastric secretions are obtained by aspiration via a tube passed through the mouth or nose, down the throat, and into the stomach. Gastric specimens are collected in sterile containers.

Cerebrospinal Fluid

Cerebrospinal fluid (CSF) is a clear, colorless liquid that circulates within the cavities surrounding the brain and spinal cord. Cerebrospinal fluid has many of the same constituents as blood plasma. Cerebrospinal fluid specimens are obtained by a physician, most often through lumbar (spinal) puncture. Common tests performed on CSF include cell counts, glucose, chloride, and total protein. An increased white blood cell count in CSF is most often associated with bacterial or viral meningitis. Cerebrospinal fluid is generally collected in three special sterile tubes labeled in correct order of collection. Laboratory protocol dictates which tests are to be performed on each particular tube, unless indicated by the physician. Cerebrospinal fluid should be delivered to the lab "stat" and analysis started immediately.

Other Body Cavity Fluids

In addition to CSF and amniotic fluid, there are various other **body cavity fluids**, which are commonly collected and analyzed. All body cavity fluids are collected in sterile containers. The type of fluid should be indicated on the specimen label. Commonly analyzed body fluids include the following:

Synovial fluid: aspirated from joint cavities
Pleural fluid: aspirated from the pleural cavity, which surrounds the lungs
Peritoneal fluid: aspirated from the abdominal cavity
Pericardial fluid: aspirated from the cavity surrounding the heart

Tissue Specimens

Tissue specimens from biopsies may also be sent to the laboratory for processing. Most tissue specimens arrive at the laboratory in formalin or another suitable solution and need only to be accessioned and sent to the proper department. However, with more biopsies being performed in outpatient situations, a phlebotomist in specimen processing may encounter specimens that have not yet been put into the proper solution. It is important for the phlebotomist to check the procedure manual to determine the proper handling for any unfamiliar specimen (*eg*, tissues for genetic analysis should *not* be put in formalin). Improper handling may ruin a specimen for a procedure that is, in all probability, expensive as well as uncomfortable for the patient and not easily repeated.

SPECIAL NONBLOOD TESTS

Gastric Analysis

A gastric analysis test examines gastric acid secretions to determine gastric function in terms of stomach acid production. A basal tube gastric analysis involves aspirating gastric secretions via a tube passed through the mouth and throat (oropharynx) or nose and throat (nasopharynx) into the stomach, following a period of fasting. This determines acidity prior to stimulation. Once this basal sample of gastric secretions has been collected, a gastric stimulant, most commonly histamine or pentagastrin, is administered intravenously and several more samples are collected at timed intervals. The role of the phlebotomist in gastric analysis testing is to assist in labeling specimens and to draw specimens for serum gastrin determinations.

Skin Tests

Although nurses most commonly perform skin testing, some laboratories do offer skin testing services, especially for outpatients. In addition, skin tests, especially for tuberculosis, are a part of employee screening programs. Skin tests do not involve the withdrawal of blood or body fluid, rather they most often involve the intradermal (within the skin) injection of an allergenic substance (substance that causes an allergic reaction) to determine if the patient has come in contact with a specific allergen (most commonly an antigen) and developed antibodies against it. Many disease-producing microorganisms will function as allergens and stimulate an antibody response in susceptible individuals. Intradermal skin testing can be performed to determine a patient's immune status associated with such microorganisms.

Common skin tests include:

Tuberculin test: also called PPD test because of the "purified protein derivative" used in testing for tuberculosis. It is probably the most common skin test.

Schick test: for susceptibility to diphtheria

Dick test: for susceptibility to scarlet fever (caused by *Streptococcus pyogenes*)

Histoplasmosis (Histo) test: for past or present infection by the fungus *Histoplasma capsulatum*

Coccidioidomycosis (Cocci) test: for an infectious fungus disease caused by *Coccidioides immitis*

TEST PROCEDURE

1. A site is selected on the volar surface of the forearm below the antecubital crease. Areas with scars, bruises, burns, rashes, excessive hair, or superficial veins should be avoided.
2. The site is cleaned with 70% isopropyl alcohol and allowed to dry.
3. 0.1 ml of diluted antigen is drawn into a tuberculin syringe using a $\frac{1}{2}$ inch, 26- to 27-gauge needle.
4. The arm is held in the same manner as for venipuncture and the skin is stretched taut with the thumb.
5. The syringe is held at a very low angle (approximately 20 degrees) and the needle is slipped just under the skin.
6. The syringe plunger is pulled back slightly to make certain a vein has not been entered.
7. The contents of the syringe are slowly expelled, creating a distinct, pale elevation of the skin 6 to 10 mm in diameter, commonly called a "bleb" or "wheal."
8. The needle is removed and the arm remains extended until the site has time to close. Pressure is *not* applied to the site nor is a bandage applied. (A bandage might absorb the fluid and also cause irritation, distorting the test results.)
9. The reaction is read in 24 to 72 hours, depending on the antigen tested.

Interpretation of the test is based on the presence or absence of **erythema** (redness) and/or **induration** (hardness).

Negative: area (zone) of erythema and induration less than 5 mm in diameter (most tests)
Doubtful: area of erythema and induration between 5 and 9 mm in diameter.
Positive: area of erythema and induration 10 mm or greater in diameter.

Sweat Chloride

Evaluation of the chloride content in sweat is used in the diagnosis of cystic fibrosis, primarily in children and adolescents under the age 20. Cystic fibrosis is caused by a disorder of the exocrine glands, affecting primarily the lungs, liver, and pancreas. Children with cystic fibrosis have abnormally high levels (two to five times normal) of chloride in their sweat.

Lab evaluation of sweat chloride involves transporting pilocarpine (a sweat-stimulating drug) into the skin by means of electrical stimulation (iontophoresis) from electrodes placed on the skin. Sweat is collected, weighed to determine the volume, and analyzed for chloride content.

Throat Culture Collection

Throat cultures are most often collected to aid in the diagnosis of streptococcal (strep) infections. Throat specimens on inpatients are usually collected by nursing staff. However, it is not uncommon for a phlebotomist to be asked to collect a throat culture specimen on an outpatient. A throat culture is collected in the following manner, using a culture kit (Fig. 14–2) containing a sterile polyester-tipped swab, covered transport tube, and transport media:

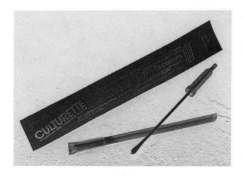

Figure 14–2 Culturette transfer media for culturing microorganisms. (Courtesy of Becton Dickinson Microbiology Systems.)

1. The patient is instructed to open his or her mouth wide while tilting the head back.
2. A small flashlight or other light source can be directed at the back of the throat to illuminate areas of inflammation. A tongue blade can be used to depress the tongue.
3. Both tonsils, the back of the throat, and any areas of ulceration, exudation, or inflammation should be brushed with the sterile swab, being careful not to touch the swab to the lips or tongue.
4. Because proper collection will often cause the patient to gag or cough, the phlebotomist may wish to wear a mask or stand to the side of the patient.
5. Once the specimen is collected, the swab is placed back into the collector tube. The ampule containing transport media is then crushed between the fingers and the swab embedded in the released media. The cover is secured and the specimen is properly labeled and sent to the lab immediately.

Nasopharyngeal Culture Collection

Nasopharyngeal (NP) cultures are often collected to detect the presence of the microorganisms that cause diphtheria, meningitis, whooping cough, and pneumonia. Nasopharyngeal specimens are collected using a sterile Dacron or cotton-tipped flexible wire swab. The swab is inserted gently into the nose and passed into the nasopharynx. Once in the nasopharynx, the swab is gently rotated, then carefully removed, placed into transport media, labeled, and transported to the lab.

Study & Review Questions

1. Additional information necessary on a nonblood specimen label is:
   a. party to be charged
   b. patient's age
   c. physician
   d. type of sample

2. Which type of urine specimen is used to detect the presence of infection?
   a. 2-hour
   b. 24-hour
   c. midstream
   d. clean catch

3. Which nonblood specimen is most frequently analyzed in the lab?
   a. CSF
   b. pleural fluid
   c. synovial fluid
   d. urine

4. Which of the following fluids comes from the lung area?
   - a. gastric
   - b. peritoneal
   - c. pleural
   - d. synovial

5. Skin tests are performed to determine if a patient has ever come in contact with:
   - a. an anticoagulant in an evacuated tube
   - b. a particular antigen that causes antibody production
   - c. an antihistamine-producing cell
   - d. antibodies used in blood testing

6. The most common skin test performed today is:
   - a. Cocci
   - b. Dick
   - c. Shick
   - d. PPD

Suggested Laboratory Activities

1. Assemble, identify, and label the various containers used for nonblood specimens.
2. Practice proper patient instruction for 24-hour urine collection by role-playing with a fellow student.
3. Perform a reagent strip analysis on an actual urine specimen.
4. Practice skin test procedure on a fellow student, substituting sterile saline for the antigen.
5. Collect a specimen for a throat culture from a fellow student.

BIBLIOGRAPHY AND SUGGESTED READINGS

Fischbach F: *Laboratory Diagnostic Tests* (4th ed.). Philadelphia: JB Lippincott Company, 1992.

National Committee for Clinical Laboratory Standards, GP8-P: *Collection and Transportation of Single Collection Urine Specimens*. Villanova, PA: NCCLS Proposed Guideline, 1985.

National Committee for Clinical Laboratory Standards, GP13-P: *Collection and Preservation of Timed Urine Specimens*. Villanova, PA: NCCLS Proposed Guideline, 1987.

National Committee for Clinical Laboratory Standards, GP16-P: *Routine Urinalysis*. Villanova, PA: NCCLS Proposed Guideline, 1991.

Quality Assurance and Specimen Handling

15

"The test results are only as good as the specimen collected."
—Unknown

OBJECTIVES

On successful completion of this chapter, the reader should be able to:

1 Define quality assurance and state the reasons for implementing such a program.
2 List the components of a quality assurance program and the 10 steps in monitoring and evaluating the process.
3 Define indicators and threshold as used in monitoring quality assurance programs.
4 Differentiate quality control from quality assurance.
5 List areas in phlebotomy subject to quality control.
6 Describe special handling methods for specimens that are light- or temperature-sensitive.
7 Identify steps for processing blood samples.
8 Describe the criteria for specimen rejection.

KEY TERMS

aerosol
aliquot
analyte
central processing
centrifugation
floor book
JCAHO
procedure manual
quality assurance (QA)
quality control (QC)
QA indicator
reference log book
threshold values
total quality management

McCall: PHLEBOTOMY ESSENTIALS. © 1993
J. B. Lippincott Company.

QUALITY ASSURANCE IN PHLEBOTOMY

As members of the health care team, phlebotomists should understand the significance of their role in the clinical laboratory and the reasons for assuring quality in their area of responsibility. Laboratory testing is an important part of patient diagnosis and medical care. Doctors rely on test results and assume the process is carefully monitored from beginning to end with the quality remaining consistent. That is why it becomes necessary to set policies and procedures to ensure that sample procurement and handling are accurate. These established policies and procedures fall under an overall process called **quality assurance (QA)**.

Reasons for Participating

The Joint Commission on Accreditation of Healthcare Organizations (JCAHO) requires hospital-wide participation in a QA program. Such a program is necessary to meet government agency requirements and to receive third party payer reimbursement. However, the overriding reason for participating in a QA program is to ensure that the highest quality medical care is delivered to the patient. **JCAHO** is a voluntary, nongovernmental agency charged with, among other things, establishing standards for the operation of hospitals and other health-related facilities and services. By 1994, JCAHO will require hospitals to have an institution-wide total quality management/continuous quality improvement (TQM/CQI) plan in place. This means all departments of a health care facility must institute ongoing evaluations of their activities and *customer expectations.*

Total quality management is based on a continuous effort to identify opportunities for improving services. The four principles involved in TQM are: 1) customer satisfaction; 2) constant improvement; 3) employee participation; and 4) orientation to process. TQM stresses constant, gradual change in operation through improvement and innovation. To make long-term improvements, every employee must continually participate in a QA program and remain flexible when change, which is inevitable, occurs.

Quality Assurance Defined

Quality assurance is defined as a program that guarantees quality patient care by tracking the outcomes through scheduled audits in which areas of the hospital look at the appropriateness, applicability, and timeliness of patient care. Guidelines are developed for all processes used and when these guidelines are formally adopted, they become the QA program.

In the late 1980s, JCAHO developed a 10-step monitoring and evaluation process, which can be used for assessing the appropriateness of care (Box 15–1).

Identifying QA Indicators

One of the most important aspects of setting up a QA evaluation process is establishing indicators that monitor all aspects of patient care. These **QA indicators** must be measurable, well-defined, specific, objective, and clearly related to an important

---

Box 15–1. The Ten-Step Monitoring and Evaluation Process

1. Assign responsibility
2. Delineate scope of care
3. Identify important aspects of care
4. Identify indicators related to these aspects of care
5. Establish thresholds for evaluation related to the indicators
6. Collect and organize data
7. Evaluate care when thresholds are reached
8. Take actions to improve care
9. Assess the effectiveness of actions and document improvements
10. Communicate relevant information to the organization-wide quality assurance program.

---

aspect of care. Indicators can measure quality, adequacy, accuracy, timeliness, effectiveness, customer satisfaction, and so on. They are designed to look at areas of care that tend to cause problems. For example, an indicator on the quality assessment form shown in Figure 15–1 might be stated as follows: "Blood cultures will not exceed the national contamination rate." A contamination rate that increased beyond a preestablished threshold listed on the form would signify a problem.

Establishing Thresholds and Evaluating Data

Established levels or **threshold values** must be set for all clinical indicators. If this level of acceptable practice is reached, it may trigger intensive evaluation of the practice to see if there is an actual problem that needs to be corrected to improve care. During the evaluation phase, data is collected and organized. Data sources could include such information as patient records, lab results, incident reports, patient satisfaction reports, and direct patient observation. A corrective action plan is established if the data identifies a problem or opportunity for improvement. The plan identifies who and what will change and when that change is expected to occur. Even when the problem appears to be corrected, monitoring and evaluation continue, to ensure that care is consistent and that quality continually improves.

Quality Control Defined

Quality control (QC), a component of a QA program, is a form of procedure control. This means that if standards are followed during a given procedure, results will be consistent. Phlebotomy QC involves checking all the operational procedures to make certain they are performed correctly. In the phlebotomy area of the lab, it is the responsibility of the phlebotomy supervisor to oversee QA and ensure that standards are being met. It is the phlebotomist's responsibility to meet those standards at all times.

QUALITY ASSESSMENT AND IMPROVEMENT TRACKING
CONFIDENTIAL A.R.S. 36-445

#: _____

STANDARD OF CARE/SERVICE: _____

DEPARTMENTS/POPULATION: LABORATORY-MICROBIOLOGY/ALL PATIENTS
DATA SOURCE(S): CULTURE WORKCARDS
DATA COLLECTOR: P. BABINA

IMPORTANT ASPECT OF CARE/SERVICE: LAB SVCS/BLOOD COLLECTION
FREQUENCY REVIEW: 3 MONTHS   100% SAMPLE
METHODOLOGY: RETROSPECITVE
TYPE: OUTCOME
PERSON RESPONSIBLE FOR:
SIGNATURES:
DIRECTOR: _____
MEDICAL DIRECTOR: _____
VICE PRESIDENT/ADMINISTRATOR: _____
DATA ORGANIZATION: P. BABINA
ACTION PLAN: J. BENSON
FOLLOW-UP: J. BENSON
DATE MONITOR BEGAN: 1990
FOLLOW-UP: 3RD QTR.

INDICATORS		THRESHOLD			CRITICAL ANALYSIS/ EVALUATION	ACTION PLAN
		EXP.	ACT.	PREV.		
Blood culture contamination rate will not exceed 3% from three groups of drawing personnel.		3%			N= 1385 Patient Centered Care draws: Nursing line draws are out of compliance but show improvement from January to March.	A communication has gone out to Nursing reminding to follow established protocols for drawing. Microbiology has implemented new protocol disallowing a line draw unless two consecutive venipunctures have failed or protocol is overridden by physician order. PCC tecs have been reinserviced on proper technique.
LAB	JAN	3%	1.1%			
	FEB		1.8%			
	MAR		1.7%			
PCC	JAN	3%	5.6%			
	FEB		4.8%			
	MAR		3.2%			
LINE DRAWS	JAN	3%	5.6%			
	FEB		7.9%			
	MAR		0.0%			

QICONFID

Figure 15-1 TQM form.

AREAS IN PHLEBOTOMY THAT ARE SUBJECT TO QUALITY CONTROL

Patient Preparation Procedures

Quality control actually starts before the specimen has been collected. To obtain an acceptable specimen, the patient must be prepared properly. In a hospital setting, this means the nurse should check a book of instruction called the **floor book** (or user manual) that has been given to the unit by the laboratory. The floor book describes preparation of the patient and special instructions for specimen collection. More concise versions of this book are designed to be carried by the phlebotomist to assist in answering questions concerning unusual requests. Being informed and updated regularly helps the phlebotomist and specimen processors be well versed in testing protocol and better able to answer inquiries.

Specimen Collection Procedures

IDENTIFICATION

Identification (as described in Chapter 9) is the most important aspect of specimen collection. Methods are being continually improved to ensure error-free patient ID. Examples are the barcode readers and accompanying labels (Fig. 15–2), and the new Bloodloc Safety System (Novatek Medical Inc., Greenwich, CT) described in Chapter 12.

LABELING

Labeling must be exact. Labeling requirements, as outlined in Chapter 10, should be strictly followed. Inaccuracies, such as transposed letters or missing information, will result in the specimen being discarded. With computer labels, the phlebotomist may be assured of correctly printed patient information, but this correct label must still be placed on the right patient's specimen.

TECHNIQUE

Proper phlebotomy techniques must be carefully taught by a professional who understands the importance of following standard procedures, as well as the reasons for using certain equipment or techniques. No matter how experienced phlebotomists may be, a periodic review of their techniques is necessary for QA.

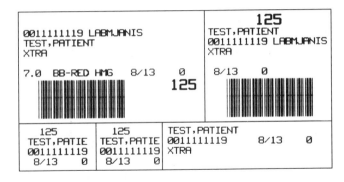

Figure 15–2 Barcode label.

COLLECTION PRIORITIES

Specimen collection priorities must be stressed. The importance of knowing how to recognize which specimen request is the most critical can save the patient unnecessary medication or additional testing. It may even shorten the patient's stay in the hospital, because in many instances therapy is based on test values that are assumed to have been collected at the proper time.

CONTINUING EDUCATION

Continuing education is mandatory to maintain proficiency and consistency. It is usually the responsibility of the supervisor to present new methods and procedural changes to the phlebotomists on a regular basis. The phlebotomists must read laboratory literature to keep abreast of current practices outside of their institution. Continuing education is also necessary for phlebotomy recertification by agencies such as the National Certification Agency (NCA).

Documentation

Different means of recording QA have been developed to document problems and assist in standardizing procedures in the collection and handling of laboratory specimens.

THE FLOOR BOOK

As mentioned previously, the floor book is an example of a QA document. It typically contains in chart form the type of specimen and minimum amount needed, special handling of the specimen, what the reference values for the test are, the days testing is available, and the normal turnaround time (TAT) (Fig. 15–3).

REFERENCE LABORATORY BOOK

Test orders that cannot be performed on site are sent to another laboratory called a reference laboratory. All samples sent out must be logged in a **reference log book**, which includes patient ID, date sent out, and date the results were received. There is also a reference manual that explains how to handle specimens to be sent to a reference laboratory and how to complete requisitions and package samples for mailing or transporting.

LABORATORY PROCEDURAL MANUAL

A complete procedure manual must be made available to all employees of the laboratory. Accrediting agencies such as JCAHO demand that this manual be updated annually. A procedural manual states in detail the step-by-step procedure for each test or practice performed in the laboratory. It will also include updates to procedures and notification of these changes to the nursing staff (Fig. 15–4).

QUALITY ASSURANCE FORMS

Accreditation standards for agencies, such as JCAHO, require the facility to show documentation on all quality control checks.

		HEMATOLOGY		
TEST	TEST VOLUME	VACUTAINER COLOR (TOP)	NORMAL VALUES	NOTES
APT test	1 mL feces or gastric fluid	Plastic container	Negative	Suitable for grossly bloody specimens only
Acid hemolysin	0.4 mL (RBC) 2.5 mL serum	Lavender and red (non-Corvac)	0%–5%	
Acid phosphatase stain	3 mL blood	Green		
Acid phosphatase w/tartrate stain (TRAP)	3 mL blood	Green		
Alpha naphthol butyrate stain (nonspecific esterase)	3 mL blood	Green		
Blood smear— differential	.03 mL blood	Lavender or fingerstick	See individual tests	See page 27
Body fluid HCT	1 mL	Fluid		
Bone marrow				Schedule in advance (4-6281)
Coulter count	1 mL blood	Lavender or lavender microtainer	See page 27	Includes WBC, RBC, HGB, HCT, MCV, MCH, MCHC
Differential	1 mL blood	Lavender		See page 28
Eosinophil count	0.5 mL blood	Lavender	150–350 /uL	See page 28
Epinephrine/ endotoxin stimulation test				Schedule in advance (4-6281). Consultation form required
Fetal hemoglobin (APT) (qualitative)	1 mL feces or gastric fluid	Red Non-Corvac or plastic container	Negative	Suitable for grossly bloody specimens only

Figure 15–3   User manual. (Courtesy of University Medical Center, Tucson, AZ.)

Equipment check forms.   Special forms for recording equipment checks on tube additives, vacuum strength, and expiration dates are available for verification of new lot numbers. Refrigerator temperatures, which must be recorded daily, are often the responsibility of the phlebotomist. Control checks on the centrifuge require periodically documenting the tachometer readings and maintenance performed.

Internal reports.   Confidential incident reports (Fig. 15–5) or specimen collection reports must be filled out when a problem occurs. These forms identify the prob-

Good Samaritan
Regional Medical Center
1111 East McDowell Road
P.O. Box 2989
Phoenix, AZ 85062
602.239.2000

SAMARITAN

DATE: February 23, 1990

TO: Nursing Staff

FROM: Michael A. Saubolle, Ph.D.
                Director, Microbiology Section
                Department of Pathology

SUBJECT: Blood Cultures

The Laboratory will introduce three new blood culture bottles (BACTEC NR 26 PLUS [aerobic], 27 PLUS [anaerobic] and a pediatric PED PLUS [aerobic] bottle) beginning in early March, 1990. These new bottles have been adapted to already contain resins for inactivation of antibiotics and to utilize higher-volume 10 ml blood inocula (rather than the older 5 ml blood draws). The pediatric PED PLUS bottle also contains resins, but accepts blood inocula of less than 5 mls and may be used when larger volumes are unobtainable.

Both types of bottles have been studied in multicenter evaluations and have been found to increase isolation rates of diagnostically significant blood isolates by up to 31 percent. They are especially useful for culturing blood from patients already receiving antibiotics and for increased recognition of pathogens such as staphylococcus, enterics and pseudomonas.

Recommended routine blood culture schedules are listed below:

Adult: each culture is defined as a draw from a single venipuncture and normally
            includes 2 bottles:

            a NR 26 PLUS (aerobic) bottle - 10 ml of blood inoculated
            a NR 27 PLUS (anaerobic) bottle - 10 ml of blood inoculated

Pediatric: each culture is defined the same as for adults and normally includes 2
            bottles:

            a PED PLUS bottle (aerobic; 1 ml minimum and 5 ml maximum inoculum)

            a NR 7A* (anaerobic; 1 ml minimum and 5 ml maximum inoculum)

            * If less than 2 ml of blood is available, the PED PLUS aerobic bottle should be
            inoculated first; the anerobic 7A bottle may be skipped if additional blood is not
            available.

            Note: the PED PLUS and 7A bottle combinations can also be used for culture of
            blood from adults in whom adequate volumes of blood are not obtainable.

Figure 15-4   Procedure manual update and notification to nursing staff.

LINCOLN

EMPLOYEE ACTION RECORD

_____   _____   _____
      EMPLOYEE NAME   DEPARTMENT   DATE

THIS FORM IS USED TO DOCUMENT DISCUSSION CONCERNING A COMMENDATION OR ACTION TAKEN TO IMPROVE INAPPROPRIATE PERFORMANCE BY AN EMPLOYEE. THE INFORMATION CONTAINED ON THIS FORM WILL BE INCLUDED IN THE EMPLOYEE'S PERSONNEL FILE.

( ) COMMENDATION   ( ) CORRECTIVE ACTION   ( ) OTHER

I. DESCRIBE ISSUE OR INCIDENT (PROVIDE DATES AND DETAILS):

_____
_____
_____
_____
_____

II. PROVIDE SPECIFIC INFORMATION DISCUSSED WITH THE EMPLOYEE REGARDING SECTION I.:

_____
_____
_____
_____
_____

III. PROVIDE THE AGREED-UPON PLAN FOR TAKING CORRECTIVE ACTION, IF APPLICABLE (INCLUDE THE DATE FOR FOLLOW-UP AND NEXT ACTION TO BE TAKEN, IF NECESSARY):

_____
_____
_____
_____
_____

IV. EMPLOYEE COMMENTS:

_____
_____
_____
_____
_____

(ATTACH ADDITIONAL SHEETS IF NECESSARY)

_____   DATE   EMPLOYEE (SIGNATURE DOES NOT NECESSARILY   DATE
DEPARTMENT MANAGER   INDICATE AGREEMENT.)

_____   DATE
VICE PRESIDENT

WHITE COPY: HUMAN RESOURCES   YELLOW COPY: DIRECTOR   PINK COPY: EMPLOYEE

JCL: 04/91 N-115

Figure 15–5   Incident form. (Courtesy of John C. Lincoln Hospital, Phoenix, AZ.)

lem, state the consequence, and describe the corrective action. For example, an incident form would be filled out when a tube of blood was mislabeled.

SPECIMEN HANDLING

Proper handling throughout the collection process, including transportation and processing, is important for maintaining specimen integrity, as well as protecting the phlebotomist and others from accidental exposure to potentially infectious substances. Improper handling can render the most skillfully obtained specimen useless. However, the fact that a specimen has been improperly handled is not always easily discerned. To assure delivery of a quality specimen for analysis, it is imperative that the phlebotomist be adequately instructed in this area. Policies and procedures should be established to cover specimen handling techniques. In addition, all specimens should be handled according to the Universal Precautions guidelines written by the Centers for Disease Control and Prevention (CDC) and enforced by the Occupational Safety and Health Administration (OSHA) as outlined in Chapter 6.

General Guidelines

Proper handling of specimens begins with the initiation of the test request and includes patient preparation, equipment selection, and "order of draw," all covered earlier in the text. This chapter deals with proper handling after the specimen is collected until it is delivered to the proper lab area for testing.

Handling of Routine Specimens

ADDITIVE TUBE MIXING

Additive tubes should be gently inverted five to ten times as soon as they are drawn. Vigorous mixing may cause hemolysis and should be avoided. Potassium, magnesium, and certain enzyme tests are examples of tests that cannot be performed on hemolyzed specimens. Inadequate mixing may cause anticoagulant tubes to form clots, which may lead to erroneous results, especially for hematology studies. Inadequate mixing of gel separation tubes may prevent the additive from functioning properly and clotting may be incomplete. Nonadditive tubes do not require mixing.

TRANSPORTING SPECIMENS

Blood specimen tubes should be transported carefully so as not to break them or cause the blood to hemolyze. Tubes should be transported with the stopper up, which aids in clot formation of serum tubes, reduces agitation which can cause hemolysis, and prevents contact of the contents of the tube with the tube stopper. Blood in contact with tube stoppers can be a source of contamination to the specimen and contributes to **aerosol** (a fine mist of the specimen) formation during stopper removal.

Non-blood specimens should be transported in leak-proof containers with adequately secured lids. Specimens transported through pneumatic tube systems should be protected from shock and sealed in zipper type plastic bags to contain spills.

Specimens arriving in the lab from off-site locations should be transported as above.

In addition, special care should be taken to protect specimens from the effects of extreme heat or cold.

Specimens Requiring Special Handling

SPECIMENS REQUIRING PROTECTION FROM LIGHT
Some test components are broken down in the presence of light, causing falsely decreased values. The most common of these is bilirubin. Other tests sensitive to light include Vitamin B12, carotene, serum and red cell folate, and urine specimens for porphyrins. Specimens can be easily protected from light by wrapping them in aluminum foil. Light-inhibiting, amber-colored microcollection containers are available for collecting bilirubin specimens from infants.

SPECIMENS THAT NEED TO BE CHILLED
Certain metabolic processes continue even after a specimen is drawn. Chilling the specimen slows down this process. Specimens requiring chilling should be completely immersed in a slurry of crushed ice and water. Large cubes of ice without water added prevent adequate cooling of the entire specimen. Placing the specimen in contact with a solid piece of ice can cause parts of the specimen to freeze, causing hemolysis and possible breakdown of analytes. ("**Analyte**" is a general term for a substance undergoing analysis.) Examples of specimens requiring chilling are blood gases, ammonia, lactic acid, renin, protime, partial thromboplastin time, and glucagon tests.

SPECIMENS THAT NEED TO BE KEPT WARM
Some specimens need to be transported at or near body temperature of 37°C. Two examples are specimens for cold agglutinins and cryofibrinogen. Specimens that need to be kept warm should be transported in a 37°C heat block.

Some tests such as the activated clotting time require that the tube for the test be kept warm prior to drawing the blood for the test. Manual activated clotting time (ACT) methods require the tube to be kept in a 37°C heat block during performance of the test, as well as prior to the test procedure. Automated methods such as the Hemochron system (International Technidyne, Edison, NJ) have a warming unit, which is part of the machine.

Time Constraints for Specimen Delivery
All specimens should be transported to the lab promptly. Ideally, routine blood specimens should arrive at the lab within 45 minutes of collection and be centrifuged within 1 hour.

Guidelines recommended by NCCLS document H18-A set the *maximum* time limit for separating serum and plasma from the cells at *2 hours* from time of collection. Less time is recommended for certain specimens, particularly potassium and cortisol specimens.

Prompt processing of specimens is easily achievable with an on-site lab as in a hospital setting but is not always possible when specimens come to the lab from off-site locations, such as doctors' offices.

Specimens that cannot reach their destination within the allotted time period should

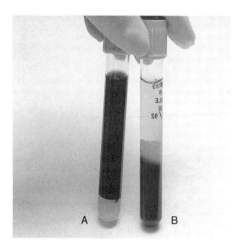

Figure 15–6   Hemogard SSTs: A. prior to being centrifuged; B. after being centrifuged.

be allowed to clot (if applicable), should be centrifuged, and the serum or plasma separated and transferred to a suitable container for transport.

If the specimens are drawn in serum separator tubes (SSTs) or plasma separator tubes (PSTs), they need only be centrifuged once they have clotted if applicable (Fig. 15–6). Once centrifuged, the separator gel will prevent glycolysis for up to 24 hours. Applicable temperature requirements should be maintained until the specimens reach the laboratory.

Exceptions to the Preceding Guidelines

Specimens for glucose determination drawn in sodium fluoride tubes are stable for 24 hours at room temperature and up to 48 hours when refrigerated at 2°C to 8°C. Hematology tests drawn in lavender stopper (EDTA) tubes are performed on whole blood specimens and should never be centrifuged. EDTA specimens are stable for 24 hours. However, it is important to make smears from EDTA blood within 1 hour of collection to preserve the integrity of the blood cells and prevent artifact formation, due to prolonged contact with the anticoagulant. "Stat" or "medical emergency" specimens take priority over all other specimens and should be transported and processed immediately.

SPECIMEN PROCESSING

OSHA Regulations

OSHA regulations require the wearing of protective equipment when processing specimens. Protective equipment includes gloves, fully buttoned lab coats or aprons, and protective face gear such as masks and goggles with side shields or chin-length face shields.

Central Processing

Most laboratories have a specific area commonly called **central processing** (or specimen processing) where all specimens are received and prepared for testing. Here, the specimens are identified, logged (accessioned), and sorted by department and type of processing required. Specimens not requiring centrifugation such as urine and hematology specimens are then distributed to the proper department. Specimens for tests requiring serum or plasma must be centrifuged and labels generated for the tubes (aliquot tubes) that will receive the serum or plasma obtained through centrifugation. "**Aliquot**" is defined as a portion of the specimen used for testing. Great care must be taken to match each specimen with the corresponding aliquot tube.

PLASMA SPECIMENS

Specimens for tests performed on plasma are collected in tubes containing anticoagulants and may be centrifuged immediately.

SERUM SPECIMENS

Specimens for tests performed on serum must be completely clotted prior to **centrifugation**. If clotting is not complete when the specimen is centrifuged, the resultant serum may clot and interfere with the performance of the test. Complete clotting normally takes around 30 to 45 minutes at room temperature. Specimens from patients on anticoagulant medication, such as heparin or dicumarol, as well as specimens from patients with high white blood counts may take longer to clot. Chilled specimens may also take longer to clot. Serum separator tubes and other tubes containing clot-activating glass particles usually clot within 15 minutes. Thrombin tubes normally clot in 5 minutes. There are also several commercially available clot activators, which can be added to the tube after the specimen is drawn. Proper mixing of clot activator tubes will ensure proper clotting.

SPECIAL PRECAUTIONS FOR HANDLING SPECIMENS

Stoppers should remain on tubes awaiting centrifugation. Removing the stopper from a specimen can cause a loss of CO_2 and an increase in pH, leading to inaccurate results for tests such as pH, CO_2, and acid phosphatase. Leaving tubes unstoppered also exposes the specimen to possible contamination and evaporation. Evaporation leads to inaccurate results due to concentration of analytes. Sources of contamination can be as simple as a drop of sweat, which interferes with electrolyte results, or powder from gloves, which may interfere with calcium determinations (some powder contains calcium).

CENTRIFUGATION

Specimen preparation. Once blood specimens have fully clotted, they may be centrifuged. A centrifuge is a machine that spins the blood at high revolutions per minute (rpms) using the centrifugal force created to separate cells and plasma/serum (Fig. 15–7). Tubes should remain stoppered during centrifugation to prevent contamination, evaporation, aerosol formation, and changes in pH.

If stoppers are removed to add separation devices, the tubes should be restoppered or covered with suitable closure devices. Use of applicator sticks to "rim" or release a clot is a potential source of contamination, as well as hemolysis, and is no longer recommended.

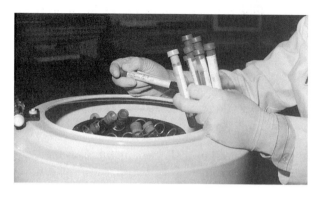

Figure 15–7 Specimen processor loading a centrifuge.

Centrifuge operation. It is imperative that tubes with equal volume of specimen be placed opposite one another or "balanced" in the centrifuge. An unbalanced centrifuge may break specimen tubes, ruin the specimen, and cause the contents to form aerosols. The lid to the centrifuge should remain closed during operation and should not be opened until the machine has come to a complete stop without using the brake.

Centrifuge each tube only once. Repeated centrifugation can cause hemolysis and analyte deterioration. In addition, once the serum or plasma has been removed, the volume ratio of plasma to cells changes. Because a centrifuge generates heat during operation, specimens requiring chilling should be processed in a temperature-controlled centrifuge.

STOPPER REMOVAL

The stopper has to be removed to obtain the serum or plasma needed for testing. Stoppers can be removed using commercially available stopper removal devices. When not using such a device, the stoppers should first be covered with a 4 × 4 gauze or tissue to catch any aerosol that may be released. The stopper should be pulled straight up and off and not "popped." Becton Dickinson has begun to manufacture a new type of stopper on their evacuated tubes. This new tube stopper system called Hemogard (Becton Dickinson, Franklin Lakes, NJ) (Fig. 15–8) is designed to protect personnel from splatters and aerosols caused by blood that remains on the stopper or around the outer rim of the tube.

ALIQUOT PREPARATION

Serum or plasma should be transferred into the aliquot tubes using disposable pipets, such as the FILTER SAMPLE Dispense Filter (Porex Medical, Fairburn, GA). Pouring specimens into aliquot tubes is not recommended due to the possibility of aerosol formation or splashing. OSHA's Final Rule for Occupational Exposure to Bloodborne Pathogens, published in December 1991, states, "All procedures involving blood or potentially infectious materials shall be performed in such a manner as to minimize splashing, spraying, splattering, and generation of droplets of these substances." The Dispense Filter by Porex is considered such an engineering control because it is a closed system. After serum has been aspirated through the filtration system into the sampler, it can then be dispensed through a restricted opening in the transfer pipet into instrumentation or aliquot tubes if more than one department needs the same specimen (Fig. 15–9).

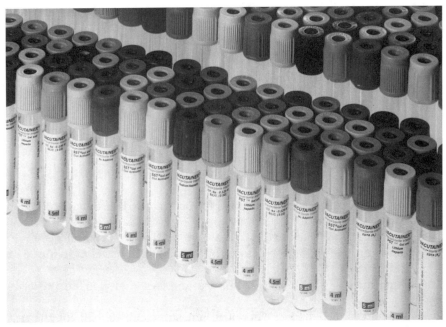

Figure 15–8 Examples of hemogard closure tubes. (Courtesy of Becton Dickinson, Franklin Lakes, NJ.)

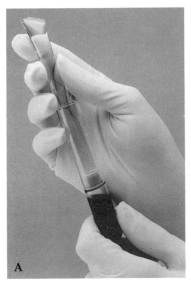

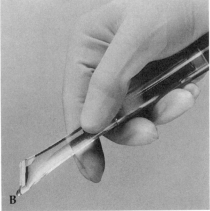

Figure 15–9 *A.* Transferring serum into a self-contained Porex FILTER SAMPLE Dispense Filter; *B.* Dispensing serum from a filter sampler. (Courtesy of Porex Medical, Fairburn, GA.)

After the serum or plasma is transferred into the aliquot tube, the tube is covered or capped and dispatched to the proper department.

CRITERIA FOR SPECIMEN REJECTION

Specimens received by the lab may be rejected for analysis for the following reasons:

1. Inadequate, inaccurate, or missing specimen identification (*eg*, a urine specimen that is not labeled).
2. Additive tubes containing an inadequate volume of blood (*eg*, a partially filled coagulation tube).
3. Hemolysis (*eg*, a hemolyzed specimen intended for potassium determination).
4. Wrong tube (*eg*, a CBC collected in a red top tube).
5. Outdated tube (*eg*, a CBC collected in a tube that expired the week before).
6. Improper handling (*eg*, a lavender top drawn for a CBC which has clots in it due to improper mixing).
7. Contaminated specimen (*eg*, a urine for culture and sensitivity in an unsterile container).
8. Insufficient specimen, referred to as "quantity not sufficient" (QNS) for the test ordered (*eg*, a specimen for an erythrocyte sedimentation rate submitted in a microtainer).

Study & Review Questions

1. Quality assurance programs are necessary:
   a. because they are mandated by regulatory agencies
   b. to receive third party reimbursements
   c. for careful monitoring of patient care
   d. all of the above

2. What book describes in detail the steps to follow for specimen collection?
   a. floor book
   b. OSHA safety manual
   c. policy manual
   d. quality control procedures

3. Which of the following specimens should be protected from light?
   a. BUN
   b. CBC
   c. bilirubin
   d. glucose

4. The machine used to separate the serum or plasma from blood samples is called a/an:
   a. Autolet
   b. centrifuge
   c. glucometer
   d. hemostat

5. After obtaining a renin level, the blood must be transported:
   a. as "stat"
   b. away from light
   c. in ice
   d. at body temperature

6. Contamination with perspiration could falsely elevate which blood levels?
   a. amylase
   b. calcium
   c. chloride
   d. magnesium

7. Which of the following instances would NOT be a reason for a specimen to be rejected for analysis?
   a. a CBC collected in a lavender top tube
   b. a specimen for potassium determination that is hemolyzed
   c. a protime specimen in a partially filled tube
   d. a specimen lacking an identification label

8. According to NCCLS guidelines, serum for analysis should not be in contact with cells for longer than:
   a. 30 minutes
   b. 60 minutes
   c. 90 minutes
   d. 120 minutes

Suggested Laboratory Activities

1. Perform quality control checks on various lab equipment (*ie*, check tube volume).
2. Make a list of the types of specimens requiring special handling and practice proper specimen handling techniques.
3. Practice proper specimen processing techniques. Balance tubes in a centrifuge, demonstrate proper tube stopper removal, and prepare an aliquot tube.
4. Identify examples of specimens that may be rejected for testing.
5. Look up special handling instructions found in a reference laboratory manual for a list of "send out" tests supplied by your instructor.

BIBLIOGRAPHY AND SUGGESTED READINGS

Bishop ML, Duben-Engelkirk JL, Fody EP: *Clinical Chemistry: Principles, Procedures, Correlations* (2nd ed.). Philadelphia: JB Lippincott Company, 1992.

"Continuous Quality Improvement: An Analysis of the New Paradigm in Healthcare," *Journal for Healthcare Quality*, Sept/Oct 1992.

JCAHO: Accreditation Manual for Hospitals. Oakbrook Terrace, IL, 1991.

National Committee for Clinical Laboratory Standards, H5-A2: *Procedures for the Domestic Handling and Transport of Diagnostic Specimens and Etiologic Agents* (2nd ed.). Villanova, PA: NCCLS, January 1985.

National Committee for Clinical Laboratory Standards, H18-A: *Procedures for the Handling and Processing of Blood Specimens.* Villanova, PA: NCCLS, December 1991.

National Committee for Clinical Laboratory Standards, H21-A: *Collection, Transport and Preparation of Blood Specimens for Coagulation Testing and Performance of Coagulation Assays.* Villanova, PA: NCCLS, December 1986.

Communication and Computers

16

OBJECTIVES

On successful completion of this chapter, the reader should be able to:

1　Describe the basic concepts of communication.
2　List barriers in verbal communication.
3　Define kinesics and proxemics and describe how they affect the communication process.
4　Describe the importance of appearance for phlebotomists.
5　Define active listening.
6　Contrast normal communication with health communication.
7　Describe proper telephone protocol in the laboratory.
8　List four classifications of computers.
9　Define three processes used by all computers.
10　List components of a computer and the types of applications used.
11　Describe frequently used programs in a laboratory information system.
12　Trace the flow of specimens through the laboratory with an information management system.
13　List information found on a computer label.

McCall: PHLEBOTOMY ESSENTIALS. © 1993
J. B. Lippincott Company.

INTRODUCTION

Phlebotomy is both a technical and people-oriented profession. Almost everyone agrees that the phlebotomist is the public relations agent for the laboratory. Often patients' perception of a health care facility is derived from the employees they deal with on a one-to-one basis, such as a phlebotomist. Favorable impressions are based on professionals properly responding to patient needs. This occurs when there is good communication between the two.

COMMUNICATION DEFINED

Communication is a skill. Defined as the means by which information is exchanged or transmitted, communication is one of the most important processes that take place in the health care system. This dynamic process involves three components: verbal skills, the ability to listen, and nonverbal skills.

Verbal Communication

Expression through the spoken word is the most obvious form of communication. It involves a sender (speaker), a receiver (listener), and, when complete, a process called feedback. It is through feedback that the receiver is given the chance to correct any miscommunication caused by personal bias or **barriers**. Normal human behavior sets up many barriers to accurate verbal communication. These biases or personalized filters are major obstructions to hearing and understanding what has been said. Examples of listening barriers are language limitations, culture diversity, emotions, age, and physical disabilities, such as hearing loss. To handle emotional barriers, such as an angry patient, the phlebotomist may try asking irrelevant questions, which will distract the patient from the procedure long enough to complete their venipuncture. To avoid creating suspicion and distrust for patients from other countries, the phlebotomist should be aware of cultural differences and avoid cliches that could be misunderstood.

Listening

It is more difficult to communicate than to speak because effective communication requires that the listener participate. It is always a two-way process. The ordinary person can absorb verbal messages at about 500 to 600 words a minute. The average speaking rate is only 125 to 150 words a minute. Therefore, the listener, in order not to be distracted, must use the extra time for active listening. Active listening means taking positive steps through feedback to ensure that the listener interprets what the speaker is saying exactly as the speaker intended it. Listening forms the foundation for interpersonal communication, and is particularly valuable in building rapport with patients. Phlebotomists should learn to watch the speaker, as well as listen, because nonverbal communication affects what they hear.

Nonverbal Communication

It has been stated that 80% of language is unspoken. Unlike verbal communication formed from words which are one-dimensional, nonverbal communication is multidimensional and involves the following elements.

KINESICS

Nonverbal communication is also called "**kinesics**," the study of body motion or language, such as facial expression, gestures, and eye contact. Body language, most often done unintentionally, plays a major role in communication because it is continuous and more reliable than verbal communication. In fact, if the verbal and nonverbal messages do not match, it is called a "**kinesic slip**." When this happens, it has been shown that people tend to trust what they see rather than what they hear. As a health professional, the phlebotomist can learn much about patients feelings by observing nonverbal communication, which seldom lies. The patient's face often tells the health professional what the patient will not reveal verbally. For instance, when a patient is anxious, nonverbal signs seen may be tight eyebrows, intense frown, narrowed eyes, or downcast mouth. Researchers have found that certain facial appearances, such as a smile, are universal expressions of emotions. Worldwide, we all recognize the meaning of a smile; however, strong cultural customs often dictate when it is used.

To communicate effectively with a person, it is important to establish good eye contact. A patient or client may be made to feel unimportant and more like an object rather a human being if no eye contact is established.

PROXEMICS

Proxemics is defined as the study of an individual's concept and use of space. This subtle but powerful part of nonverbal communication should be understood in order to relate better to the patient in a health care facility. Every individual carries around him or her an invisible "bubble" defined as personal territory. The size of this bubble depends on the individual's needs at the time. Naturally occurring territorial zones fall into four categories: intimate distance (a radius of 1 to 18 inches); personal distance (a radius of $\frac{1}{2}$ to 4 feet); social distance (a radius of 4 to 12 feet); and the public distance (a radius of more than 12 feet). These "zones of comfort" are very obvious in human interaction. Entering personal or intimate zones is necessary in the health care setting, and if not carefully handled, the patient may feel threatened, insecure, or out of control. Fortunately, it is becoming more acceptable in certain instances to merge into each others' bubbles without discomfort, such as in the relationships of teacher and student or health care worker and client.

APPEARANCE

Most health care facilities have dress codes because it is understood that appearance makes a statement. The impression the phlebotomist makes as he or she approaches the patient sets the stage for future interaction. The right image portrays a trustworthy professional. A phlebotomist's physical appearance should communicate cleanliness and confidence. Lab coats, which completely cover the clothing underneath, should be clean and pressed. Shoes should be conservative and polished. Close attention should be paid to personal hygiene. Bathing and the use of deodorant should be a daily routine. Strong perfumes or colognes should be avoided. Hair and nails should be clean and look natural. Hair, if long, must be pulled back and fingernails should be short. Phlebotomists who deal with patients that are ill or irritable will find a confident and professional appearance helpful in doing their job.

TOUCH

Touching can take a variety of forms and convey many different meanings. For example, "accidental touching" could happen in a crowded elevator. "Social touching" could take place when a person grabs the arm of another while giving advice. "Therapeutic touching" is designed to aid in healing. This special type of nonverbal communication is a very important ingredient to the well-being of humans, and even more so in DIS-eased (not at ease) humans. Numerous studies have shown the importance of touch in healing.

Because medicine is a contact profession, touching privileges are granted and expected of health care workers under certain circumstances. Whether a patient or health care provider is comfortable with touching is based on his or her cultural background. Because touch is a necessary part of the phlebotomy procedure, it is important for a phlebotomist to realize that often patients are much more aware of your touch than you are of theirs; there may even be a risk of the patient questioning the appropriateness. Generally speaking, patients respond favorably when touch portrays a thoughtful expression of caring.

HEALTH COMMUNICATION

It is not easy for the patient or the health professional to face disease and suffering every day. For many patients, being ill is a terrifying experience; having blood drawn only contributes to their anxiety. Patients reach out for comfort and reassurance through conversation. Consequently, a phlebotomist must understand the unusual aspects of "health communication" and its importance in comforting the patient.

Communication between the health professional and patient is more complicated than normal interaction. Not only is it often emotionally charged but it also involves, in many instances, other people who are very close to the patient and tend to be very critical of the way the patient is handled. Recognizing some of the elements in health communication, such as empathy, control, trust, and confirmation, will aid the phlebotomist in successfully interacting with the patient.

Elements in Health Communication

EMPATHY

Defined as identifying with the feeling or thoughts of another person, **empathy** is an essential element in interpersonal relations. It involves putting yourself in the place of another and attempting to feel like that person. Some people have a high degree of empathy. Empathetic health professionals help patients handle the stress of being in a health care institution. A health professional should communicate true feeling to the patient and seek to understand that person's point of view. When a health professional recognizes the needs of the patient and allows the patient to express his or her emotions, this helps to validate the patient's feelings and gives the patient a very necessary sense of control.

CONTROL

An important element of health communication is control. Feeling in control is essential to an individual's sense of well-being. People like to think that they can influence the way they respond to happenings in their lives. Many patients perceive themselves as unable to cope physically or mentally with events in a hospital because it is a foreign environment that makes them feel fearful and powerless.

Consequently, a hospital is one of the few places where an individual gives up control over most of the personal tasks he or she normally performs. Due to this loss of control, the response of the patient is typically to act angry, which characterizes them as a "bad patient," or to act extremely codependent and agreeable, which characterizes them as a "good patient." Phlebotomists should be aware of the patient's feelings and learn ways to restore a sense of control to the patient. For instance, when a patient says he or she is not going to have blood drawn, a phlebotomist should allow him or her to express that statement of control and even agree with the patient. If patients are allowed to exert that right, they will often change their minds and let the phlebotomist do the procedure because then it is their decision. Sharing control with the patient may be difficult and often time-consuming, but awareness of the patient's needs is important. To allow patients more control of their environment actually improves their health.

TRUST

Another variable in the process of communication is trust. Trust, as defined in the health care setting, is the unquestioning belief by the patient that health professionals are performing their job responsibilities as well as they possibly can. As is true with most professionals, health care workers tend to emphasize their technical expertise while completely ignoring the elements of interpersonal communication, which are essential to a trusting relationship with the patient. Having blood drawn is just one of the situations in which the consumer must trust the health professional. Developing trust takes time and phlebotomists spend very little time with each patient. Consequently, during this limited interaction, they must do everything possible to win the patient's confidence by consistently appearing knowledgeable, honest, and sincere.

CONFIRMATION

Confirmation deals with how health care workers respond to the patient during daily interactions. Confirming responses help the patient feel recognized as a person in spite of the depersonalizing environment of a hospital. The right response contributes to reducing the feelings of separation from loved ones in a health care facility. Confirming responses such as, "Yes, I hear what you are saying" make the patient feel that his or her opinion is appreciated. For more clarification and a way of drawing out the patient's true feelings, the health provider could say, "Tell me more or help me to understand what you mean."

A familiar communication problem occurring in busy hospitals is the labeling of patients, such as "the burn case in room 322." This form of communication is dehumanizing and is a subtle way of "disconfirming" patients. Each patient needs to be accepted as a unique individual with special needs. For instance, if the results of a blood test take a long time to get put on the chart, a patient may feel uncertainty and needlessly think something is very wrong. The patient needs confirmation by a caring health professional that the delay is a standard procedure and is expected for that particular test.

In summary, by recognizing the previously mentioned elements of empathy, control, trust, and confirmation the phlebotomist can enhance communication with patients and assist in their recovery. Understanding these communication elements will help when used with other means of communication such as the telephone.

TELEPHONE COMMUNICATION

The telephone is presently a fundamental part of communication. It is used 24 hours a day in the laboratory. To phlebotomists or laboratory clerks, it becomes just another source of stress, bringing additional work and uninvited demands on their time. The constant ringing and interruption to the workflow often causes laboratory personnel to overlook the effect their style of telephone communication has on the caller. To maintain a professional image, proper protocol should be reviewed by every person given the responsibility of answering the phone. They should be taught how to answer, put someone on hold, or transfer calls properly.

Proper Telephone Protocol

To increase good communication, the following telephone techniques should be followed:

1. *Answer promptly.* If the phone is allowed to ring too many times, the caller assumes the people working in the laboratory are inefficient or insensitive. When answering the phone, state your name and your department.
2. *Be helpful.* When a phone rings, it is because someone needs something. Due to the nature of the health care business, the caller may be emotional and need a calm, pleasant voice on the other end to answer the request. To assist callers and facilitate the conversation, ask how you can assist them. Keep your statements and answers simple and to the point to avoid confusion.
3. *Prioritize calls.* Callers should be informed if they are interrupting another call. Always ask if they can be put on hold in case it is an emergency that must be handled immediately. Coordinating several calls takes an organized person. Disconnecting a caller while transferring irritates the caller.
4. *Be prepared to record information.* Documentation is necessary when answering the phone at work to ensure that accurate information is transmitted to the necessary person. Have a pencil and paper close to the phone. Listen carefully, which means clarifying, restating, and summarizing the information received.
5. *Know the laboratory policies.* People who answer the telephone need to be familiar with the policies to avoid misinformation. Answers should be consistent. This helps establish the laboratory's credibility, as a caller's perception of the lab involves more than obtaining accurate test results.
6. *Diffuse hostile situations.* Some callers are angry because of lost results or errors in billing. Agreeing with a hostile caller will immediately diffuse the caller. After the caller has been calmed down, an inquiry can be handled.

7. *Try to assist everyone.* It is possible to assist callers and show concern even if you are not actually answering their questions. Validate their request by giving a response that tells the inquirer something can be done. Sincere interest in the caller will enhance communication and contribute to the good reputation of the laboratory.

Today, in many areas of health care, the telephone, a valued communication tool, is being replaced in part with a more objective and efficient means of communication: the computer.

COMMUNICATION THROUGH COMPUTERS

As computers become more common in the United States, their use as an essential tool for the health care community increases. The computer can now be found throughout all departments of a hospital, group practice, or health maintenance organization. Various types of hardware and software are being used to manage **data** (information collected for analysis or computation), monitor patients' vital signs and most recently, aid in diagnosis. With this type of sophisticated support, we see health care and computer technology becoming increasingly codependent. There is no doubt that today's health care workers will encounter computers in the job environment, requiring computer literacy for people entering any area in health care. A person may be called "computer literate" if he or she can:

1. Understand the basic components and functions of a computer.
2. Perform basic operations to complete required tasks.
3. Willingly adapt to the changes that computers are making on the quality of life.

Computer Classifications

Today's computers can be categorized according to type, function, and size. Computers classified by size are either microcomputers, minicomputers, mainframes, or supercomputers.

- *Microcomputer* or *personal computer* (PC): These computers are very popular with the general public and they serve a necessary function in business. They are easy to use and versatile. Microcomputers have been found in health care facilities for some time now because they are practical and inexpensive. Examples of this type of computer are International Business Machines (IBM) PS/2, Apple's Macintosh, and the powerful laptops made by Compaq, Apple, and others.
- *Minicomputer:* This classification is characterized by the amount of storage, the processing speeds, and the variety of equipment available, which all exceed the microcomputer. They are stand-alone computers that have the capability of maintaining a complete database system for processing patient accounts or laboratory information systems. Examples are Digital Equipment Corporation (DEC) VAX, the Hewlett Packard 9000, and Stratus AX2000.
- *Mainframe:* This classification of computers has a more powerful computer processing unit (CPU) and more disk storage. These systems are capable of processing enormous amounts of information at fast speeds, making them more appropriate for businesses,

such as insurance companies, banks, government agencies, and centralized hospital networks. These types of computers are manufactured by Bull of France and IBM, among others.

- *Supercomputer:* These computers, developed by companies such as Cray and Hitachi, are the largest of all systems. They are capable of processing more information at a greater speed using highly complicated applications than any other computer system in the world. Because of the heat generated by such speeds, they often require cooling that can be as elaborate as liquid nitrogen. Supercomputers are multimillion dollar expenditures and are, therefore, rarely encountered. Presently, they are being used in national defense, research in health care, and for the development of artificial intelligence, a concept that will undoubtedly be used extensively in health care.

Computer Components

Whether operating a small microcomputer or interacting with a supercomputer, the user will employ the three basic components of any system. All computers must have a means to "**input**" information, a way to "process" information, and a method to "**output**" information.

INPUT

There are several ways to move information into a computer. The most common form used is a keyboard, much like a typewriter keyboard with additional keys for computer functions. Other methods of input include the light pen, designed to read information on a computer screen, and scanners programmed to read bar codes.

PROCESS

After information has been input, it is processed through a unit called the **central processing unit (CPU)**. This CPU, made up of many electrical components and microchips, has three elements. The control unit manages or oversees the processing and completion of each task required by the operator. The arithmetic logic unit (ALU) performs mathematical processes and makes decisions based on logical comparisons of input data. The third element, memory, can be of two types: **random access memory (RAM)** and **read only memory (ROM)**. Random access memory is the temporary storage of data that will be lost when the computer is shut off. If the data needs to be kept for a later date, the operator must transfer it to a hard disk or floppy diskette. Read only memory storage is installed by the manufacturer; its purpose is to instruct the computer on how to begin the necessary operation requested by the user. Because ROM has been referred to as both hardware and software, it was recently decided to lessen the confusion and call it "firmware."

OUTPUT

Output describes the return of processed information to the user or to someone in another location. Just as there are several ways to input information, there are several means by which users can receive the processed data. One of the most common ways is through a printer. When the data is printed on paper, it is said to be hard copy. Another output device is the monitor or **cathode ray tube (CRT)**, which looks like a television screen and displays text as it is entered and during the processing.

Elements of the Computer

There are three elements that make up computer systems. These elements are called hardware, software, and storage.

Hardware is the equipment that is used to process data and includes the CPU and peripherals (all additional equipment attached to the CPU) used for the input or output of information. Examples of hardware peripherals are keyboards, monitors, bar code readers, joysticks, printers, and modems (devices that transfer data to other computers over telephone lines). A monitor (CRT) and keyboard combination is called a "terminal" and are necessary peripherals for minicomputers, mainframes, and supercomputers.

Software is the programming (coded instructions) required to control the hardware in the processing of data. Two basic types exist: systems software and applications software. Systems software controls the normal operation of the computer. Applications software refers to programs prepared by software companies or in-house programmers to perform specific tasks required by users. Software applications come in five basic types: spreadsheets, communication systems, database systems, word processing, and graphics. Packages that perform more than one application, such as word processing, spreadsheet, and database are called integrated software. The advantage of integrating applications is that it allows the different functions to be merged easily into one document.

Storage of information outside the CPU is necessary because RAM, as mentioned previously, is limited temporary storage, which will be lost when the computer is turned off. Storage outside the CPU is called secondary storage. Examples of permanent secondary storage devices for documents and programs are diskettes, hard disks, magnetic tapes, and compact disks (CDs).

Computers and the Laboratory

As discussed previously, computers are accurate processors of information at incredible speeds. For this reason, computer systems in health care are considered more efficient and cost-effective than relying on manual methods. Systems have been designed that will manage patient data and interface with automated analyzers and the main hospital information system. Competition between companies who sell laboratory information management systems (LIMS) is based on the ease of input, the format of output, and the availability of customized software. Extensive research goes into selecting the right computer system for specific laboratory needs. After selecting a vendor, it will take several months to bring a system "on-line" (operational). Usually one or two people are put in charge of the system's daily operation; they are called "system managers." These individuals have the responsibility to train other personnel in the laboratory and keep them updated as changes are made to the software. They must readily develop troubleshooting skills as they solve day-to-day problems that develop after the system is installed.

General Computer Skills

General skills that the phlebotomist will learn, regardless of the LIMS that is used, are as follows:

- *Logging on* (Fig. 16–1): Each person that is allowed on a system is given a password. This password will uniquely identify each person who is trying to "log on" (become

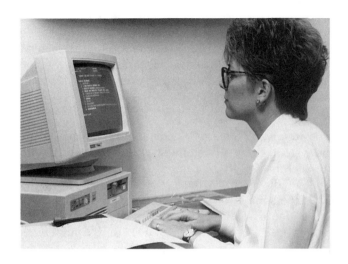

Figure 16–1 Health care worker at a microcomputer workstation.

a system user). Most systems require a user name to be entered before the password. When the log-on sequence is completed, a "**menu**" will be displayed listing the options the user may choose from at this point.

- *Cursor movement:* After logging on, the flashing indicator on the screen called the **cursor** indicates the starting point for your input. When entering patient information in a LIMS, the cursor will automatically reset itself at the correct point for data input after the Enter key has been pressed.
- *Entering data:* Once the necessary information has been input, the Enter key must be pressed for information to be processed. If an error is made in spelling or selection, it can be easily deleted by back spacing before pressing the Enter key. If the wrong data is entered, it is possible to correct errors even at this point.
- *Correcting errors:* This procedure is necessary to correct mistakes realized after the Enter key has been pressed. The procedure to delete orders is program-dependent and must be learned with each system. Some LIMS software uses order verification, an additional step in the process to allow a review of the information before being accepted.
- *Verifying orders:* After all patient data has been entered, it will appear on the monitor as a complete order. At this point, the user can review the data again and choose to modify, delete, or accept it. When all orders have been entered, the user can request an inquiry of the orders as still another check.
- *Inquiring about orders:* Requesting order inquiry will allow the user to retrieve any or all of the test orders associated with a patient.
- *Deleting orders:* If after the user has entered an order, and finds it is not correct, he or she can request the computer to delete or reject it. The command "delete" can also be used when an order is canceled.

Laboratory Information Management Systems (LIMS)

The objectives of LIMS are to file results efficiently, accumulate statistics to determine workload, generate report forms, and monitor quality assurance in the laboratory work. There are several types of systems on the market at this time, for example, Cerner, CHC, and Sunquest. Each type of information system allows the user to define its own parameters for terms and conditions that make the system unique to that facility. Several programs within the system allow the users to do specific tasks seemingly at the same time, such as: 1) admit patients, 2) request test orders, 3) print labels, 4) verify collection, and 5) inquire about results.

TECH CODE

In laboratory settings, users are given both a **tech code** and a password. Passwords are used to gain access to the system. Passwords should be kept strictly confidential as the security associated with each password determines what system functions can be accessed. Passwords are also logged with every transaction on the system, allowing the system manager to identify the person performing each transaction. Tech codes, on the other hand, are used to further identify each person *entering data* on the system, mainly for the purpose of accruing workload. Tech codes do not need to be confidential. Often phlebotomists do not verify their own collections. Rather, a data entry clerk may verify all collections and must have access to the list of tech codes so that he or she can associate the proper phlebotomist with each draw.

MNEMONIC CODES

The LIMS uses **mnemonic** (memory-aiding) codes often in the form of abbreviations to request the appropriate program or function necessary to enter data. For example, in the Sunquest Laboratory Information System, to enter tests ordered on a patient, a phlebotomist would type the mnemonic RE (requisition entry) at the function prompt. The "requisition entry" program can be called many different names but is basically the same procedure for any of the systems. During this data entry phase, an "**accession number**" is given to each requested order. This number is generated by the LIMS when the specimen request is entered into the computer and is used to identify that specimen as long as it is in the laboratory.

One of the mnemonic codes used in identifying specimen types is always printed whenever a label is generated. For example, if the code on the label reads "1 Blue," the phlebotomist knows that a blue top tube is required. This demonstrates one of the benefits of computerized label generation: the label aids the phlebotomist in acquiring the proper specimen in a timely fashion (Fig. 16–2).

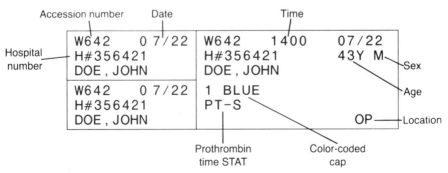

Figure 16–2 Computer label.

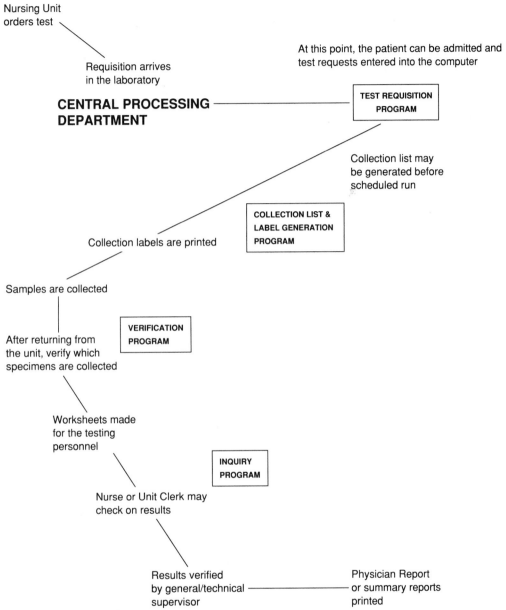

Nursing Unit
orders test

Requisition arrives
in the laboratory

At this point, the patient can be admitted and
test requests entered into the computer

**CENTRAL PROCESSING
DEPARTMENT**

**TEST REQUISITION
PROGRAM**

Collection list may
be generated before
scheduled run

**COLLECTION LIST &
LABEL GENERATION
PROGRAM**

Collection labels are printed

Samples are collected

After returning from
the unit, verify which
specimens are collected

**VERIFICATION
PROGRAM**

Worksheets made
for the testing
personnel

**INQUIRY
PROGRAM**

Nurse or Unit Clerk may
check on results

Results verified
by general/technical
supervisor

Physician Report
or summary reports
printed

Figure 16–3   Example of workflow chart.

A diagram of steps used by the Sunquest LIMS in the processing of a typical specimen from arrival into the lab and through reporting of results is shown in Figure 16–3.

Laboratory Computerization in the Future

As we move into the 21st century, rapid advances in technology will play a
major part in health care. Laboratory medicine will change drastically with the advent

of very sophisticated computerized instrumentation that can perform chemistry, hematology, and coagulation tests at the bedside, or "point-of-care" (any hospital area where it is clinically indicated). These portable, easy-to-use testing instruments will be very attractive to physicians who need continuous monitoring of their patients. Most of the self-contained, internally calibrated devices can be operated with minimum training. Test results are obtained and evaluated immediately by comparing them through computer modems to existing data in the patient's records. These instruments will be minimally invasive (requiring only a small amount of blood from a skin puncture) or, as presently being used in research, totally noninvasive. This point-of-care or "near-patient" technology is designed to reduce cost while enhancing patient care. It appears that personnel, such as patient care technicians or phlebotomists, may be given this testing responsibility.

Study & Review Questions

1. Which of the following is an example of proxemics?
   a. eye contact
   b. zone of comfort
   c. facial expressions
   d. personal hygiene

2. Which of the following is NOT one of the major elements in health communication?
   a. confirmation
   b. empathy
   c. deliberation
   d. trust

3. The best way to handle a "bad" patient is to:
   a. refuse to collect specimens from the patient
   b. help the patient to feel in control of the situation
   c. tell the patient that you will report him or her to your superiors
   d. talk sharply to the patient and let him or her know that you are the one in control

4. Which of the following is proper telephone protocol?
   a. wait for the phone to ring three or four times so as not to appear anxious
   b. do not identify yourself in case there are problems later
   c. be careful of the tone of voice used and keep answers simple
   d. listen carefully but do not take notes because it takes too much time

5. A computer, such as the Macintosh, often found in the home is called a:
   a. mainframe
   b. microcomputer
   c. minicomputer
   d. supercomputer

6. Peripherals on a computer include all of the following EXCEPT:
   a. bar code reader
   b. joystick
   c. modem
   d. CPU

7. To log on to most computer systems requires the use of a(n):
   a. accession number
   b. bar code reader
   c. modem
   d. password

8. Mnemonics are:
   a. memory-aiding codes
   b. hardware
   c. programs
   d. questions

Suggested Laboratory Activities

1. Practice verbal and nonverbal communication by role-playing with a fellow student.
2. Practice proper telephone communication skills.
3. Practice working with a computer.
4. Using a simulated hospital computer system, practice admitting patients, requesting tests, and verifying test collection.
5. Identify the coded information on a computer label.

BIBLIOGRAPHY AND SUGGESTED READINGS

Chambers DW, Abrams RG: *Dental Communication*. East Norwalk, CT: Appleton-Century-Crofts, 1986.

Montagu A: *Touching: The Human Significance of the Skin* (3rd ed.). New York: HarperCollins, 1986.

Northouse PG, Northouse LL: *Health Communication: Strategies for Health Professionals* (2nd ed.). East Norwalk, CT: Appleton & Lange, 1992.

Purtilo R: *Health Professional/Patient Interaction* (3rd ed.). Philadelphia: WB Saunders Company, 1984.

Laboratory Mathematics

17

On successful completion of this chapter, the reader should be able to:

1 Name basic metric units and prefixes.
2 Convert metric units to English units.
3 Describe how to convert larger metric units to smaller units.
4 Define military time and convert 24-hour time to 12-hour time.
5 Convert Fahrenheit temperature to Celsius temperature.
6 Convert Roman numerals to Arabic (common) numbers.
7 Calculate percentages and prepare a 5% and 10% solution.
8 Calculate adult and infant blood volumes.

KEY TERMS
blood volume
Celsius
Centigrade
Fahrenheit
decimal system
gram
liter
meter
metric system
military time

McCall: PHLEBOTOMY ESSENTIALS. © 1993
J. B. Lippincott Company.

INTRODUCTION

Aside from basic proficiency in addition, subtraction, multiplication, and division, it is helpful for the phlebotomist to understand systems of measurement, associated terminology, and calculations commonly encountered in the medical laboratory.

THE METRIC SYSTEM

The **metric system** is the system of measurement used in the health care industry. The metric system derives its name from its fundamental unit of distance, the **meter** (M or m). In the metric system, the meter is the basic unit of linear measure; the **gram** (G or g) is the basic unit of weight, and the **liter** (L or l) is the basic unit of volume.

The metric system is a **decimal system** (a system based on the number 10). In a decimal system, units larger or smaller than the basic units are arrived at by multiplying or dividing by 10 or powers of 10.

In the metric system, prefixes added to the basic units indicate larger or smaller units. Prefixes are the same whether the units are meters, grams, or liters. Table 17-1 shows prefixes commonly used in the medical laboratory.

Metric units can be converted to larger units by moving the decimal point to the left, according to the appropriate multiple.

Example: convert 100 grams to kilograms.

From Table 17-1, we determine that 1 kilogram is equal to 1,000 or 10^3 grams. The multiple is three. Therefore, to convert 100 grams to kilograms, move the decimal point three places to the left:

$$100 \text{ g} = 100.0 = .1 \text{ kg}$$

To convert metric units to smaller units, move the decimal point to the right the appropriate multiple.

Example: convert 100 grams to milligrams.

Table 17–1.
Commonly Used Measurement Prefixes

| Prefix | Multiple | Unit of Measure | | |
		meter	gram	liter
kilo- (k)	1,000 (10^3)	km	kg	kl
deci- (d)	1/10 (10^{-1})	dm	dg	dl
centi- (c)	1/100 (10^{-2})	cm	cg	cl
milli- (m)	1/1,000 (10^{-3})	mm	mg	ml
micro- (μ)	1/1,000,000 (10^{-6})	μm	μg	μl

From Table 17-1, we see that 1 mg is equal to 10^{-3} gm. The multiple is a minus three. Move the decimal point three spaces to the right:

100 g = 100.000 = 100,000 mg.

A red blood cell is approximately 8 μm in diameter. What is its size in centimeters?

Often it is necessary to convert our English system of units to metric units. Table 17-2 lists English units and their metric equivalents commonly encountered in the health care setting.

To convert from English units to metric units, multiply by the factor listed. Metric units can be converted back to English units by dividing by the same factor or multiplying by the factor in the metric conversion chart.

> *Example:* Convert 200 pounds to kilograms (kg).
> 1 pound is equal to 0.454 kg.
> Therefore,
> multiply 200 × .454 to arrive at 90.8 kg.

Table 17-3 shows the common equivalents for converting metric units to English units.

To convert metric units to English units, simply multiply by the factor involved. To convert English units back to metric units, divide by the same factor or multiply by the factor in the English unit conversion chart.

> *Example:* Convert 15 ml to teaspoons.
> 1.0 ml is equal to 1/5 tsp.
> Therefore,
> multiply 15 × 1/5 = 15/5 = 3 tsp
> (or 15 × .2 = 3.0 tsp)

Table 17–2.
English–Metric Equivalents

	English		*Metric*
Distance	yard (yd)	=	0.9 meters (m)
	inch (in)	=	2.54 centimeters (cm)
Weight	pound (lb)	=	0.454 kilograms (kg) or 454 grams (g)
	ounce (oz)	=	28 grams (g)
Volume	quart (qt)	=	0.95 liters (l)
	fluid ounce (fl oz)	=	30 milliliters (ml)
	tablespoon (tbsp)	=	15 milliliters (ml)
	teaspoon (tsp)	=	5 milliliters (ml)

Table 17–3.
Metric–English Conversion Equivalents

	Metric		*English*
Distance	meter (m)	=	3.3 feet / 39.37 inches
	centimeter (cm)	=	0.4 inches
	millimeter (mm)	=	0.04 inches
Weight	gram (g)	=	.0022 pounds
	kilogram (kg)	=	2.2 pounds
Volume	liter (l)	=	1.06 quarts
	milliliter (ml)	=	.03 fluid ounces
	milliliter (ml)	=	.20 or $\frac{1}{5}$ tsp

Note: A milliliter (ml) is approximately equal to a cubic centimeter (cc) and the two terms are often used interchangeably.

MILITARY TIME

Most hospitals use **military** (or European) **time**, which is based on a clock with 24 numbers instead of 12 (Fig. 17-1). Twenty-four-hour time eliminates the need for designating AM or PM. Each time is expressed by four digits. The first two digits represent hours, and the second two digits represent minutes. Twenty-four-hour time be-

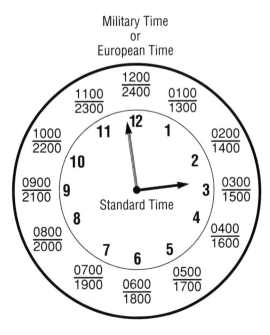

Figure 17–1 Clock showing 24-hour (military) time.

gins at midnight (0000) and ends at 2359. 1 AM is 0100; 2 AM is 0200, and so on. Noon is 1200; 1 PM is 1300.

To convert regular (12-hour) time to 24-hour time, *add* 12 hours to the time from 1 PM on.

> *Example:* 1:00 PM becomes 1:00 + 12 = 1300 hours
> 5:30 PM becomes 5:30 + 12 = 1730 hours

To convert 24-hour time to 12-hour time, *subtract* 12 hours after 1 PM.

> *Example:* 1300 hours becomes 1300 − 1200 = 1:00 PM

Your requisition says that a specimen must be drawn at 1530. What time would that be in 12-hour time?

TEMPERATURE MEASUREMENT

Two different temperature scales (Fig. 17-2) may be used in the health care setting. The **Fahrenheit** (F) scale is often used to measure body temperature, while the **Celsius** (C), also known as the **Centigrade** scale, is used to measure temperatures in the laboratory.

Fahrenheit

The freezing point of water is 32°F, and the boiling point is 212°F. Normal body temperature expressed in Fahrenheit is 98.6°F.

Celsius

The freezing point of water is zero (0°C) and the boiling point is 100°C. Normal body temperature expressed in Celsius scale is 37°C.

The following formulas can be used to convert from one temperature scale to the other:

Celsius temperature = 5/9 (°F − 32)

Fahrenheit temperature = 9/5 (°C) + 32

A specimen must be transported at body temperature (98.6°F). The thermometer in the heat block reads 30°C. Is the heat block warm enough to transport the specimen?

ROMAN NUMERALS

In the Roman numeral system, letters represent numbers. Roman numerals may be encountered in procedure outlines, doctor's orders or prescriptions, and in the identification of values or substances such as coagulation factors.

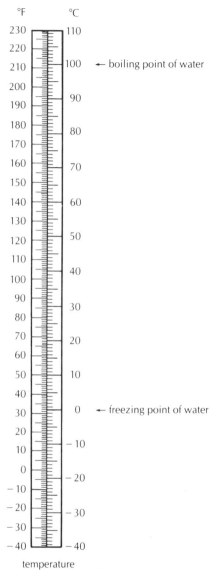

°F   °C

100 ← boiling point of water

0 ← freezing point of water

temperature
conversion
scale

Figure 17–2   Thermometer showing both Fahrenheit and Celsius degrees (Memmler RL, Cohen BJ, Wood DL).

The basic Roman numeral system consists of the following seven capital (or lower-case) letters:

I   (i) = 1
V (v) = 5
X (x) = 10
L (l) = 50

C   (c) = 100
D   (d) = 500
M   (m) = 1,000

Guidelines for Interpreting Roman Numerals

1. When numerals of the same value follow in sequence, the values should be added. There should never be more than three of the same numeral in a sequence.

   > *Example:* III = 1 + 1 + 1 = 3
   > XX = 10 + 10 = 20

2. When a lower value numeral precedes a numeral with a higher value, the lower value should be subtracted from the higher value. Numerals V, L, and D are never subtracted. No more than one lower value number should precede a higher value number.

   > *Example:* IV = 5 − 1 = 4
   > IX = 10 − 1 = 9

3. When a numeral is followed by one or more numerals of lower value, the values should be added.

   > *Example:* XI = 10 + 1 = 11
   > VII = 5 + 1 + 1 = 7

4. When a lower value numeral comes between two higher value numerals, it is subtracted from the numeral following it.

   > *Example:* XIX = 10 + 10 − 1 = 19
   > XXIV = 10 + 10 + 5 − 1 = 24

5. Roman numerals are written from left to right in order of decreasing value (except for numerals that are to be subtracted from subsequent numerals).

   > *Example:* XXVII = 10 + 10 + 5 + 1 + 1 = 27
   > MCMXCII = 1,000 + (1,000 − 100) + (100 − 10) + 1 + 1 = 1,992

6. A line over a Roman numeral means multiply the numeral by 1,000.

   > *Example:* $\overline{V}$ = V × 1,000 = 5,000

Your book says that factor VIII is the antihemophilic factor. What common (Arabic) number is this factor?

PERCENT

Percent means per 100 and is represented by the symbol "%." Two values are involved when a number is expressed as a percent. They are the number itself and 100.

For example: 10% means 10 per 100 or 10 parts in a total of 100 parts.

To change a fraction to a percent, multiply by 100 and add a percent sign to the result.

> *Example:* Change 3/4 to a percent.
>
> $$3/4 \times 100/1 = 300/4 = 4\overline{)300}\,^{75} = 75\%$$

Your paper says that you got 45 out of 50 questions correct. What is your grade expressed as a percent?

SOLUTIONS AND DILUTIONS

Concentration of laboratory reagents is often expressed as a percentage. For example, a solution of 70% isopropyl alcohol is used in skin cleansing prior to blood collection. And a 10% dilution of bleach (5.25% sodium hypochlorite) is used to disinfect counter tops and other surfaces.

A 10% dilution of bleach means that there are 10 parts of bleach in a solution containing a total of 100 parts. The above dilution also can be expressed as a ratio, showing the relationship between part of the solution and the total solution. A dilution of 10 parts in a total of 100 parts is the same as 1 part in a total of 10 parts, or a 1:10 (1 to 10) dilution.

A 10% dilution of bleach can be prepared by adding 10 ml bleach to 90 ml water, resulting in a total of 100 ml of bleach solution. The same percentage dilution would result from adding 1 ml bleach to 9 ml water or 20 ml bleach to 180 ml water.

BLOOD VOLUME

Blood volume in adults is generally stated as 5.0 quarts or 4.75 liters (L). Because people are not the same size, common sense tells us that they should not all have 5 quarts of blood. Actual blood volume is based on weight. Blood volume can be calculated for any size person from infant to adult, as long as the weight of the person is known.

Adult Blood Volume

Adult blood volume is 70 milliliters per kilogram of weight.
Example: Calculate the amount of blood volume for a man who weighs 250 lbs.

1. Change the weight in pounds to kilograms.

    Because 1 lb = .454 kg; you need to multiply 250 lb × .454
    to arrive at 113.5 kg.

2. Next, multiply the number of kilograms by 70 because there are 70 milliliters of blood for each kg of weight.

    113.5 kg × 70 ml/kg = 7,945 ml

3. Because blood volume is reported in liters rather than milliliters, divide the total number of ml by 1,000. (1 liter = 1,000 ml)

Blood volume = 7,945 ml/1,000 ml = 7.945 L or 7.9 L

Infant Blood Volume

It is very important to be able to estimate the blood volume of an infant, especially if the infant is in an intensive care unit where blood samples may be taken several times a day. A very small infant can become anemic if not monitored closely. Removal of more than 10% of an infant's blood volume in a short amount of time can lead to serious consequences including cardiac arrest.

An infant's blood volume is 100 ml per kilogram.

Example: Calculate the blood volume of a baby who weighs 5.5 lbs.

1. Change the weight from pounds to kilograms using the same formula as for adults.

5.5 lbs × .454 = 2.5 kg

2. Multiply 2.5 kg by 100 for total blood volume in milliliters.

2.5 kg × 100 = 250 ml

3. Change blood volume in ml/kg to liters.

250 ml/1,000 ml = 0.25 L

Suggested Laboratory Activities

1. Practice converting English units to metric units.

2. Fill one of each of the various sizes of tubes with water using a teaspoon, tablespoon, and so on, and record the results.

3. Practice converting 12-hour time to 24-hour time.

4. Compare a Centigrade thermometer with a Fahrenheit thermometer. Record the actual temperature of the classroom or lab in both Fahrenheit and Centigrade.

5. Prepare a 1:10 solution of bleach.

6. Perform the calculations needed to determine an infant's blood volume.

BIBLIOGRAPHY AND SUGGESTED READINGS

Bishop ML, Duben-Engelkirk JL, Fody EP: *Clinical Chemistry: Principles, Procedures, Correlations* (2nd ed.). Philadelphia: JB Lippincott Company, 1992.

Campbell J, Campbell J: *Laboratory Mathematics: Medical and Biological Applications* (3rd ed.). St. Louis: Mosby/YearBook Publishers, 1984.

Highers M, Forrester R: *Mathematics for the Allied Health Professions*. East Norwalk, CT: Appleton & Lange, 1987.

Glossary

ABO blood group system: A genetically determined blood group system that recognizes four blood types: A, B, AB and O, based on the presence or absence on the red blood cells of what are identified as the A and B antigens.

accepting assignment: When a provider agrees to accept a fixed amount from an insurer as payment in full for a given service.

accession number: A unique number given to each test request.

accreditation: The process by which a professional or governmental agency evaluates an educational institution according to accepted criteria or standards to assure that graduates are qualified for professional employment.

activated coagulation time (ACT): Also referred to as activated clotting time, this procedure tests the activity of the intrinsic coagulation factors and is used to monitor heparin therapy.

additive: Any substance such as an anticoagulant, antiglycolytic agent, separator gel, cell preservative, or clot activator added to a blood collection tube. Additives do not include tube or closure coatings.

aerobic: With oxygen.

aerosol: A substance released in the form of a fine mist.

agglutinate: Clump together.

agglutinins: Antibodies present in the plasma of a person's blood that will react against and agglutinate RBCs carrying antigens of a different blood type.

agranulocytes: WBCs lacking easily visible granules.

albumin: A plasma protein manufactured by the liver which functions to help regulate osmotic pressure of the blood.

aliquot: A portion of a sample used for testing.

Allen test: A test performed to ascertain collateral blood flow to the hand prior to performing radial ABGs.

alveoli: Thin-walled saclike chambers within the lungs where the exchange of O_2 and CO_2 between the air and blood takes place.

ambulatory care: Care provided outside of inpatient institutions or "care for the walking client."

anabolism: The process by which the body converts simple compounds into complex substances needed to carry out the cellular activities of the body.

anaerobic: Without oxygen.

analyte: A general term for a substance undergoing analysis.

anatomic position: A way of referring to the body or body parts in which the patient is standing erect, arms at the side with palms and eyes facing forward.

ancillary blood glucose testing (ABGT): Instant or "rapid" glucose testing commonly performed using small, portable glucose analyzers. Also called bedside glucose testing.

anemia: An abnormal reduction in the number of RBCs in the circulating blood.

aneurysm: A localized dilation or bulging in the wall of a blood vessel, usually an artery.

antecubital fossa: The area of the arm located anterior to and below the bend of the elbow where the major veins for venipuncture are located.

antecubital veins: Major superficial arm veins located in the antecubital fossa.

anterior: Also called ventral, refers to the front.

antibody: Protein substance manufactured by the body as a response to a foreign protein or antigen and directed against it.

antibiotic susceptibility: Procedure to determine the ability of an antibiotic to slow or stop the growth of a specific microorganism.

anticoagulant: A substance that prevents blood from clotting.

antigen: A substance that causes the formation of antibodies that are directed against it.

antimicrobial therapy: Use of chemical substances to kill or stop the growth of microorganisms.

antiseptics: Germicidal solutions that are used to clean the skin prior to venipuncture or skin puncture.

anuclear: Without a nucleus.

aorta: The largest artery in the body, arising from the left ventricle of the heart and approximately 1 inch (2.5 cm) in diameter.

approval: A process similar to accreditation.

ARD: Antimicrobial Removal Device; a bottle containing a resin which removes antimicrobials/antibiotics from the blood.

arrhythmia: An irregularity in the heart rate, rhythm, or beat.

arterial blood gases (ABGs): Evaluation of arterial blood to provide valuable information about a patient's oxygenation, ventilation, and acid–base balance which is needed for the diagnosis and management of respiratory disease.

arteries: Thick-walled vessels that carry blood away from the heart.

arterioles: The smallest branches of arteries.

arteriosclerosis: A disease condition that involves thickening, hardening, and loss of elasticity of artery walls.

arteriospasm: Involuntary contraction of an artery.

ASAP: As soon as possible.

ASCP: American Society of Clinical Pathologists; certifying agency and professional organization for laboratory personnel.

ASMT: American Society for Medical Technology; professional organization for laboratory personnel.

ASPT: American Society for Phlebotomy Technicians; certifying agency and professional organization for phlebotomists.

assault: An intentional threat or movement that could make a person feel in danger of harmful physical contact.

atherosclerosis: A form of arteriosclerosis involving changes in the intima of the artery due to an accumulation of lipid material.

atria: The upper chambers on each side of the heart which receive blood before it enters the ventricles.

atrioventricular (AV) node: A structure located in the lower right atrium of the heart, that slows conduction of the electrical pulse generated by the sinoatrial node, creating a slight delay before electrical impulses are carried to the ventricles.

atrioventricular valves: Valves at the entrance of the ventricles.

AV bundle (bundle of His): A group of cardiac muscle fibers that form part of the electrical impulse-conducting system of the heart.

A-V shunt: Arterial–venous passage artificially constructed to divert blood flow.

avascular: Containing no blood vessels.

bacteremia: Bacteria in the blood.

bactericidal: Kills bacteria.

bacteriostatic: Prevents or inhibits the growth of bacteria.

barriers: Anything that interferes with communication, such as personal bias or culture diversity.

basal state: Early in the morning while the body is still at rest and approximately 12 hours after the last intake of food, exercise, or activity.

basilic vein: The large vein on the inner side of the arm in the antecubital fossa. The third-choice vein for venipuncture.

basophils: The least numerous of the WBCs, comprising less than 1% of the WBC population. The granules of basophils are large, stain dark blue and often obscure the nucleus.

battery: An intentional, unconsented-to physical contact by one person with another person.

bedside manner: Behavior by a phlebotomist that puts the patient at ease while the phlebotomist performs his or her duties.

bevel: The point of the needle that has been cut on a slant for ease of entry.

biconcave: Indented from both sides.

biohazard: Anything that is potentially harmful to the environment and man.

bleeding time (BT): The time required for blood to stop flowing from a standardized incision. The BT is dependent on platelet plug formation in the capillaries and is measured to determine platelet and vascular function.

Bloodborne Pathogen Standard: OSHA's regulations for all employees with occupational exposure to pathogens found in the blood.

blood pressure: A measure of the force exerted by the blood on the walls of blood vessels.

blood volume: An individual's calculated amount of blood based on their weight. In adults it is calculated on 70 ml of blood per kilogram of weight and in infants, on 100–110 ml per kilogram of weight.

B-lymphocytes: WBCs that give rise to plasma cells which produce antibodies.

body cavities: Large hollow spaces that house various organs of the body.

body plane: A flat surface determined by making a real or imaginary cut through a body in the normal anatomic position.

body substance isolation (BSI): Recently proposed modification of routine patient care practices augmented by elements of disease specific precautions for bloodborne pathogens, used for all patients.

brachial artery: Main artery of the arm, which is located in the medial anterior aspect of the antecubital fossa near the insertion of the biceps muscle.

bradycardia: A slow rate, less than 60 beats per minute.

breach of confidentiality: An unauthorized release of information concerning a patient.

bundle of His: Part of the electrical conduction system, located between the ventricles, it conducts impulses from the AV junction to the right and left bundle branches.

calcaneus: Heel bone.

calcium (Ca): A mineral needed for proper bone and teeth formation, nerve conduction, and muscle contraction, and essential to the clotting process.

cannula: A temporary surgical connection between an artery and a vein used for dialysis and blood drawing.

CAP: College for American Pathologists.

capillary action: Process by which blood is drawn up by contact only into a small tube.

capillaries: Tiny vessels, one cell layer thick, that connect the arterioles and venules and allow the exchange of oxygen and nutrients between the cells and the blood.

Caraway tubes: Disposable, glass microcollection tubes.

carbaminohemoglobin (HbCO₂): Hemoglobin combined with CO_2.

cardiac cycle: One complete contraction and subsequent relaxation of the heart with each cycle lasting approximately 0.8 seconds.

cardiac output: The volume of blood pumped by the heart in 1 minute, approximately 5 liters per minute.

cardiopulmonary resuscitation (CPR): Revival of heart and lung activity after they have stopped functioning.

catabolism: The process by which complex substances in food are broken down into simple substances.

catheter: A tube passed through the body for injecting or withdrawing fluids from body cavities or blood vessels.

CDC: Centers for Disease Control and Prevention, a division of the U.S. Public Health Service which investigates diseases that have epidemic potential.

Celsius: A temperature scale on which melting point is 0 degrees and boiling point is 100 degrees. Normal body temperature expressed in Celsius (or Centigrade) is 37 degrees. Also known as the Centrigrade scale.

central processing: Also called specimen

processing, where all specimens are received and prepared for testing.

Centigrade: *See* Celsius.

centrifugation: A process of separating substances of different densities by using a centrifuge or machine that spins specimens requiring separation at high speeds.

cephalic vein: The second choice vein for venipuncture located in the lateral aspect of the arm in the antecubital fossa.

cerebrospinal fluid (CSF): A clear, colorless liquid that circulates within the cavities surrounding the brain and spinal cord with many of the same constituents as blood plasma.

certification: A process which indicates the completion of defined academic and training requirements and the attainment of a satisfactory score on a national examination.

chain of custody: Special protocol that must be strictly followed; requires documentation that the specimen is accounted for at all times.

chain of infection: A related series of events which lead to infection.

Chordae tendineae: Thin threads of tissue which attach the AV valves to the walls of the ventricles.

circulatory system: Also called the cardiovascular system, consists of the heart, blood, and blood vessels along with the lymph, lymph vessels, and nodes (lymphatic system).

civil law: The law of private rights between persons or parties.

clean-catch: Method of obtaining a urine sample so that it is free of contaminating matter from the external genital areas.

CLIA '88: Clinical Laboratory Improvement Amendments signed into federal law in 1988, mandating that all laboratories be regulated using the same standards regardless of their location, type, or size.

clot activator: Clot-enhancing substance, such as siliceous earth, silica, or celite.

coagulation: Blood clotting process.

collapsed vein: An abnormal retraction of the vessel walls.

collateral circulation: A process that allows tissue to be supplied with blood from an accessory vessel.

combining form: A word root along with a combining vowel which can be attached to a suffix or another word root.

combining vowel: A vowel (usually an "o") which joins a word root to a suffix or another word root in order to ease pronunciation.

compatibility: Able to be mixed together with favorable results, such as in blood transfusions.

concentric circles: Beginning from the center and moving outward in ever-widening even circles.

continuing education units (CEUs): Credits given for workshops and seminars offered to continually upgrade skills and knowledge.

coring: Removal of a portion of the skin or vein.

coronary arteries: The first branches off of the aorta, just beyond the aortic semilunar valve, which supply blood to the heart muscle.

cost shifting: Term used to describe how providers attempt to make up for reduced reimbursements from government-paid programs, by charging more to other payers.

CPU: Central Processing Unit; handles Input/Output, *ie,* manipulation and calculation of data.

crossmatch: A compatibility test performed before a unit of blood is determined to be suitable for transfusion.

CRT: Cathode Ray Tube; monitor or screen for displaying computer output.

culture & sensitivity (C&S): The process by which organisms are grown on media, identified, and an antibiotic susceptibility (sensitivity) test performed to determine which antibiotics will be effective against the organism.

cursor: A flashing marker on the CRT that indicates where the next key stroke will appear.

cyanotic: Pertaining to cyanosis or blue/gray discoloration of the skin due to lack of oxygen.

data: Information collected for analysis or computation.

decimal system: System based on the number 10. In a decimal system, units larger or smaller than the basic units are arrived at by multiplying or dividing by 10 or powers of 10.

dermis: Corium or true skin, a layer composed of elastic and fibrous connective tissue.

diabetes insipidus: A condition characterized by increased thirst and increased urine production caused by inadequate secretion of ADH.

diabetes mellitus: A condition in which there is impaired carbohydrate, fat, and protein metabolism due to a deficiency of insulin.

diagnostic related groups (DRGs): A system of disease classification used to determine PPS rates for reimbursement purposes.

diastole: The relaxation phase of the cardiac cycle.

diastolic pressure: The pressure on the arteries during relaxation of the ventricles; averages 80 mm Hg and is an estimate of systemic vascular resistance.

differential: Determination of the number and characteristics of cells on a smear by staining and examining the cells under a microscope.

discard tube: Also called "clear tube." A tube used to collect and discard approximately 5 ml of blood in order to prevent IV or tissue fluid contamination of a specimen.

disinfectants: A solution containing an agent intended to kill or irreversibly inactivate microorganisms (but not necessarily their spores). Disinfectants are used on surfaces and instruments, and are generally not safe for use on human skin.

distal: Farthest from the center of the body, origin, or point of attachment.

diurnal variation: Normal daily changes in lab values.

dorsal cavities: Internal spaces located in the back of the body.

edema: An accumulation of fluid in the tissues.

electrocardiogram (EKG or ECG): An actual record of the electrical currents that correspond to each event in the heart muscle contraction.

electrolytes: Substances that conduct electricity when dissolved in water, such as potassium or sodium.

electrical safety: Rules related to the safe use of electrical equipment.

embolism: Obstruction of a blood vessel by an embolus.

embolus: A blood clot, part of a blood clot, or other mass of undissolved matter circulating in the blood stream.

empathy: Objective insight into the emotions and feelings of another person.

endocardium: A thin membrane lining the heart which is continuous with the lining of the blood vessels.

engineering controls: One of the primary methods used to control the transmission of HBV, HIV, and other bloodborne pathogens by removing or isolating the hazard or isolating the worker from exposure.

entitlements: A right earned by individuals through employment, such as Social Security or Worker's Compensation.

epicardium: The thin outer layer of the heart, continuous with the lining of the pericardium.

epidermis: The outermost and thinnest layer of the skin.

eosinophils (eos): Granular leukocyte whose granules are beadlike and stain bright orange–red with the eosin acid stain.

erythema: Redness.

erythrocyte: A mature, anuclear, biconcave disk-shaped blood cell which is responsible for transporting oxygen to the cells of the body and carbon dioxide away from the cells. Also called red blood cell (RBC).

erythropoietin: Hormone secreted by the kidneys which stimulates red cell production.

essentials: Educational standards set forth by accrediting agencies.

evacuated tubes: Premeasured vacuum tubes that receive the patient's blood during the venipuncture procedure.

external respiration: The process by which O_2 from the air enters the bloodstream in the lungs, and CO_2 leaves the bloodstream and is breathed into the air from the lungs.

extrinsic: A pathway initiated by the release of thromboplastin (factor III) from injured tissue and the activation of factor VII, pro-convertin.

extravascular: Outside the bloodstream.

Fahrenheit: A scale used to measure body temperatures, based on the freezing point of water (32 degrees) and the boiling point (212 degrees).

fasting: Abstinence from eating or drinking except water for approximately 12 hours prior to collection of the specimen.

feather: The thinnest area of a blood smear where the differential is performed.

femoral artery: Major systemic artery located superficially in the groin, lateral to the pubis bone.

fibrin: A filamentous protein formed by the action of thrombin on fibrinogen.

fibrin degradation products (FDP): Small fragments of partially digested fibrin found in the bloodstream.

fibrinogen: Also called factor I, a protein found in plasma that is essential for clotting of blood.

fibrinolysis: Process initiated by the activation of the clotting mechanism which releases substances that lead to the dissolution of the fibrin clot.

fistula: A tube passing from a cavity or vessel to a free surface or another cavity. Also the term used to describe an artificial joining of an artery and a vein.

flanges: Extensions on the sides of an evacuated tube holder to aid in tube placement and removal.

flea: Small metal bar which is inserted into the tube after collection of a capillary blood gas specimen to aid in mixing the anticoagulant by means of a magnet.

floor book: Also called User Manual, a manual of instruction provided to the unit by the laboratory which describes preparation of the patient and special instructions for specimen collection.

fomites: Any substance that adheres to and transmits infectious material.

frontal plane: Also called coronal plane, divides the body vertically into front and back portions.

FUO: Fever of unknown origin.

gastric analysis: A laboratory test that examines gastric acid secretions to determine gastric function in terms of stomach acid production.

gauge: A standard for measuring the diameter of the lumen of a needle.

germicide: An agent that kills pathogenic microorganisms.

glucose: Blood sugar.

glucose monitoring: A means of observing and recording the blood sugar for the purpose of maintaining a normal level.

glycolysis: Normal body reaction in which glucose is hydrolyzed or broken down by an enzyme.

gram: The basic unit of weight in the metric system, approximately equal to a cubic centimeter or milliliter of water.

granulocytes: WBCs with easily visible granules.

great saphenous vein: The longest vein in the body, located in the leg.

guaiac test: Also called occult blood; tests for blood in stool.

hardware: CPU, monitor, and all peripherals, such as barcode readers, modems, and joysticks.

HazCom: The abbreviation for the Hazardous Communication Standard, enacted in 1986 by OSHA, that requires employers to maintain documentation on all hazardous materials.

health maintenance organization (HMO): Group practice that is reimbursed on a prepaid, rather than a fee-for-service, basis.

hematocrit: Percentage by volume of red blood cells in whole blood.

hematoma: A swelling or mass of blood (usually clotted) caused by blood leaking from a blood vessel during or following venipuncture, or arterial puncture.

hemoconcentration: A condition in which the plasma portion of the blood filters into the tissues causing an increase in nonfilterable blood components such as RBCs, enzymes, iron, and calcium.

hemoglobin (Hb or Hgb): An iron protein

pigment found in red blood cells that carries O_2 and CO_2 in the blood stream.

hemolysis: The destruction of RBCs and the liberation of hemoglobin into the fluid portion of the specimen causing the serum or plasma to be pink (slight hemolysis) to red (gross hemolysis) in color.

hemostasis: Process by which the body stops the leakage of blood from the vascular system.

hemostatic plug: Fibrin clot.

heparin lock: A special winged needle set that can be left in a patient's vein for up to 48 hours, used to administer medication and draw blood.

hepatitis: Inflammation of the liver, from toxic or viral origin.

homeostasis: A "steady state" condition in which the body maintains its internal environment in a state of equilibrium or balance.

hyperglycemia: Condition in which the blood sugar (glucose) is increased, as in diabetes mellitus.

hypoglycemia: A condition in which the blood sugar (glucose) is abnormally low, as in hyperinsulinism.

identification card: ID cards given to clinic patients from which specimen labels can be imprinted using an Address-o-graph machine.

immunoglobulins: Antibodies that are released into the blood stream where they circulate and attack foreign cells.

ID band: Identification bracelet.

induration: Hardness.

indwelling line: Tubing inserted into a main vein or artery used primarily for administering fluids and medications.

infection: Invasion of a body by a pathogenic microorganism resulting in injurious effects or disease.

inferior: Also referred to as caudal; beneath, lower, or toward the feet.

inflammation: Tissue reaction to injury, such as redness or swelling.

informed consent: Agreement by the patient to medical treatment after having received adequate information about the procedure, risks, and consequences.

inpatient care: Care performed in a health care setting where patients stay overnight.

input: Data that is entered into the CPU.

intravascular: Within the vascular system.

intrinsic: Pathway involving coagulation factors circulating within the bloodstream, initiated with activation of Factor XII.

integumentary system: The skin and its appendages; the hair and nails, also referred to as the largest organ of the body.

internal respiration: The process by which O_2 leaves the bloodstream and enters the cells, and CO_2 from the cells enters the bloodstream.

interstitial fluid: Fluid found between cells or in spaces within an organ or tissue.

intracellular fluid: Fluid found within cell membranes.

iontophoresis: Introduction of various ions into the skin by electrical stimulation from electrodes placed on the skin.

ischemia: Temporary lack of blood flow to the heart due to obstruction.

isolation procedures: An infection-control procedure that separates patients with certain transmissible infections or diseases from other patients.

Ivy Bleeding Time: A bleeding time test modified by Ivy in 1941, performed on the volar (inner) surface of the forearm using a blood pressure cuff to maintain constant pressure.

JCAHO: Joint Commission on Accreditation of Healthcare Organizations, a voluntary, nongovernmental agency charged with, among other things, establishing standards for the operation of hospitals and other health-related facilities and services.

keloid: Fibrous tissue growth at scar area of the skin.

kinesics: The study of body motion or language, such as facial expression, gestures, and eye contact.

kinesic slip: When nonverbal messages don't match verbal messages.

lancet: A sterile, disposable, sharp pointed instrument used to pierce the skin to obtain droplets of blood used for testing.

lateral: Toward the side.

leukemia: An increase in WBCs characterized by the presence of a large number of abnormal forms.

leukocytosis: An abnormal increase in WBCs in the circulating blood.

leukopenia: An abnormal decrease of WBCs in the circulating blood.

leukocyte: Also called white blood cell (WBC), round cell containing a nucleus whose main function is to combat infection and remove disintegrating tissue.

licensure: A similar process to certification, but offered by a governmental agency, granted through examination to a person who can meet the requirements for education and experience in that field.

lipemic: Cloudy serum or plasma caused by increased lipid content.

liter: The basic unit of volume in the metric system which is equivalent to 1,000 ml.

Luer adapter: In the Luer-Lok system, a device for connecting syringe to the needle and when locked into place gives a secure fit.

lumen: The internal space of a vessel or tube.

lymphocyte: A nongranular leukocyte, the second most numerous of the WBCs, comprising approximately 15% to 30% of the WBC population.

lymphostasis: A stoppage of lymph flow caused by lymph node removal.

lysis: Rupturing of red blood cells.

malpractice: A claim of improper treatment or negligence brought against a professional person by means of a civil lawsuit.

material safety data sheets (MSDS): Written required information on all products with a hazardous warning on the label.

medial: Toward the midline or middle.

median cubital: The vein located in the middle of the antecubital fossa area of the arm. The first-choice vein for venipuncture.

Medicaid: A program funded by the state and federal government for providing medical care to the poor.

medical emergency (Med Emerg): Designation replacing "stat" for requesting tests that are needed in critical or "life or death" situations.

medical record number: The unique num-

ber given to a patient for purposes of identification.

Medicare: A federally funded program enacted in 1965 that provides health care to people over the age of 65 and the disabled, regardless of financial status.

median cutaneous nerve: A major arm nerve that lies along the path of the brachial artery and in the vicinity of the basilic vein.

megakaryocyte: A large cell which is formed in the bone marrow and is the precursor to platelet cells.

menu: A listing on the computer screen of options from which the user selects the program or process he or she needs.

meter: The basic unit of linear measurement in the metric system, equal to 39.37 inches.

metric system: A decimal system of weights and measures based on the basic meter, gram, and liter units.

metabolism: The sum of all the chemical reactions necessary to sustain life.

microbes: Microscopic organisms or organisms not visible to the naked eye.

microcollection tubes: Capillary collection tubes made of plastic with color-coded stoppers which correspond to the blood collection tubes used in venipuncture.

microhematocrit tubes: Disposable, narrow-bore glass or plastic tubes that fill by capillary action and are primarily used for hematocrit (packed cell volume) determinations on micro samples.

midstream collection: Specimen obtained during the middle of the urination rather than the beginning or end.

military time: Also called European time; based on a clock with 24 numbers instead of 12, eliminating the need for designating a.m. or p.m.

milliliter (ml): A unit of volume measurement which is approximately equal to a cubic centimeter (cc); the two terms are often used interchangeably.

mnemonics: Memory-aiding codes such as the abbreviations used to request the appropriate computer program or function necessary to process data.

monocytes (monos) The largest of the leukocytes, comprising from 1% to 7% of the WBC population.

modes of transmission: The route by which an organism is transferred from one host to another.

myocardial infarction (MI): Heart attack or death of heart muscle due to obstruction of the coronary artery.

myocardium: The thick, muscle layer of the heart.

NAACLS: National Accrediting Agency for Clinical Laboratory Sciences.

nasopharyngeal (NP) culture: A sample collected using a special NP swab inserted gently through the nose into the nasopharynx area to detect the presences of the microorganisms such as those which cause diphtheria, meningitis, whooping cough, and pneumonia.

Natelson tubes: Microcollection tubes that are approximately 147 mm in length and fill by capillary action to a capacity of approximately 250 μ.

NCA: National Certification Agency; certifies all levels of clinical laboratory personnel.

NCCLS: National Committee for Clinical Laboratory Standards, a national, nonprofit organization formed by representatives from the profession, industry, and government that develops guidelines and sets standards for all areas of the laboratory.

needle sheath: Covering or cap of a needle.

negligence: The violation of a duty to exercise reasonable skill and care in performing a task.

neutrophils: Normally the most numerous of the WBCs, averaging 65% of the total WBC count with granules that are fine in texture and stain lavender.

noninvasive: Not penetrating the skin.

nosocomial: Pertaining to a hospital or place of care for the sick.

nosocomial infection: An infection acquired in a health care institution.

occlusion: Obstruction.

occult blood: *See* guaiac test.

occupational exposure: An anticipated skin, eye, mucous membrane, or parenteral contact with blood or other potentially infectious materials that may result from the performance of the employee's duties.

on-line: When a computer system is operational.

OSHA: Occupation Safety and Health Administration; a U.S. government agency that regulates the safety and health of workers.

osteochondritis: Inflammation of the bone and cartilage.

osteomyelitis: Inflammation of the bone, especially the bone marrow, caused by bacterial infection.

outpatient care: *See* ambulatory care.

output: Any data that flows from the CPU to peripherals.

ova & parasite (O & P): A stool sample for diagnosis of intestinal parasites.

oxyhemoglobin (HbO$_2$): Hemoglobin combined with O$_2$.

palmar surface: Palm side of the hand.

palpate: To examine by feel or touch.

parenteral: Any route other than the alimentary, *ie*, intramuscular, intravenous, or subcutaneous.

patency: State of being freely open, as in a patient's veins.

pathogen: A substance or microbe capable of producing disease.

patient identification: The process by which a health care worker verifies the fact that a patient is the same as the one described on a requisition or work order.

Patient's Bill of Rights: The rights or privileges a patient has while in a hospital or other health care facility which are clearly defined in a document originally published in 1975 by the American Hospital Association.

peak level: Drug level collected when the highest serum concentration of the drug is anticipated, around 15–30 minutes after administration of the drug.

pediatric tubes: Small evacuated tubes designed to be used on small veins.

pericardial fluid: Fluid aspirated from the cavity surrounding the heart.

pericardium: A thin, fluid-filled sac surrounding the heart.

peritoneal fluid: Fluid aspirated from the abdominal cavity.

personal protective equipment (PPE): Disposable gloves, lab coats or aprons, and/or protective face gear, such as masks and goggles with side shields required by OSHA to be worn when handling body fluids.

petechiae: Small, non-raised red spots which appear on a patient's skin under certain conditions such as when a tourniquet is applied.

phagocytosis: A process by which the bacteria and antigens are surrounded and engulfed by WBCs.

phlebitis: Inflammation of a vein.

phenylketonuria (PKU): A hereditary disease caused by the inability of the body to metabolize phenylalanine due to a defective enzyme. Mental retardation results if not treated early.

phlebotomy: The procedure for withdrawing blood from the body.

plasma: A clear, pale yellow fluid that is nearly 90% water (H_2O).

plantar surface: Bottom or sole of the foot.

platelet adhesion: The process by which platelets stick to injured surfaces.

platelet aggregation: The process by which platelets degranulate and stick to one another.

platelet plug formation: Platelet aggregation and adhesion to a blood vessel following an injury.

pleural fluid: Fluid aspirated from the pleural cavity which surrounds the lungs.

point-of-care testing: Testing done at the patient's bedside or virtually anywhere the patient happens to be, using portable or hand-carried instruments.

polycythemia: An overproduction of red blood cells.

polymorphonuclear (PMN): A term used to describe a type of WBC whose nucleus has several lobes or segments.

posterior: Also called dorsal, refers to the back.

postprandial (PP): After a meal.

potassium (K): A mineral that is essential for normal muscle activity and the conduction of nerve impulses.

pneumatic tube system: A unidirectional, continuously operating vacuum system that transfers specimens in plexiglas carriers from the patient units to the laboratory.

Preferred Provider Organization (PPO): An independent group of doctors and hospitals that offer their services to employers at discounted rates.

prefix: A word part that precedes a word root and modifies its meaning.

pre-op: Before an operation or surgery.

primary hemostasis: First part of the coagulation process which involves formation of a platelet plug.

prothrombin: Protein in circulating blood called factor II which is involved in coagulation.

procedural manual: A document required by JCAHO that states in detail the step-by-step procedure for each test or practice performed in the laboratory.

professionalism: The conduct and qualities that characterize a professional person.

Prospective Payment System (PPS): A program begun in 1983 to standardize the Medicare/Medicaid payments made to hospitals by reimbursing hospitals a set amount for each patient procedure.

proxemics: The study of an individual's concept and use of space.

proximal: Nearest to the center of the body, origin, or point of attachment.

psychoneuroimmunology (PNI): A new field of medicine which deals with the study of interactions between the brain, the endocrine system, and the immune system.

pulmonary circulation: The system that carries blood from the heart to the lungs to remove carbon dioxide and returns oxygenated blood to the heart.

pulse: A measurement of pressure created as the ventricles contract and blood is forced out of the heart and through the arteries.

pumping: Vigorous opening and closing of the fist.

QA Indicator: A monitor for all aspects of patient care; indicators must be measurable and cover high-volume procedures and high-risk situations.

quality assurance: A complete program that guarantees quality client care by tracking the outcomes through scheduled audits in which the hospital looks at the appropriateness, applicability, and timeliness of patient care.

quality control (QC): A form of procedural control which is a component of a quality assurance program.

quantity not sufficient (QNS): Insufficient amount of substance required for testing.

radial artery: An artery located on the thumb side of the wrist, which is usually the first choice and therefore most common site for arterial puncture.

Random Access Memory (RAM): Temporary storage of data in the CPU that will be lost when power is discontinued unless transferred to permanent storage.

Read Only Memory (ROM): Firmware installed by the manufacturer. Its purpose is to instruct the CPU on how to begin the necessary operations requested by the user.

Reciprocity: Granting of corresponding privileges, such as a state recognizing another state's license.

reference values: Normal values for lab tests, usually established using basal state specimens.

reference laboratory: An off-site laboratory to which specimens are referred for testing procedures not routinely done in-house.

reflux: A backward flow of blood into the patient's veins from the collection tube during the venipuncture procedure.

resheathing: To recap or replace the sheath on a needle.

reticulocytes: Immature RBCs in the blood stream that contain nuclear remnants.

Rh antigen: A substance that when present on the surface of RBCs causes the formation of antibodies that interact specifically with it.

Rh immunoglobulins: A substance that if given before as well as shortly after an Rh-negative mother delivers an Rh-positive baby, will prevent sensitization by destroying any Rh factor in the mother's bloodstream.

risk management: A department in organizations that identifies risk and oversees the protection of employees, employers, and patients from the chance of injury or loss associated with the risk.

sagittal plane: Divides the body vertically into right and left portions.

sclerosed: Hard, cordlike, and lacking resilience.

secondary hemostasis: Second stage of coagulation that involves formation of a tougher "fibrin" clot formed of RBCs, platelets, and fibrin.

semen analysis: Laboratory test used to assess fertility and to determine the effectiveness of sterilization following vasectomy.

semilunar valves: The crescent-shaped valves that control blood exiting the ventricles of the heart.

septicemia: Blood poisoning or pathogenic bacteria in the blood.

serum: A clear, pale yellow fluid that remains after blood clots and is separated. It has the same composition as plasma except it does not contain fibrinogen.

sexually transmitted diseases (STDs): Diseases such as syphilis, gonorrhea, and genital herpes which are usually transmitted by sexual contact.

sinoatrial (SA) node: A node, also called the pacemaker, located in the upper wall of the right atrium which generates an electrical impulse that initiates contraction of the heart.

skin antisepsis: Destruction or inhibition of multiplication of microorganisms on the skin through use of antiseptics or germicides.

skin puncture: Collecting blood after puncturing the skin with a lancet or similar skin puncture device.

skin test: Intradermal injection of an allergenic substance to determine if a patient has come in contact with a specific allergen (antigen) and developed antibodies against it.

sodium (Na): An extracellular ion in the blood plasma that helps maintain fluid balance.

software: Programs; for example, word processing, graphics, and games.

solutes: Dissolved substances.

STAT (stat): A term derived from the Latin word "statim" meaning immediately.

steady state: A stable condition; no exercise, suctioning, or respirator changes, for at least 30 minutes prior to obtaining blood gases.

subcutaneous layer: A layer of connective as well as adipose tissue that connects the skin to the surface of muscles.

suffix: The end of a word (word ending), that follows a word root and either changes the meaning of the word root or adds to it.

superior: Also referred to as cranial: higher, above, or toward the head.

supine: Lying on the back, face upward.

susceptible host: A person who has little resistance to an infectious disease.

sweat chloride: A test that uses iontophoresis to stimulate sweat production in order to evaluate chloride content in sweat. The test is used to diagnose cystic fibrosis primarily in children and adolescents under the age of 20.

sweeps: Hospital rounds which occur at regular intervals throughout the day.

synovial fluid: Fluid aspirated from joint cavities.

syncope: Fainting.

systemic circulation: The system that carries oxygenated blood from the heart, along with nutrients, to all the cells of the body, and then returns to the heart carrying waste products from cellular metabolism.

systole: The contraction phase of the cardiac cycle.

systolic pressure: The pressure in the arteries during contraction of the ventricles, usually around 120 mm Hg.

tech code: Code given to computer users which uniquely identifies the user within the laboratory and is recorded with all entries on the system.

test requisition: The form on which a test is ordered and sent to the lab.

therapeutic drug monitoring (TDM): Process used by the physician to determine an effective drug dosage as well as manage individual patient drug treatment.

third party payer: A fiscal intermediary, most often an insurance company that pools individual contributions for a common group objective, protection from financial disaster.

threshold values: Acceptable level for a quality assurance indicator.

thrombin: An enzyme formed from prothrombin which reacts with fibrinogen to form fibrin during the clotting process.

thrombocytes: Also known as platelets; the smallest of the formed elements in the bloodstream.

thrombocytopenia: Decreased platelets.

thrombocytosis: Increased platelets.

thrombophlebitis: Inflammation of a vein, particularly in the lower extremities along with thrombus formation.

thrombus: Blood clot in a blood vessel.

T-lymphocytes: Specialized WBCs that play an important role in immunity by directly attacking infected cells.

tolerance test: A test of the body's ability to absorb and utilize a particular substance.

tort: A civil wrong or other breach of contract, *ie,* negligence or battery.

Total Quality Management (TQM): An institution-wide plan to assure quality care, mandated by JCAHO to be instituted by 1994, requiring all departments in the hospital to have ongoing evaluations which focus on quality of process rather than outcome.

transfusion reaction: A response to an incompatible blood transfusion resulting in antigen/antibody reactions that cause agglutination or lysis of the RBCs.

transport media: The medium or agent used to carry infective material to a laboratory for culturing.

transverse plane: Divides the body horizontally into upper and lower portions, often called a cross section.

trough level: Drug level collected when the

lowest serum concentration of the drug is expected, usually immediately prior to administration of the next scheduled dose.

tuberculosis (TB): Infectious airborne disease affecting the respiratory system caused by the bacteria *Mycobacterium tuberculosis.*

tunica adventitia: The outer layer of blood vessels made up of connective tissue which is thicker in arteries than veins.

tunica intima: The inner layer or lining of blood vessels made up of a single layer of endothelial cells.

tunica media: The middle layer of blood vessels made up of smooth muscle tissue which is much thicker in arteries than veins.

turn-around-time (TAT): Specified amount of time for sample to be drawn, processed, and for test results to be sent to the floor / unit.

Typenex ID band: A special three-part identification bracelet for a blood recipient which contains the same information and unique ID number for client confirmation on all three parts.

universal precautions: A set of rules established by CDC and adopted by OSHA to control infection from body fluids in the health care setting.

urinalysis: Laboratory test which includes physical examination, chemical, and microscopic analysis of urine.

UTI: Urinary tract infection.

vasoconstriction: Constriction of a blood vessel to decrease the flow of blood to an area.

veins: Vessels that return blood to the heart. Veins carry deoxygenated blood, except the pulmonary vein, which carries oxygenated blood from the lungs back to the heart.

vena cava: The largest vein in the body.

venesection: Slicing a vein in the forearm and collecting the specimen in a cup or bowl.

venipuncture: Collection of blood by penetrating a vein with a needle, syringe, or other collection apparatus.

venous stasis: Stagnation of the normal blood flow.

ventral cavities: Internal space located in the front of the body.

ventricles: Lower chambers of the heart. Also known as the delivering chambers of the heart because they pump blood into the arteries.

venules: The smallest veins at the junction of the capillaries.

virulence: Infectious or capable of overcoming the defensive mechanism of the host.

winged infusion set: Also called butterfly; consists of a stainless steel needle connected to a 5- to 12-inch length of tubing.

word root: Foundation of all medical terms.

zones of comfort: In communication, the different distances around a person which are comfortable for intimate, personal, social, and public discourse.

Answers to Study and Review Questions

Appendix A

Chapter 1
1. a
2. d
3. a
4. b
5. d
6. c
7. c
8. b

Chapter 2
1. c
2. a
3. a
4. d
5. b
6. a
7. d
8. c

Chapter 3
1. a
2. a
3. c
4. a
5. d
6. b
7. d
8. a

Chapter 4
1. b
2. c
3. c
4. d
5. d
6. d
7. c
8. d

9. b
10. c

Chapter 5
1. c
2. a
3. d
4. a
5. b
6. c
7. b
8. d
9. a
10. b

Chapter 6
1. c
2. d
3. b
4. a
5. b
6. a
7. c
8. d

Chapter 7
1. d
2. c
3. b
4. d
5. b
6. c
7. c
8. d

Chapter 8
1. a
2. b
3. c

4. c
5. c
6. d
7. b
8. d

Chapter 9
1. a
2. d
3. c
4. a
5. b
6. c

Chapter 10
1. a
2. b
3. c
4. c
5. b
6. b
7. d
8. c

Chapter 11
1. d
2. c
3. b
4. d
5. c
6. b
7. a
8. b

Chapter 12
1. c
2. b
3. d
4. c

5. a
6. b
7. b
8. a

Chapter 13
1. b
2. d
3. b
4. c
5. d
6. a

Chapter 14
1. d
2. d
3. d
4. c
5. b
6. d

Chapter 15
1. d
2. a
3. c
4. b
5. c
6. c
7. a
8. d

Chapter 16
1. b
2. c
3. b
4. c
5. b
6. d
7. d
8. a

Conversational Phrases in English and Spanish

Appendix B

*The following remarks or sentences are designed to assist the phlebotomist when conversing with a patient who speaks only Spanish. Before approaching the patient, these **basic phrases** should be said aloud several times to a person who could correct the pronunciation, if necessary. If these phrases are said incorrectly, the meanings could be changed enough to insult or bewilder the patient.*

Hello	¡Hola! (Ō·lah)
Good morning	Buenos días (BWĀ·nōs DĒ·ahs)
Good afternoon	Buenas tardes (BWĀ·nahs TAHR·dās)
Good evening	Buenas noches (BWĀ·nahs NŌ·chās)
I am from the laboratory	Soy del laboratorio (soy dāl lah·bō·rah·tō·RĒ·ō)
My name is	Me llamo (mā YAH·mō)
I am here to take a blood sample	Estoy aquí para tomarle una prueba de sangre (ās·TOY ah·KĒ PAHR·ah tō·MAHR·lā UN·ah prū·Ā·bah dā SAHN·grā)
What is your name?	¿Cual es so nombre? (kwahl ās sō NŌM·brā? OR ¿Como se llama? (CŌ·mō sā YAH·mah?
May I see your wristband?	¿Me permite ver su identificación? (mā pār·MĒ·tā vār sū ē·dān·tē·fē·cah·sē·ŌN?)
Mr. or Sir	Señor (sā·NYOR)

Mrs. or Madame	Señora (sā·NYŌ·rah)
Ms. or Miss	Señorita (sā·nyō·RĒ·tah)
Okay	Muy bien (MŬ·ē byān)
You are the person I need	Usted es la persona que necesito (ūs·TĒD ās lah pār·SŌN·ah kā na·sā·SĒ·tō)
I am going to put a tourniquet on your arm	le voy a poner un torniquete en su brazo (lā voy ah pō·NĀR ūn tor·nē·KĀ·tā ān sū BRAH·sō)
Please	Por favor (por fah·VOR)
close your hand	cierra su mano (SYĀ·rah sū MAH·nō)
open your hand	abra su mano (AH·brah sū MAH·nō)
straighten your arm	ponga derecho su brazo (PŌN·gah dā·RĀ·chō sū BRAH·sō) OR estire su brazo (ās·tĒ·rā sū BRAH·sō)
bend your arm	doble su brazo (DŌ·blā sū BRAH·sō)
relax	relajese (rā·lah·CHĀ·sā) NOTE: the "ch" in this word is pronounced gutturally
sit there	sientese aquí (syān·TĀ·sā ah·KĒ)
Your doctor ordered this	Su doctor ordeno esto (sū dōc·TOR or·DĀ·nō ĀS·tō)
You need to ask your doctor	Necesita preguntarle a su doctor (nā·sā·SĒ·tah prā·gūn·TAHR·lā ah sū dōc·TOR)
Have you eaten?	¿La comido? (lah cō·MĒ·dō)
It will hurt a little	le dolerá un poco (lā dō·lā·RAH ūm PŌ·kō)

I will get the nurse

Buscaré a la enfermera
(būs·cah·RĀ ah lah ām·fār·MĀ·rah)

Thank you

¡Gracias!
(GRAH·syahs)

Have a good day

Qué le vaya bien
(kā lā VĪ·yah byān)

Someone will be back in a few minutes

Alguien regresará en un momento
(ahl·GWĒ·ān rā·grā·sah·RAH ān ūm
mō·MĀN·tō)

Index

Page numbers followed by *f* indicate figures; those followed by *t* indicate tabular material.

ABO blood group system, 79–80, 80t
Accession number, 252
Accreditation, 5, 265
Activated coagulation time (ACT) test, 185–186, 186f, 265
Additives
  for evacuated tubes, 117–118, 118t
  mixing of, 158f, 163, 234
Adhesives, allergies to, 136
Adrenal glands, 51f
  disorders of, 53
  functions of, 52
Aerobic collection, 190, 265
Age, 129
Agranulocytes, 78–79, 265
Aliquot
  definition of, 265
  preparation of, 237, 238, 239f, 240
Allen test, 209f, 210, 265
Allergies, 136
Altitude, 129
Ambulatory care, 14
American Society for Medical Technology (ASMT), 6, 266
American Society of Clinical Pathologists (ASCP), 5, 6, 266
American Society of Phlebotomy Technicians (ASPT), 5, 6, 266
Ammonium oxalate, 118
Amniotic fluid, 219

Anabolism, 43, 265
Anaerobic collection, 190, 265
Analyte, 237, 265
Anatomy
  cavities in, 42–43, 43f, 267
  directional terms in, 41
  planes in, 41, 42f, 267
  position in, 41
Ancillary blood glucose testing (ABGT), 195–196, 196f, 265
Antecubital fossa, 73, 265–266
Anterior direction, 41, 42, 266
Antibiotic sensitivity, culture and sensitivity test for, 218
Anticoagulants
  for arterial blood sample, 213
  reflux of, 138
  for tubes, 117–118, 118t
  for whole blood specimens, 81
Antiglycotic agents, 118
Antimicrobial removal device (ARD), 191, 266
Antimicrobial therapy
  effect on blood culture, 191
Antisepsis
  skin, 190, 275
Antiseptics, 112
  allergies to, 136
  definition of, 265
  contamination from, 140
Appearance
  in communication, 245
Approval, 5–6, 266

Arrhythmia, 67
Arterial blood gases (ABGs). *See also* Arteries, puncture of
  Allen test in, 209f, 210
  complications with, 212
  definition of, 266
  equipment and supplies for, 207–208
  preparation for, 208
  procedure for, 208–212, 211f
  sampling errors in, 212–213
  site selection for, 203–206, 204f
  specimen rejection in, 213
Arteriospasm, 212
Artery(ies)
  of arm, 204f
  brachial, 75, 204f, 205
  coronary, 66
  femoral, 75, 75f, 205–206, 206f
  of leg, 75f, 206f
  pulmonary, 73f
  puncture of, 139, 203–206
  radial, 75, 203, 204f, 205
  of vascular system, 69–70
ASCP. *See* American Society of Clinical Pathologists
ASMT. *See* American Society for Medical Technology
ASPT. *See* American Society of Phlebotomy Technicians
Assault, 10
Assignment, 15
Atria, 65, 266
Autologous blood donation, 189